A HUNDRED YEARS

OF MEDICINE

A HUNDRED YEARS

OF

Medicine

by

C. D. Haagensen

and

Wyndham E. B. Lloyd

SHERIDAN HOUSE

NEW YORK

TYPOGRAPHY, PRINTING, AND BINDING IN THE U. S. A. BY
KINGSPORT PRESS, INC., KINGSPORT, TENNESSEE

PREFACE

I T I S H O P E D that this historical essay may prove to be of value not only to the layman, for whom it is primarily intended, but also to those medical practitioners and students who have not found time for any specialized study of the history of medicine.

This book cannot claim to be comprehensive. In many respects it is necessarily incomplete. The available material is unmanageably abundant. To have included everything in detail would have made the book unwieldy, whereas to have condensed excessively would have made it unreadable. I have therefore presumed to select some of the important and more interesting aspects of the subject while omitting others which may be equally important but which are too technical to be readily described to the non-medical reader.

The arrangement of this book has been determined largely by the fact that important medical advances are not made in a single day but are generally the result of a laborious series of steps made by a number of different workers over long periods of years. Consequently the importance of each contribution to medicine can best be understood by tracing it separately from its origins rather than by attempting to survey the whole field of advance in strict chronological order. Furthermore, by treating each subject separately it is possible to appreciate the train of thought more clearly at a great saving of space and repetition.

I have refrained from using technical terms without explaining their meaning and hope that the ordinary English words which in some places have been substituted for the technical ones will not irritate those with medical knowledge.

Except for those great ones who make it, history is necessarily secondhand. The author is therefore gratefully indebted to many different writers for the material from which this book is made. In a work of this kind it is impossible to give a reference for every statement made, consequently apologies and thanks are respectfully tendered to those authors both dead and alive from whom facts have been gathered without acknowledgment.

WYNDHAM E. B. LLOYD

PREFACE

TO THE AMERICAN EDITION

IN THE AMERICAN EDITION of *A Hundred Years of Medicine* both the context and scope of the work have been much changed. Part I, which deals with the historical background of modern medicine, and Chapters X to XIV of Part II, dealing with infectious disease, remain substantially as Dr. Lloyd wrote them except that I have added features of the American scene and have omitted some of those that were of more special interest to English readers.

The remainder of this new edition has been entirely rewritten, and I am solely responsible for the opinions expressed therein. In this part of the book the emphasis has been placed upon the history of our knowledge of the chief disease entities. In a single volume only a relatively small number can be dealt with, and these perforce must be the *common* ones. Among the many interesting diseases of metabolism, for instance, only diabetes and pernicious anemia are discussed, because they are much the most frequent.

Some of these matters are necessarily rather technical. Although the simplest possible terms have been chosen, the non-medical reader may find it necessary to look up occasional anatomical and chemical terms. It is hoped that the layman whose intellectual curiosity leads him to delve into a historical work of this kind will be willing on his part to do a certain amount of such reference work. Medicine is today deeply in need of the sympathetic understanding of laymen, and this book will have served its purpose if it interests them in some of its problems.

I also hope that the first year medical student—who is likewise a beginner in medicine—will find this book a provocative introduction to his course. Knowledge of *the face of disease* clothes the dry facts of anatomy, physiology, and pathology with reality. The beginning medical student needs this contact with reality. Our historical approach to it sometimes may seem to give it a sort of detective story flavor, but our aim is to interest as well as to instruct. Meat is always better with a little sauce.

I am indebted to Archibald Malloch, to many medical associates who have read the parts of the manuscript dealing with subjects outside of my own specialty, and also to my wife, who has helped in many ways with the preparation of the book.

C. D. HAAGENSEN

New York 1942

CONTENTS

III.   Surgery During the Last Hundred Years

IV.   New Social Aspects of Medicine

ILLUSTRATIONS

PART ONE

Medicine Up to a Hundred Years Ago

THE ORIGINS OF MEDICINE

MODERN MEDICAL science must at times seem almost miraculous to the laymen. Like other sciences it has grown so enormously during the last hundred years that the layman is tempted to regard its accomplishments as beyond all understanding. This, however, is not an attitude that will bring him any closer to a proper appreciation of the difficulties, both scientific and organizational, which beset physicians today.

History is the best teacher, not only in the so-called social sciences, but in a physical science such as medicine, which is rapidly becoming an exact science. Through the historical approach we learn not only of the foundations upon which the science is built, but something of the human side of the men who laboriously sought out its basic truths. The subject is thus brought to life and made into an integrated, logical whole. A mere summary of what we know today would be inadequate.

The history of medicine in its entirety would carry us back to the remotest periods of antiquity, but we cannot travel so far within the compass of this book. Nevertheless, in order to understand the developments of medical theory and practice during the last century, we must have at least some idea of the state of knowledge which existed a hundred years ago, and of the general trend of events which preceded it.

Although there was a kind of medicine already in existence at the dawn of history, it was in general based upon magic and upon astrology rather than science. In the fourth and fifth centuries before Christ, however, Hippocrates of Cos appears to have been the first to insist upon the scientific and also the ethical aspects of medicine. It was Hippocrates who founded the profession, and from his school came directly or indirectly all the famous physicians and practical observers of the past. His teaching, essentially scientific, held unchallenged priority for many years, until the time of Galen of Pergamum (131–201 A.D.), physician to the Emperor Marcus Aurelius.

Wide and original discoveries and studies have been accredited to Galen in anatomy, physiology, the study of disease, and also of drugs. Most of the pathways that Galen had begun to cut through the jungle of ignorance remained as he left them for nearly fourteen centuries, while others were overgrown by the weeds of forgetfulness and dogma which flourished so vigorously in the Dark Ages. The knowledge of the Greeks virtually disappeared from Europe at the fall of the Western Roman Empire. The ignorance of the barbarians wantonly destroyed that knowledge which the Christians of Western Europe, finding no place for it in their lives, lost through lack of interest rather than through active hostility. Indeed, had not the vigorous peoples of Arabia absorbed, largely from the Nestorian Christians, the great ideas of the Greeks, it is doubtful how much there would have been left of the early foundations of medicine on which the present-day science has been built.

It was thanks to Arabian scholarship that the most famous of all ancient text-books of medicine came to be written: the *Canon* of the Persian philosopher who is generally known as Avicenna (979–1037 A.D.). This, his most influential work, follows the ideas of Hippocrates and Galen intermingled with those of Aristotle, worked up into a great system of medicine. Its five books deal with physiology, the study of disease, hygiene, the treatment of sickness and the compounding of physic. This great work contains many fallacies but much good sense, and remained the standard work on medicine for many years.

In the Middle Ages medicine was purely dogmatic. What the

ancients had said, what Hippocrates, Aristotle, Galen, and Avicenna had written, was assumed to be right, and there was none to dispute the oracular pronouncements of the past. If we except Roger Bacon, an experimental genius whose discoveries were premature and consequently without any wide influence, no one dared to question the truth of the old authorities until the reawakening of knowledge in the 15th, 16th and 17th Centuries. Many fallacies which were then accepted could have been shattered easily by experimental science. But experimental science was asleep.

The beginning of the modern experimental period may be said to date from Paracelsus, that strange 16th Century figure— sorcerer, philosopher, alchemist and physician—who overthrew the absolute sovereignty of Hippocrates, Galen, and Avicenna. The keynote of his teaching at the University of Basel was that men should search into the workings of nature for themselves; and he startled the world by publicly committing the *Canon* to the flames of a students' bonfire.

At the same time Vesalius was laying the foundations of modern anatomy at the University of Padua. Galen's excellent anatomical knowledge had suffered sad mutilation at the hands of the Arabians and other mediaeval scribes. Vesalius, as a result of many personally conducted dissections, put anatomical studies on a sure basis of fact with his famous *De Humani Corporis Fabrica*, published in 1543. At the same University of Padua the great Englishman William Harvey, at the beginning of the 17th Century, was trained in that thorough knowledge of anatomy which enabled him to make his far-reaching discovery of the circulation of the blood. Modern physiology, that is to say the study of the functions of the normal healthy organism, had its beginning here. Harvey insisted on the direct experimental approach to nature.

In the 17th Century students of medicine concerned themselves mainly with physics and chemistry, in terms of which they attempted to explain function and disease, and to apply these newly discovered principles to the practice of medicine. For example, we find that the vegetable drugs, the "Galenicals," were beginning to be replaced by "chemicals." But this period also produced a revival of the Hippocratic methods of *observation*, apart from any consideration of theory, in the work of the great Englishman, Thomas Sydenham. Sydenham believed that mere theories were valueless and set out to provide accurate descriptions of the signs and symptoms of diseases. He supposed, as we do now, that each disease was a definite individual species and could be classified like an animal or plant. Sydenham's influence continues to be felt even today.

After two thousand years, medicine had returned to the basic scientific approach of Hippocrates, and the way was opened for those modern developments which have made healing a matter of accurate knowledge rather than unsupported theorizing.

THEORIES OF MEDICINE

IN THE 18TH CENTURY

EIGHTEENTH CENTURY medicine, which may be thought of as a prelude to our modern epoch of startling medical advance, did not break free from dogma all at once. In spite of the revival of the Hippocratic method by Sydenham, the tendency to theorize about the nature of disease remained. Some of these theories were quite fantastic, while others, even if fallacious and unworkable, were at least credible. Some of them, though false in themselves, led directly to good results. This was particularly apparent in those systems which indicated the use of mild remedies in the place of the more vigorous measures then in vogue, measures which too often were the final blow to the weakened strength of the patients.

There had been many brilliant achievements in other sciences —in chemistry, in physics and in astronomy. Certain all-embracing theories had had widespread success. Kepler and Newton, for example, had brought the motions of the planets, the tides, and the falling apple all under one universal law. Inspired by the results of such wonderful simplicity, it was natural that physicians should seek to discover some complete and universal system of medicine. The result of this was a large crop of "systems," particularly in Germany and in Scotland, which for the most part had a very great effect in hampering positive progress.

Some hoped to follow the great mathematicians of the 17th

and 18th Centuries and to base their theories on mechanics or mathematics. A complete mathematical system, for example, was attempted by Dr. Richard Mead, the fashionable London physician, who had inherited the practice of the successful and insolent [1] John Radcliffe. It was the latter who had left a huge sum of money to be used for the foundation of a library, an astronomical observatory, and an infirmary at Oxford. Mead's teacher, Archibald Pitcairne of Edinburgh, had endeavoured to apply mechanics to physic and to base medicine on geometry.

At Halle University at this time Friedrich Hoffmann was teaching that life is based on the presence of some kind of universal fluid or ether, while Georg Ernst Stahl postulated a conscious soul whose efforts, often ill-directed, to throw off some adverse influence, constituted disease. Stahl's theory was a kind of animism which, rejecting any sort of mechanical explanation, was contrary to all the scientific ideas then in vogue.

Most famous perhaps among the Scottish physicians was John Brown of Edinburgh, the disreputable boor whose unsound theories had a tremendous effect throughout Europe up to the end of the century. The Brunonian theory, as it was called, held that the phenomena of life depend on stimulus and that diseases were of two kinds, those due to lack of stimulus (the asthenic) and those in which there was too much stimulus (the sthenic). Fortunately Brown decided that the great majority of diseases were asthenic and therefore required stimulants. Now in many diseases stimulating treatment is very desirable, so that in this respect he made a distinct advance on the drastic weakening measures employed by so many of the practitioners of that time. Brown had two sovereign remedies, the one stimulant and the other depressant. These were alcohol and opium, and to these he himself is said to have fallen a victim.

[1] "Mead, I love you," Radcliffe is reported to have said, "and I'll tell you a sure secret to make you a fortune—use all mankind ill." (Cited by Garrison, *History of Medicine*, 4th ed., Philadelphia, 1929, p. 390.)

Homeopathy, which was first put forward as a medical doctrine towards the end of the 18th Century, was the invention of a German, Samuel Hahnemann of Meissen. Homeopathy took no account of the causes of diseases but studied only the symptoms. It affirmed that symptoms could be cured by those very drugs which would produce these symptoms in a healthy person. Hahnemann furthermore added to his theory the extraordinary notion that the physiological effect of drugs is made much stronger by diluting the drugs, by pounding them and shaking them. His practice then was to give incredibly minute doses such as could generally have had little or no effect, either beneficial or the reverse. Here again the theory had considerable success simply because the very mild nature of the treatment gave the *Vis Medicatrix Naturae* the needful opportunity to effect a cure.

In general, the great theories of which we have given examples bade their exponents try one or sometimes two kinds of treatment on every one of their patients. It was an age of panaceas. We find different practitioners placing all their hopes on purges, on clysters, on bleeding, on mineral waters or on whatever remedy their systems demanded.

Among these fanatics we may perhaps mention François-J.-V. Broussais. Certainly his theory was better than many others, for he tried to do away with vague notions of mysterious "disease" and endeavored to show that any given malady was due to something wrong with some definite organ. Irritation, he declared, was the basis of life—and of disease. Disease occurred when there was some increased irritation in some particular organ. He selected the stomach as the usual seat of trouble. In practice, however, his system resulted in an orgy of blood-letting rivaling the excesses of the great Dr. Sangrado in Le Sage's romance *Gil Blas*. As late as 1833 bleeding was still so popular that it was found necessary to import forty-one and a half millions of leeches into France. Broussais' ideas were widely accepted and blood flowed in cataracts until Laennec and other more advanced clinicians and, above all, Louis, with his medical statistics, had made it very obvious that the effects of ill-judged bleeding were not only worthless but often fatal.

Despite their great vogue, the theorists contributed little of permanent value to the knowledge of the nature and cure of disease; but signs were not lacking that men's minds were beginning to stir in new directions.

PRACTICAL SCIENTIFIC PROGRESS

IN THE 18TH CENTURY

Fortunately there were, besides all these theory-mongers, many in the 18th Century who devoted themselves wholeheartedly to more scientific medicine. These were trained and highly practical observers and, if they had their theories, they did not allow their work to be hampered by any preconceived notions. It was during the 18th and early 19th Centuries that the foundations of pathology and the principles of hygiene and of sound clinical diagnosis were firmly laid.

The progress that was made during this period in medicine and surgery was the work of several different schools in different countries. Owing to the unsettled state of Europe discoveries and methods did not always travel very readily from one country to another. Consequently we find the English and various Continental schools developing along somewhat different lines.

On the Continent there was Hermann Boerhaave at Leyden, whose teaching spread to England through his many English pupils. His was the great center of medical training and he endeavored to apply all available discoveries in every scientific subject to the practical advancement of medicine.

At Padua Giovanni Battista Morgagni laid the very important foundations of morbid anatomy. He examined great numbers of bodies after death and carefully and systematically recorded everything which he found abnormal. The great importance of his work lies in the fact that he also recorded the diseases, and signs and symptoms of the diseases, in the individuals before they died. In this way he began the scientific study of the changes brought about in the body by disease—a study without which medicine could hardly have made any but purely empirical advance.

Morgagni's great work was followed up by the Scotsman Matthew Baillie, who was a pupil at William Hunter's famous Windmill Street School, to which we shall have occasion to refer later. Baillie published the results of an enormous amount of work in a systematic treatise, *Morbid Anatomy*, excellently illustrated with copper-plates.

In England Richard Mead, in spite of his mathematical theories and his conjectures about the power of the sun and moon over the human body,[1] had very definite ideas about epidemic diseases. In 1720 he published a *Short Discourse Concerning Pestilential Contagion and the Methods to be used to prevent it*. This remarkable work contains detailed instructions for quarantine, for the evacuation of towns, for the cleansing or demolition of infected houses, for cleaning the streets, for removing nuisances, and for the prohibition of assemblies. He definitely states that lack of cleanliness and overcrowding is the reason "why the poor are most obnoxious to contagious diseases." Almost the whole of his recommendations are such as would appeal to any sanitary authority today.

Notable studies of certain infectious fevers had been made in England by John Huxham and John Fothergill. The former made careful reports on such diseases as typhus and typhoid, scarlatina and diphtheria, though he did not, of course, use these names, nor did he always distinguish between the various fevers. He, too, was a pupil of Boerhaave of Leyden. Fothergill made important contributions towards the study of infectious sore-throats.

Another notable Englishman who studied at Leyden was Sir John Pringle. He gained considerable experience as physician to

---

[1] Of course there is nothing inherently foolish about this conception of disease. That seasonal and climatic variations affect some maladies is obvious enough, and it is certain that such influences are primarily controlled by the sun and the moon.

the British forces during the campaigns in Flanders and wrote a valuable work on the health of the Army. In this he studied carefully the types of the various diseases together with the climate and season of their incidence. He showed that many diseases had remediable causes and pointed out the means of removing them. Later he became President of the Royal Society and presented the Copley Medal in 1756 to the representative of Captain Cook, who had achieved a remarkable performance in preserving the health of his crew during a three-year voyage, with only one man dead of sickness. It was Pringle who inaugurated military hygiene by combating damp, filth, and bad air in Army barracks and cantonments.

The English Navy had its sanitary champion in James Lind, who did for the seamen what Pringle had accomplished for the soldiers. His successful essay on the most effectual means of preserving the health of sailors had run into three editions by 1772. His directions against gaol-fever (typhus) and scurvy met with well-merited success. To Lind is due the almost complete disappearance of scurvy from the Navy.

In surgery the 18th Century Englishmen also made very great advances, and of these the greatest was John Hunter. He was the pupil of the celebrated Percival Pott of St. Bartholomew's Hospital, whose name is recalled to medical men by Pott's fracture (of the fibula) which he himself sustained through falling from his horse, and Pott's disease (tuberculosis of the spine) which he described.

Hunter's activities were multifarious. Besides his medical discoveries on the repair of tendons, on digestion, on teeth, on transplantation, inflammation, wounds, shock, and many other subjects, he also made important excursions into human anatomy, physiology, and the comparative anatomy of beasts, insects, and plants. He collected a magnificent private museum of over 13,000 specimens. After Hunter's death in 1793, his executors offered to sell the collection to the government. But Pitt, then Prime Minister, said, "What! Buy preparations! Why, I have not money enough to purchase gunpowder." The collection was eventually acquired by the state, however, for the sum of £15,000, and placed under the care of the Corporation of Surgeons.

Hunter's importance lies in his methods as well as in his individual discoveries. He inaugurated a new era in surgery by the application of the principle of experimental verification. Before his time surgery had been based solely on anatomy, and little or no heed had been paid to pathology, that is to say the causes and sequence of changes—the natural history of disease. The work of the great morbid anatomist Morgagni had had no practical application. It was Hunter's great achievement that he showed the importance first of applying the available knowledge to surgery, and second of making experiments to try the accuracy of his conclusions.

A typical instance of the use to which he put his discoveries is his experiment with a deer in Richmond Park. He had ligated the artery which supplied blood to one of the antlers of a buck. This antler, deprived of its blood-supply, became cold; but, so far from dying, in a few days the antler had regained its blood-supply, not because the tying had been badly done, but through the enlargement of subsidiary connecting arteries above and below the ligature. Shortly after this he was able to apply the same process in the treatment of those pulsating swellings of arteries known as aneurysms, which generally prove fatal if they are not arrested. Previously surgeons had been forced to cut down on the aneurysm and remove its contents after tying the artery above and below. This was often disastrous. The alternative had been amputation. Hunter was able to show that better results could be obtained by tying the artery higher up in a healthy part of the limb without danger of the limb suffering from want of blood.

Personally, John Hunter seems to have been a rude and quarrelsome man: in fact, as he himself had prophesied, he met his death from an attack of angina pectoris, to which he was subject, brought on by a fit of rage.

Among Hunter's pupils was one who was destined to have a

most profound effect upon medical thought and medical practice. This was Edward Jenner, who, starting from the belief popular in Gloucestershire that cow-pox and smallpox were antagonistic to one another, conceived the prodigious idea of vaccination against smallpox. His great discovery, which was published in 1798, was hailed with enthusiasm on the Continent and in America and many thousands of persons had been vaccinated before the close of the year 1800.

Methods of clinical diagnosis received a tremendous impetus from two other discoveries of the first importance; namely, the methods of *percussion* and *auscultation*. Both of these methods came from the Continent, the one from Vienna, the other from France.

Percussion is a way of finding out the gross physical conditions inside the body, particularly in the chest, by studying the varying sounds which occur when the body is tapped with the fingers. Leopold Auenbrugger, of Vienna, made this important contribution to medicine. In 1761, he published his *Inventum Novum*, which set forth the principles of the method. The ridicule and sarcasm which this brought upon his head delayed the general application of the invention for nearly fifty years. Finally in 1808 his book was translated into French and rapidly attained fame throughout Europe. The method itself depends upon the principle that the chest (and abdominal) wall is a kind of drum which, when lightly struck in different places, gives out notes which differ according to whether there is gas, liquid, or solid lying inside at the place where the wall is struck.

Auscultation means simply the study of the sounds which go on inside the body and is chiefly applied to the heart and lungs. The significance of these sounds was discovered by René T.-H. Laennec, a great Parisian clinician, early in the 19th Century. It was in 1819 that he invented the stethoscope. With this instrument he made so careful an examination of the sounds he heard in the heart and lungs of patients both healthy and sick that he put the study of these sounds for the first time upon a really firm foundation. The methods of Auenbrugger and Laennec together are responsible directly for much of the knowledge which has since been gained about the diagnosis of disease in the chest.

It was not until after the close of the Napoleonic Wars that these ideas were put into practice in the British Isles. The first English translation of Laennec's great work was made by John Forbes in 1821. He also translated in 1824 Auenbrugger's important work on percussion, which had long remained unknown to English physicians. The famous Dublin school of medicine began to adopt the methods of Laennec at this time. Its leader, William Stokes, brought the use of the stethoscope to the notice of the profession and published much valuable work on heart-disease.

In the United States these improved methods of physical diagnosis were popularized chiefly by a group of young Boston physicians who took post-graduate training in Paris, and whose contributions we shall describe in a later chapter.

From France, too, came the first statistical studies of disease. Of course there had been statistics of births and deaths before this time, but the great Parisian clinician Pierre-C.-A. Louis (1787–1872) was the first to show the value of purely medical· statistics. By collecting the records of numbers of cases of different diseases he was able to show convincing proof of the efficacy, worthlessness, or disastrous results of their treatment. Thus he helped to stem the torrent of blood-letting in which Broussais and others indulged, for he brought forward figures to show that in pneumonia, at least, bleeding was worse than useless. To Louis belongs the credit of showing that statistics are an important adjunct to the advancement of medical knowledge.

In German medicine at the beginning of the 19th Century we find numbers of different schools of thought, some of which made great advances while others indulged in such overwhelming masses of verbiage that it is almost impossible to discover any meaning at all in their systems. One group, following the zoologists and botanists, tried to formulate a dogmatic classification which, in the state of medical knowledge existing at the time, could not be very successful. This school was led by Johann Lucas Schönlein, who did valuable work in introducing the use of the microscope and examination of the blood. Schönlein made also one very significant discovery when he showed that the skin disease known as *favus* was due to a parasitic fungus. This was an isolated discovery—the first of the microscopical parasites of which many more were to be found in the course of the next hundred years.

At Vienna a new school of medicine was growing up. Here Josef Skoda made considerable advances in the use of auscultation for the diagnosis of chest diseases. Though he believed that diagnosis could be perfected, when it came to treatment he confessed himself impotent and took a completely defeatist attitude. "*Nichts tun is das beste bei der innern Medizin,*" was his philosophy.[1]

The treatment at the disposal of the physicians of these times was necessarily inadequate. Before the discovery of the parasitic nature of many diseases there could be no specific remedies except the few drugs that were known by experience to be effective. Quinine for malarial fevers and mercury for syphilis were used with good effect. Most drugs, however, could only be used to relieve symptoms and could not strike at the cause of the disease, for this was unknown.

[1] "The best treatment is to do nothing."

18TH CENTURY SURGERY
AND ITS LIMITATIONS

Surgery, also, as practised in the 18th Century, was limited by the rudimentary knowledge of the causes of disease. If we look at the surgical writings, the notes and reports of hospitals, the textbooks and other publications of the 18th Century, we are at once struck by the fact that the operations of those days were for the most part emergency procedures necessitated by trauma or infection. Broken bones were set, wounds probed and sutured, crushed or gangrenous limbs amputated, abscesses lanced. The operations for thyroid disease, appendicitis, gall bladder disease, and cancer that make up the bulk of a surgeon's work today were unknown.

Although these limitations of the scope of the surgeon's art were of course partly due to the fact that many of the surgical diseases that we know today were not then understood, they arose chiefly from the two great surgical handicaps. The first was the lack of a means of controlling pain, and the second was the lack of a method of controlling infection.

It will be readily understood that in the days when operations were done without anaesthetics, it was highly desirable that they should be done as rapidly as possible. The patient's agony called for speed, which took precedence over everything. The great surgeons of the past justly prided themselves on the dexterity and rapidity with which they could perform operations.

It must be realized that there were only a few surgeons who

would undertake big operations, and these were found only in the great towns. Operating must have been a ghastly business and he who could perform feats of skill amid the agonizing scenes in the operating theater must have had nerves of steel. Some surgeons might alleviate the frightful distress by dosing the patients with opium or alcohol, but even this could not make the pain bearable.

Operation therefore was generally only undertaken with the object of saving life. The patient was not usually cured even if he survived the surgeon's care, because such procedures as amputations, for example, which constituted a large part of all the operations performed, could hardly be said to be cures. They were usually undertaken in emergencies where they were the only hope for the patient's life. Many of the greatest surgeons were fully of the opinion that the knife should be used only as a last resort and that wholesale removal of parts of the body was an admission of ignorance and failure.

The absence of anaesthetics, apart from the patient's point of view, had the further disadvantage that the surgeons were prevented from embarking upon new operations of a more severe or intricate kind, such as can now be attempted with success. It was not until the coming of anaesthetics that painstaking attention to detail could take the place of the lightning legerdemain of the older school of operators and that conservative measures could be practised at comparative leisure.

But the greatest handicap of the surgeons of a hundred years ago and before was infection. Almost every accidental wound brought to a hospital for treatment, and every operative wound made in a hospital, became infected. A high percentage of these infections were serious ones. Under these circumstances surgery was limited to minor procedures on the surface of the body, and to opening abscesses and amputating limbs that had to be dealt with. The surgeons dared not invade the great cavities of the body, the chest, the head, and the abdomen.

Good descriptions of the actual practice of surgery a hundred years ago are fortunately available to us. In 1818 three young Dutch surgeons set out on a tour of Continental clinics. One of them wrote an interesting account of what they saw, excerpts from which have recently been published by Deelman. The American surgical scene of the time has been well set forth in a series of case reports from the New York Hospital recently published by Pool and McGowan. They were taken from the recently found "Surgical Register" for the hospital covering the period from 1808 to 1833.

18TH CENTURY HOSPITALS:

HOSPITALISM AND ITS CAUSES

THE OLDER hospitals of Europe had their origin in religious foundations, and their functions differed essentially from those of today. They were not medical but ecclesiastical. They were for the care rather than the cure of their inmates. Excluding monasteries and friaries there were more than 750 charitable institutions in mediaeval England. It was from some of these that the oldest of present-day hospitals grew, but there were others that retained their original characters as homes for the aged and infirm. Of the former type is the great hospital of St. Bartholomew in the City of London, while a good example of the latter kind is the hospital of St. Cross, near Winchester.

Many of the more famous hospitals of England were built in the 18th Century to fill the growing need for purely medical care of the sick. St. Thomas's Hospital had previously been founded in 1693, while St. Bartholomew's was rebuilt in 1739. The philan-thropist Thomas Guy, who spent next to nothing on himself but gave away magnificently, began the building of the hospital that bears his name, and, when he died in 1724, left the bulk of his fortune, amounting to over £200,000, for its completion and en-dowment. It was to be further supported by donations which gave the benefactors "free letters" by which they could obtain entry for any sick person whom they might choose. The Westminster Hospital, St. George's Hospital, and The London Hospital were all founded between 1719 and 1740, while Edinburgh and Glasgow and other large towns also built for themselves similar institutions.

All these were general hospitals: they took in anyone, whatever his complaint might be. There were a few, but very few, hospitals for special diseases. In London, for example, a special smallpox hospital was opened in 1746; the Children's Hospital was opened in 1769. The Royal Sea-Bathing Infirmary for scrofula (the King's evil) was started in 1791, largely through the action of the famous Dr. John Coakley Lettsom. He had, however, been anticipated by Russell who, observing that scrofula seldom or never attacked fishermen, began an institute for sea-bathing at Brighton. The great "sea-water Russell" himself describes how "children sent to him for treatment delicate and pale, over-clothed and glandular, had been returned to their parents after sea-bathing bare-necked, their hair shaved, the tumours of the neck cured, and the countenances healthy." The Royal London Ophthalmic Hospital was established as the first special hospital for diseases of the eyes in 1804.

In America also, during the 18th Century, general hospitals were built in several of the important cities. The Pennsylvania Hospital in Philadelphia was opened in 1752. The New York Hospital was opened in 1776, and Bellevue Hospital in the same city in 1794. The Charity Hospital in New Orleans (originally St. John's Hospital) was established in 1736. All of these institutions played an important role in the development of American medicine.

The general character of the buildings of these early hospitals can be seen from those still in use today, with the addition of modern plumbing, for example the older blocks of buildings at St. Bartholomew's. But though the buildings were the same, the hospitals were far from being the clean and sanitary institutions that they are now. The new buildings of the time rapidly lapsed into unparalleled squalor, largely because of overcrowding, lack of cleanliness, and inadequate water supplies.

A sidelight on the filthiness of the rooms may be gained from the fact that Dr. Lettsom, when a student, seemed to think his teacher, the poet Mark Akenside, excessively fussy because he prohibited spitting in the wards. Benjamin Rush, an eminent Philadelphia physician of this period, who had served in the hospitals on both sides of the Atlantic, labelled them "the sinks of human life."

The famous Englishman John Howard, who did so much to reform hospitals and prisons, has left a good description of the conditions in 18th Century hospitals. In the Greek hospitals in Constantinople, for example, he found the sick lying on the floors in a neglected condition. Of St. Thomas's Hospital in London he wrote, "There were no water-closets." In Westminster Hospital, he reported, "A sum is paid every year for the destruction of bugs and blankets. A very sickly boy had not had his clothes taken off for a fortnight."

The surgical wards were veritable forcing-houses for sepsis. They could hardly have been organized in a way better calculated to favor the spread of septic diseases. There were four horrible sicknesses which were so much more prevalent in hospitals than outside them that they were called "hospital diseases." These were erysipelas, pyaemia, septicaemia and gangrene, mysterious pestilences that came upon the patients and killed them like flies. There seemed neither rhyme nor reason for these deaths. It appeared to be simply a matter of misfortune. The fatalities bore little or no relationship to the care or skill with which the operations had been performed. The scourges came in waves, and, once established in a ward, would travel from patient to patient with heart-rending swiftness. Sir James Simpson in his statistical investigations on hospitalism showed that in large metropolitan hospitals 1 in 2.4 patients who underwent amputation died, for the most part of sepsis; while outside, in private and country practice, only 1 in 9.2 died. The mortality from amputation was therefore about four times as great in hospitals as in private homes.

In those times wounds were seldom known to heal in the clean and straightforward way in which they mostly do today. Suppuration was the rule, healing "by first intention" a rarity. Some, indeed, taught that pus formation was one of the essential processes of healing, and they talked of "laudable pus." A simple fracture mended wonderfully well, but when the fracture was compound, that is to say when the skin was broken, the outlook was black. The surgeon waited gloomily, fearing the dreaded shivering attack which ushered in the fatal poisoning of the blood.

The methods of treatment varied with different surgeons. There was the "open" method, in which the wound was left uncovered in order to promote the formation of a scab, for it was noted that when a healthy scab had once formed, then the wound would heal without accident. Other surgeons, believing the air to be the bearer of disease, closed up the wound with airtight dressings such as gold-beater's skin. Where the wound was already infected, this treatment, which shut in the poisons, led to frequent disaster. Perhaps one of the most successful methods was that practised by James Syme, the great Edinburgh surgeon and the teacher of Lister: the drainage of the wounds by leaving the long ends of the ligatures hanging out. In this way he sought to drain out the poisons into the dressings of the wound; but such drainage must have been at best imperfect.

The last of the pre-antiseptic surgeons were agreed upon one point at least: namely, that sepsis was favored by dirt and by having other "dirty" (suppurating) wounds in the same ward, and by overcrowding the patients. None realized that, in general, it was they themselves who were unconsciously poisoning their patients every time they used the probe or the knife. The probe was a favorite instrument for the examination of wounds; it was never sterilized and, at the most, was washed after its use on each patient. Who could devise a better means of carrying infection? And these conditions continued until late in the 19th Century.

The surgeons themselves wore their oldest frock-coats in the operating theater. These were often heavily encrusted with dried blood and pus. In some instances the surgeons even attached a certain sense of superiority to them. These loathsome coats might be used for six months, a year, or more, without being changed. When we consider that frequently the pieces of whipcord used for the tying of arteries were kept hanging on the buttonhole of such a coat, we can only be astonished that every operation did not end in disaster.

The hospital nurses of the 18th Century demand some brief description. They were generally of the charwoman type, unreliable and incompetent. Miss Nightingale quoted a London doctor regarding the nurses in his hospital: "All drunkards without exception, sisters and all, and there are but two nurses whom the surgeon can trust to give the patients their medicine."

It is needless to say that there were many vigorous champions of these nurses, who absolutely denied the charges of tippling. Their denials may perhaps be accorded the weight they deserve when we read Lord Granville's ingenuous observation: "The nurses are very good now, perhaps they do drink a little, but so do the ladies' monthly nurses, and nothing could be better than them: poor people, it must be so tiresome sitting up all night." Dickens' portrait of Sarah Gamp in *Martin Chuzzlewit* is a vivid description of a nurse of this type.

The hospitals of these olden times were terribly overcrowded. The beds were packed close to one another in large open wards, and it was not unusual to have more than one patient in each bed. The example of the Hôtel Dieu, the great hospital opposite Notre Dame Cathedral in Paris, is no doubt an extreme one, but it throws some light on the conditions that existed in some places. In 1786 the leading Parisian surgeon of the day, Jean-Louis Petit, complained that the Hôtel Dieu ought to be rebuilt outside the city, where, he said, "one would no longer see six unhappy patients heaped in a bed annoying and frightening each other, infecting each other, one throwing himself about and shrieking when the others have need of repose. One would no longer see a dying patient confess himself beside five others who hear every word he says; another receive the last Sacrament on a mattress where a patient in the agony of death voids his excrements with his last breath, or a patient who cannot retain the effect of a purgative or an emetic lying beside a madman who in his frenzy forms a deplorable contrast with the priest who recites the prayers for the dead."

The dispensaries or out-patient departments of the hospitals in great cities, where the poor had no other means of obtaining ambulatory medical care, were similarly overcrowded. Indeed we do not have to go back to the 18th Century to find glaring examples of this. In 1878 Robert Bridges, who later became Poet Laureate, wrote a revealing description of the crowded conditions in the casualty department of St. Bartholomew's Hospital. During his house-officership he worked in this department for three months between the hours of 9 and 12 on four mornings of the week. He dealt with a total of 7735 patients, of whom 5330 were new cases! Many of these had only trifling complaints, but some were seriously and others mortally ill. Bridges realized full well that the task of "filtering" out the sick patients when he had no time to examine them properly was impossible. He did the best he could to distinguish the old women who wanted cod liver oil to burn in lamps or confection of senna for jam tarts, from those who were really sick, devoting an average of 1.28 minutes to each patient. But he concluded that the system was for him an "intolerable" one. It is of interest that this righteous protest against superficial and hurried medical methods was one of three medical papers that Bridges wrote before he gave up medicine for poetry.

Hospital care was not transformed in a day. Many 18th Century traditions hung on until much later, and fostered in the public that fear of hospitals which persists even today.

THE SANITARY CONDITIONS OF THE
PEOPLE A HUNDRED YEARS AGO

THE STATE of public hygiene on the eve of the great era of medical discovery was one to invite overcrowding of the hospitals, especially by the poor of the great cities. And yet, in reading descriptions of the sanitary conditions of the people a hundred years ago we must remember first of all that these conditions were in many ways better than they had been during many preceding centuries. Second, we must bear in mind that such accounts often described the worst slums that could be found, and cannot therefore be accepted as representative of the state of the people as a whole. This is not to say that the hygiene of the people was good; indeed, much of what we read appears horrible beyond belief.

If we wish to find out some of the worst features in the lives of the people in England at that time we cannot do better than turn to the admirable report of the Poor Law Commissioners for 1842 on the *Sanitary Condition of the Labouring Population of Great Britain,* which had been prepared by Edwin Chadwick. Here we find described conditions that seem absolutely inconceivable to us today.

The book deals particularly with the towns. Largely as a result of recruitments from the country for the new factories, towns had been growing fast—too fast indeed for any proper scheme of housing to be devised. In the big towns it was the speculative builder who supplied the houses for the rapidly increasing additions to the population. In order to obtain the highest possible yield for their money the builders set about leasing and buying land and cramming as many people as was possible on to a given acreage at the least possible cost.

The streets were made as narrow as was feasible. The houses were built back to back without drainage or foundations, and constructed of the flimsiest and cheapest materials available. There was nothing to stop the builder from doing exactly as he pleased; and what he pleased was generally as far removed from any kind of town planning as it is possible to imagine. There was, in fact, according to the Health of Towns Commission, actual encouragement to build bad houses, because, if the house was bad enough, it escaped payment of taxes, "partly through the inefficiency of the law and partly through the difficulty of enforcing it." There were, of course, notable exceptions. Certain enlightened landlords made conditions before granting leases and insisted on substantial buildings, wide streets, and sometimes even sewers. This was far from general, however, and the results of such thoughtless building were worse than the most pessimistic landlord could have expected.

In the older towns like Edinburgh and Glasgow overcrowding was as bad as in the newer towns. Large families lived in rooms that had been originally intended for cellars, without light, air or drainage. Here might be found twelve or eighteen persons in as many square feet. The absence of drainage or sewers produced conditions too revolting to be fully described. Many of these badly built dwellings had low passages leading into square courts which were used entirely as dung receptacles of the most disgusting kind. Indeed, part of the rent of the houses was paid for by the sale of these heaps for manure.

We read of open drains in Stirling which were flushed only when there was a hard shower. The filth from the gaol was washed down the public streets at intervals. Blood flowed from the slaughter-house down the highways. Often the lower parts of the houses themselves were used as dung-heaps or pigsties. There were no public toilets and the stairs and streets were often used as such.

In Manchester the streets were barely passable from mud or tolerable from stench. There were, according to the Poor Law Commissioners, many "open cesspools, obstructed drains, ditches full of stagnant water, dunghills, pigsties, etc., from which the most abominable odours were emitted." That the streets in these and many other towns were not drained would have been of little consequence had they been properly scavenged; but attempts at street-cleaning were of the most inadequate and perfunctory kind.

In many places the sewers that did exist were hopelessly unsuitable and never originally intended for house-drainage, or indeed for anything more than to carry water off from the streets. Through carelessness or ignorance they were often constructed with flat bottoms so that they were rapidly silted up; frequently they were built without regard to geographical levels so that from time to time, especially during floods, the contents of the sewers were regurgitated into the houses. This was particularly likely to happen when the drains opened into a tidal river. Nauseous gases too often found their way from untrapped sewers into dwelling-houses. Where efficient main sewers existed there was more likely to be a considerable charge for connecting a house to the main rather than a penalty for omitting to do so.

In places where house-drainage was connected up with sewers, these generally ran directly into the local river, canal, or stream with the natural result that such water became a stinking open drain. The Thames had become horribly polluted. "What was the use of praying to be delivered from plagues and pestilences so long as the common sewers ran into the Thames?" reasoned Florence Nightingale. "The Serpentine, itself, intended . . . as an ornamental water, became an open sewer which drained Kilburn, Paddington and Bayswater," writes a historian of the period.

The absence in many places of an adequate supply of water had a very pronounced effect in increasing or keeping up an intense squalor. Water is important not only because it is necessary for the flushing of sewers and the cleaning of streets, but also because it induces cleanly domestic habits.

In certain districts the shortage was pitiful. In Hampstead and Hendon water was bought by the pailful, while in Edinburgh many persons had to carry it for long distances and then perhaps to the top of a five- or six-story house. In many places the supply was intermittent and turned on for grossly inadequate periods. Generally the only supply of running water that was available for private houses was to be had at considerable expense from private water companies. A notable exception to this was Bath, where there was a plentiful supply, which, owing to the geography of the town, needed no mechanism to arrive at any part.

Often the little water that was available was of the most disgusting kind, filthy, unwholesome, malodorous and discolored. A water-supply was not an unmixed blessing where it enabled people to have their own cesspools. London, for example was riddled with these faulty contrivances, which were often liable to leak or overflow; and as a result any neighbouring water-supply might be contaminated with sewage.

Lack of ventilation and light was by no means peculiar to the cellar dwellings which we have described. The notorious window tax, though reduced in amount, still set a price on these necessities. It is true that the duties were levied only on those houses which had more than eight windows; but in many places there were large houses inhabited by several families of poor people, and these were taxed on the total number of windows.

If such abominations were to be found in the larger towns, what sort of sanitation was there likely to be in the villages? Little or none. It must be remembered, however, that conditions that are likely to create squalor in towns can be comparatively harmless in the country. If one were to apply the standards of many small villages in England today to a town of considerable size, the results would be horrible. The country villagers had no piped water-supply and no need for drains and sewers; but if they had overcrowding in their cottages, they had also the fresh air of the countryside and lived their lives for the most part out of doors. The country folk were liable to the same diseases which attacked the townsmen; but it is significant that the death-rate of the country was lower. This circumstance may be partially accounted for by the fact that many who were born in the country went to die in the towns.

There has been an unfortunate tendency to idealize the village life of those days, but the legend of the healthy villages of the 18th Century is probably no truer than that of the healthy savage of today. Goldsmith's "Sweet Auburn" must have been an insanitary place even before it became deserted. In George Crabbe's *The Village* we find a graphic account of the sorrow and squalor in the parish poor-house and "of the consequential apothecary who gives an impatient attendance in these abodes of misery. . . ."

> A potent quack long versed in human ills
> Who first insults the victim whom he kills;
> Whose murd'rous hands a drowsy Bench protect,
> And whose most tender mercy is neglect.

It has been customary to blame the Industrial Revolution for the unhealthy state of the towns and to some extent this is justified. But the industrialists were not wholly to blame. That there was "sweated labor" under vile conditions there can be no doubt. The descriptions of the badly ventilated, overheated and candle-lit workrooms of the London journeymen tailors, for example, make sad reading. The depressing effect of long hours in foul air, laden with moisture and perspiration, surely drove them to the habit of breakfasting off gin. Small wonder that numbers of them were "taken with a decline." The master tailors attributed this ill-health to drink, whereas it seems fairly clear that heavy drinking was but one of the appalling results of the conditions under which the journeymen lived.

Industry drew countless numbers of men, women and children into towns too small to hold them. Overcrowding was an inevitable result. If the new houses of the speculative builder were "unfit for human habitation" (in the language of the modern sanitary inspector) they were probably no worse and sometimes better than the normal artisan's house of the day. Of drainage and water-supply there had been none before and they were not missed.

It is necessary to view the advantages of industrialism as well as its drawbacks. Commerce, improved agriculture, and new facilities for transport had made the food of the people more plentiful, more varied, and above all, more certain. Manufacturers had given them cheap cotton—a circumstance which, next to water, did more towards keeping them clean than any other single factor. The truth of the matter is that the great evils which had been present for many hundreds of years were simply accentuated by the Industrial Revolution. There was nothing new about them. They were a legacy from the Middle Ages. It has been pointed out that the reason we hear so much of these distressing circumstances is that the masses were becoming articulate. Previously they had suffered in silence, but with leadership they could make themselves heard. The Victorian novelists, too, were to do much to draw attention to current abuses, but to convince ourselves that these things were not new we have only to read some of the novelists of the 18th Century—for example, Tobias Smollett, himself a doctor of medicine, who gives us so graphic a description of the methods of sewage disposal at Edinburgh, of the food supply of London, and the waters of Bath.

In America the growth of cities and the Industrial Revolution also brought bad sanitation, but to a lesser extent than in England. This was due to several factors. The introduction of methods for manufacturing print cotton goods in New England led to the building of many factories and to a concentration of laborers in cities during the decade of 1820 to 1830. But since the new factories were usually built on water power sites in the country or in the outskirts of towns, the tenements that grew up around them escaped to a considerable extent the overcrowding that the Industrial Revolution brought about in the older, larger, and more static English towns. Moreover, the factory system had developed in England a generation earlier, and its evils were already apparent to some.

When Dickens, who was thoroughly aware of the problems of his day, toured America in 1842, he visited tenement districts, hospitals, insane asylums, and prisons wherever he could find them. His descriptions were full of praise. The conditions under which the factory workers in Lowell lived, their pianos, circulating libraries, and literary magazine filled him with joy.

Of course there were black spots. The New York slums were the worst. Here the very poor, and hordes of immigrants, lived under horrible conditions. The best description of these slums was written by Dr. John H. Griscom, City Inspector of Health during the year 1842. He became deeply interested in the need for sanitary reform and placed the problem before the City Council. He was rewarded for his pains by not being reappointed Inspector. Griscom thereupon published his recommendations in a little book entitled *The Sanitary Condition of the Laboring Population of New York*. Here he described misery and disease in the New York slums comparable to that detailed by Chadwick in English cities. The congestion in New York slums was accentuated by the flood of immigrants. The inhabitants of the cellars suffered the most, since they were crowded together without light or air in foul holes into which sewage continually seeped. As might be expected, disease made frightful havoc among them. The system of tenantry in which the actual owner of the property escaped direct responsibility by delegating authority to a sublandlord made reform difficult.

Dickens saw some of these conditions when he visited New

York, and described them realistically. "There is one quarter, commonly called the Five Points," he wrote, "which in respect to filth and wretchedness, may be safely backed against Seven Dials, or any other part of the famed St. Giles." The scavenger pigs loose on Broadway were a touch of local color that did not escape his eye.

As late as 1865 these appalling conditions persisted in New York. A sanitary inspector reported of the Sixth Ward that "Domestic garbage and filth of every kind is thrown into the streets, covering their surface, filling the gutters, obstructing the sewer culverts. . . . In winter the filth and garbage, etc., accumulate to the depth sometimes of two or three feet." At this date about 18,000 people were still living in cellars, in which appalling conditions persisted: "At high tide the water often wells up through the floors, submerging them to a considerable depth. In very many cases the vaults of privies are situated on the same or a higher level, and their contents frequently ooze through the walls into the occupied apartments beside them."

One of the worst abuses of the period of which we write was the exploitation of child labor in factories. In the latter part of the 18th Century in England this took the form of veritable slavery. Pauper children were indentured in gangs to the eager factory owners. They worked for sixteen hours a day, frequently with irons riveted upon their ankles. They slept in relays in filthy beds that were never allowed to cool, in nearby barracks. The first British Factory Act in 1802 provided for proper clothing and food for these children and reduced their hours of work to twelve! Another generation went by before further Factory Acts brought this abuse under control.

In America also child labor was exploited, but not so cruelly as in 18th Century England. In 1837 a Pennsylvania Senatorial Committee found that one-fifth of the entire number of workers in the cotton mills of the state were under twelve years of age, and that the time spent at work ranged from eleven to fourteen hours a day. In this state in 1848 the working day was limited to ten hours, and in 1849 the minimum age of workers was raised to thirteen years. In 1842 Massachusetts limited the work day for children to ten hours. For many years to come, however, despite much legislation, children were forced to wear out their youth in the dreary mills of New England towns.

THE HEALTH OF THE PEOPLE

A HUNDRED YEARS AGO

U NDER SUCH adverse housing conditions as we have described, the general level of health of the people was low. Unfortunately, lack of dependable vital statistics makes it difficult to estimate it precisely.

We can find plenty of information about individual institutions, doctors, diseases or cases of sickness, but about the health of the public in general the data are meagre. In order to make any reliable estimate of the prevailing health conditions it is essential to know the population at any given time, the number of births in each succeeding period, the number and the causes of the deaths, and the age of each person at death. None of these can we find accurately.

The London Bills of Mortality, from 1605, were compiled by the parish clerks, who also entered the causes of death as determined by official searchers, generally persons ignorant of the elements of medicine. There were also the parish registers, but in these we find many defects. First, there are many omissions, for it is baptisms and burials, not births and deaths, that are entered here. Dissenters might not be entered, while Jews and Roman Catholics often had separate cemeteries. In many places, too, the registers were kept with the utmost carelessness. In making up the Bills of Mortality the information was taken from the parish registers, so that the same mistakes occur in both.

The first census in England was taken in 1801, but through lack of efficient control it was unreliable. Consequently it is only from information obtained later in the century that we can obtain by retrospective computation the best, but by no means accurate, estimate of the population in England.

At this early date dependable vital statistics were equally lacking in America. Here Bills of Mortality were made up by the towns on the basis of the enumeration by sextons of the burials in cemeteries. These records were necessarily inaccurate. In many parts of the country there was no method for registering births. In New York City, for instance, there was no registry of births as late as 1838.

The United States Constitution provided for a decennial census, and thus we became one of the first countries to institute a regular periodical enumeration of inhabitants. It must be admitted, however, that this provision for a census by the writers of the Constitution was made on political grounds rather than out of consideration for public health. The first census was made in 1790.

The systematic registration of vital statistics, upon which so much of our modern information about public health depends, was begun in the Scandinavian countries. Since 1686 Swedish ecclesiastical law has required the clergy to keep records of marriages, births, deaths, and of all persons moving into or leaving the parish, but these records were at first irregular and incomplete. In 1748 the Swedish Riksdag passed a comprehensive law to regulate the recording and compilation of these parish statistics. It also provided for a census. Sweden therefore has an unbroken series of vital statistics dating back to 1749, a unique contribution to public health. In Norway, the recording of parish vital statistics was begun in 1735, and the first census was made in 1769.

Meagre and uncertain as is the information we possess regarding vital statistics during the 18th Century, we can see certain tendencies which stand out quite clearly: there are movements which occurred on so large a scale that they show obviously through all possible sources of error. First and foremost is the undoubted fact that, while previously the population had not increased very quickly, an enormous increase occurred in the last half of the 18th Century throughout Europe. If we discount immigration and emigration (which were not on so large a scale as to affect the general conclusion), this can have arisen only from an increased birth-rate or a decreased death-rate, or both.

It has often been assumed that the birth-rate rose rapidly, but there is really very little good evidence for this. If we assume, however, that the population increased because of a diminished death-rate, we can point to many very good reasons for such a belief. We can show the disappearance of a number of adverse factors which had combined to kill off the people in previous times and we can point to the active measures which had been carried out to achieve this disappearance.

In the Middle Ages famine had been a destructive agent of incalculable scope. Agriculture was primitive and a failure of the crops in one area led to a scarcity of food through lack of efficient transport from other districts. The same factors led furthermore to a lack of variety of foods, especially of fresh food during the winter months. By 1830 improved methods of agriculture and better transport had to a large extent banished the fear of famine from the land.

The other great enemy was pestilence. If we inquire into the diseases which took a heavy toll of life in previous times we shall find that many of these were decreasing, some of them to vanishing-point. Some diseases may have disappeared of themselves for no very obvious cause, but with others we can point to some excellent reasons.

Leprosy was virtually extinguished, and this has been claimed as a triumph for the method of segregating the sick; but the disappearance of leprosy may well have been due to some quite different cause, for the exact method of infection is as yet unknown.

Plague, too, had disappeared from London and, except for occasional epidemics, from the Western world. The reason for this is by no means clear. Strict quarantine against the dreaded pestilence may have had much to do with it, but other reasons have been advanced. For example, it has been suggested that it might have been due to the fact that the black rat, chief carrier of the disease, was largely displaced by the brown rat of Norway, whose habits are not so domestic as his black cousin's.

Smallpox was always present in Europe and America in the 18th Century, attacking principally the very young, killing enormous numbers, particularly of infants, disfiguring and often blinding those it did not kill. No class was exempt: indeed in the previous century it had carried off the Queen of England herself. Smallpox hospitals were founded for the reception of the sick. The inoculation of mild smallpox to guard against a more virulent attack was freely practised. This certainly achieved its effect in making many people immune, but it was a highly dangerous practice and must have helped to keep the disease alive after the coming of vaccination. Jenner's discovery that inoculation with cowpox (vaccination) was effective and safe, was announced in 1798 and gave new hope against the scourge. He was a pupil and friend of John Hunter's and his great discovery resulted from his daring to use his teacher's experimental methods to test the Gloucestershire tradition that milkmaids who had contracted cowpox from milking did not get smallpox. Benjamin Waterhouse introduced vaccination in America in 1800 by vaccinating his own son, as Jenner himself had done. In the years that followed, vaccination began to be practised on an increasing scale. The results must have helped materially to swell the population by saving the lives of thousands of infants every year.

The chief diseases of London in 1819, according to a contemporary scholar, were "intermittent and remittent fevers and dysentery," in fact such diseases as would be diminished by proper drainage and a good water-supply, for hidden in this list, but unrecognized, were the diseases which are now known as malaria and typhus (gaol fever). The latter was not clearly differentiated by the physicians of the period from typhoid fever (enteric) and relapsing fever. An American, W. W. Gerhard, who had been trained in the study of fevers by Louis in Paris, first clearly differentiated typhoid from typhus in 1837. This group of diseases was endemic in Gerhard's native Philadelphia, as in the other larger American cities of the time.

Some of the observers of the day fully recognized that both typhus and relapsing fever were diseases of dirt and starvation. As we have seen, Pringle and Lind had shown the way to rid the Army and Navy of typhus fever. John Howard, the great prison-reformer, at great personal risk and with immense energy made a tour of the gaols in England and Wales. The shocking squalor of these pestilential dens is recorded in his famous book, *The State of the Prisons of England and Wales*, first published in 1777. Howard, however, was not merely an observer, for he added to his description many sound hygienic suggestions for remedying this deplorable state of affairs. His recommendations have a modern flavor: baths, soap and water, smooth floors, ovens for baking the louse-ridden clothes of the prisoners, segregation of the sick, and the provision of the services of doctors. Later these methods, with fumigation, ventilation, and lime-washing, were taken up by others and applied, for example, in hospitals. Later still, separate wards were reserved for those with infectious fevers. The energetic campaign included eventually the provision of separate fever hospitals in some of the larger towns. Typhus began slowly but surely to decline.

Howard's teachings, though successfully adopted in other spheres, were rapidly discarded in the prisons themselves. In 1812 James Neild visited the prisons as Howard had done and found them "relapsing into their former horrid state of privation, filthiness, severity, and neglect," so that he had to fight Howard's battle anew. Typhus again became a great scourge in the British Isles in the early 19th Century. The disease reached its culmination in Ireland in 1816 and 1819. During these famine years there were 700,000 cases among the six million inhabitants.

At the beginning of the 19th Century, agues, many of which were undoubtedly malaria, were also rapidly diminishing in many parts of England, though they were not finally extinguished until much later. The disappearance of these fevers almost always followed the efficient draining of marsh-lands. Such drainage was not, of course, made with this object primarily in view, but rather for the reclaiming of land or the prevention of floods. Whether the dying out of malaria in England can be attributed entirely to this cause is probably doubtful, for mosquitoes capable of conveying malaria are not uncommon in England today; but, historically speaking, we may say that the sequence of events looks temptingly like cause and effect.

In America malaria was prevalent as far north as the Canadian border during Colonial times. During the first half of the 19th Century, however, the disease gradually retreated from the northern states, for reasons that are not entirely clear. It continues to this day endemic in the southern states, chiefly along the coast and in swampy regions.

In viewing such statistics as there are for the beginning of the 19th Century we find that a large decrease in the death-rate among infants and young children seems to have occurred apart from all consideration of infectious fevers. This has been attributed, probably correctly, to better standards of living, healthier dwellings and better medical advice. When we say healthier dwellings it must be clearly understood that this is not intended to mean good housing as judged by present-day standards, but a relative improvement in the conditions of living. Many English medical writers of the early 19th Century, Bateman and Farr, for example, are almost lyrical about the improvements that had taken place in the health of London and in the whole of England and Wales within their lifetime. These advances were observed on all sides and were attributed to more hygienic habits, to cleaning and scavenging, to drainage, to greater temperance, to better agriculture, and to better medicine.

SOME COMMON INFECTIOUS DISEASES
OF A CENTURY AGO

N o w t h a t we have outlined briefly the abject conditions under which the people struggled for life at the beginning of the 19th Century, it will not be surprising to find that the towns were very hotbeds of infectious disease. "Low" or "putrid" fevers were hardly ever absent from the worst of these Augean stables. We hear much more of epidemic infectious disease than of other kinds for an obvious reason. A sudden attack of a pestilence produces a profounder stir among the people than does the toll levied continuously by more insidious diseases. An unexpected outbreak obtrudes itself where the more ordinary of the killing maladies are taken as a matter of course. We tolerate the occurrence of hundreds of deaths every week on the highways of this country, for instance, whereas a similar number of deaths in railway accidents would leave us profoundly shocked.

We hear much of typhus fever, but rather less of other diseases which carried off so many lives. The reason for this is not far to seek. Typhus was likely to attack the adolescent and adult breadwinner, while smallpox, for example, wrought havoc among infants and young children and was taken more as a matter of course. These contagions must have been readily spread by all the circumstances of squalor and overcrowding which we have mentioned, as well as by the wholesale pawning of clothes and bedding and the migrations in search of work that took place in times of scarcity. Other diseases were carried chiefly by contaminated water supplies.

There was, moreover, one terrible disease for which a magnificent welcome had been prepared and which, though it may never have invaded the West before, was expected with alarm. In the year 1831 the Asiatic cholera, which had been laying waste the continent of Asia for the past dozen years, made its dreaded appearance in Europe, where the evils of war helped to propagate the contagion. It reached Germany from Russia through three routes, by way of Poland, Danzig, and Austria. In Hungary the havoc was fearful. More than a quarter of a million persons contracted the disease and of these some hundred thousand died.

In England a rigorous quarantine was instituted and the people waited with anxiety for the appearance of the terrible disease. In October it reached Hamburg, and it was not long before some vessels from Europe evaded the quarantine and the cholera disembarked at Sunderland. The disease quickly slew some two hundred persons at this port, but had well-nigh exhausted itself in the district before it spread with undiminished violence to other towns.

Early in January of 1832 the cholera reached Newcastle and proceeded on its way to Edinburgh. Scotland began to suffer, and the disease, as was its wont, took its chief toll in regions where dirt and depression most prevailed. Glasgow acted promptly by providing a cholera hospital, by closing the theaters and places of public entertainment and by discouraging shipping. Neglect of sanitation, however, brought its own reward. The disease appeared with explosive violence in the pauper infirmary and, before the epidemic waned, Glasgow had lost more than three thousand souls.

London was attacked in February and Parliament hurriedly conferred large powers on the Privy Council to make arrangements against the danger. The *Annual Register* states that "the alarm was infinitely greater than the danger" and, indeed, it is true that England suffered less, proportionately, than France or

Hungary; nevertheless, the total deaths amounted to 21,882 in England and Wales, 20,070 in Ireland and 9,592 in Scotland.

The disease was carried to the Americas by Irish immigrants, reaching both Canada and New York in June, 1832. Early in the next month it reached Philadelphia and by August it was in Maryland and Virginia, It followed the Ohio River to the central states and eventually to the Mississippi. During the following summer it spread widely through the central and southern and western states, crossed the Rockies and reached the Pacific. The terrible toll of the disease in New York can be judged from the fact that in 1832 Bellevue (then but recently opened as a fever hospital) cared for 2,000 patients, of whom 600 died.

The importance of this epidemic, which was the first of a series of visitations, lies not in the actual mortality which it caused but in the psychological effect which it produced on the rulers and the people, to say nothing of the medical profession. There does not seem to be very much doubt that it was the fear of the cholera which was largely responsible for the acceleration of the movement towards the improvement of the hygiene of the towns. The actual mode of propagation was not discovered until much later, but it was generally agreed by medical men that, whatever the primary cause of the disease, squalor was its meat and drink.

It is well to bear in mind this agreement among doctors. The disease had been excellently described, the pathology studied, a variety of remedies had been tested, and hospitals had been provided. True, the origin, the cure, and the mode of propagation were yet unknown, but the cholera did not leave medical men as it had found them. The attention of thinking people was concentrated on the state of public hygiene in the towns, for here was an obvious and *removable* cause of disease.

Yellow fever was another of the great plagues of the western hemisphere, but except for one or two isolated occasions when it was brought to seaports, it never appeared in Europe. Its regular habitat was the West Coast of Africa and the coastal areas bordering on the Gulf of Mexico, including the West Indies. During the last half of the 18th Century there were repeated epidemics in the Atlantic seaboard towns of the United States as far north as Boston. Yellow fever thrives almost exclusively in crowded centers of population. New York and Philadelphia, being the two largest cities of Colonial times, therefore suffered most severely. The 1793 epidemic in Philadelphia was the most terrible ordeal the city has ever experienced. Accurate records were not kept, but it is estimated that about one tenth of the populace perished. All who could, fled, but many were prevented from escaping by the terrified inhabitants of the neighboring countryside who barricaded the roads leading from the stricken city. New York City had a long series of yellow fever epidemics, none of which were as severe as this great Philadelphia epidemic. In 1805, for instance, when New York had a population of 75,000, there were 600 deaths from yellow fever.

Influenza is a disease which is regrettably prevalent today. It has been epidemic for as long as we can trace it back. When we follow it back into the 18th Century it becomes inextricably mixed up with the various agues and other fevers which were not then clearly distinguished from one another. In 1803 a definite epidemic of influenza occurred throughout Europe. From 1830 to 1833 it was generally diffused over both the Eastern and Western Hemispheres. In America it occurred in 1807 and 1808, again in 1815 and 1816, and from 1824 to 1826.

The influenza of 1833 in England seems to have claimed many deaths among the rich, differing, in this respect, from the cholera of the preceding year. One observer stated that he had heard of "not less than nine lords or ladies who had been carried off by it or through its indirect agency in the course of the last week." [1] The monthly bills of mortality rose suddenly to double their previous total, but they sank again fairly soon.

This epidemic seems to have been very widespread indeed

[1] *Lancet*, 2:145, 1833.

in England, and there was no place or class exempt. One doctor of the time is reported to have rejoiced at the state of affairs, saying: "I have not a moment to spare. In the very thick of my best harvest. Best thing I ever had: quite a Godsend: everybody ill, nobody dies—so the recoveries are all cures you know." [1]

The doctors did not at first realize the seriousness of the disease. When they did so we find them eagerly discussing the pathology and treatment, without, however, coming to much agreement even about the advisibility of blood-letting. The consensus of opinion was against the belief that influenza was contagious. They declared it to be no more so than the last year's cholera. The rapidity of the spread and the way in which it jumped from one part of the country to another were against the contagion theory. Evidently at this time contagion was very much out of vogue.

That this disease was not at first considered serious may have been due to an effect on statistics which is now known to be highly characteristic of influenza. This illness kills directly only a proportion of its true victims. For example, attacks occur frequently among persons of middle age who are suffering from consumption, asthma or some other respiratory disease, or among the aged who also have a lowered resistance to infection. The result is that many deaths are recorded as being due to some other cause than influenza, although they might not have occurred if this disease had not been contracted on the top of the other ailments. The consequence of this is that an epidemic of influenza sends up the figures of the "deaths from all causes" out of proportion to the deaths from the disease itself.

Measles has been known to be widespread ever since it was first properly distinguished from other eruptive diseases. Deaths from measles were comparatively rare in the 18th Century, but for some reason the mortality had been steadily increasing at the close of the century and continued to do so throughout the nine-

[1] *Lancet*, 2:125, 1833.

teenth. Both measles and whooping-cough were gradually becoming more and more important causes of death. Smallpox was declining. This is to be accounted for, partially at least, by the increasing numbers of children who were being inoculated with cow-pox according to the teaching of Jenner. Measles generally attacks later in life than smallpox. Weakly children may die of it. If they are prevented from dying of smallpox then they may die of measles or of something else later on. Statistics therefore show an increase in the mortality of diseases other than smallpox.

Scarlet fever came also in epidemics during the 18th and 19th Centuries, though it is difficult always to be sure whether an account of a "throat distemper" refers to this or to some other disease.

Diphtheria was prevalent on the continent of Europe and in America during the 18th Century, but it did not occur to any great extent in the British Isles. There was a particularly severe epidemic in the New England states during 1735 and 1736, and a half dozen further epidemics during the remainder of the century. Everywhere except in France the disease was seen but little during the first half of the 19th Century. It then became pandemic in Europe and America. In the United States it spread throughout almost the whole country during 1856. In England it appeared in London and the southern counties in 1857 and rapidly extended over the whole country.

These are very brief histories of a number of common infectious diseases which attacked our forefathers. Some of these diseases are still with us, a perpetual reminder of the fields still open to medical research.

9

THE MEDICAL PROFESSION IN THE 18TH CENTURY—ITS ORGANIZATION AND EDUCATION

THE COMMON ills of the 18th Century man, as well as the epidemic diseases which we have described, were cared for by quacks of all sorts as well as by physicians with widely different training. For a hundred years ago the medical profession was not organized on the basis of any generally accepted standards. A man could be a physician or a surgeon or he might be a mere quack, and for the general public there was no means of distinguishing one from another.

In Tudor times in England attempts had been made to prevent unauthorized persons from practising medicine. In 1511 it was enacted that no one should practise medicine or surgery in London unless he was first examined and approved by appropriate authorities. But this arrangement did not work and the poor were neglected by the surgeons, so that a further act was passed to allow persons with botanical knowledge to attend the sick poor.

From the time of the Renaissance and onwards we find a sharp distinction drawn between the physicians and the surgeons. The physicians were considered to constitute a superior profession. In 1518 they were formed into a college which was to become in 1851 The Royal College of Physicians. Surgery, on the other hand, was a less distinguished calling and was practised by the barber-surgeons, for in the time of Henry VIII the Barbers' Company had been united with the Guild of Surgeons to become the United Barber-Surgeons' Company. The union lasted until 1745, when the surgeons broke away from this misalliance, finally, in 1800, obtaining a separate charter which incorporated them as the Royal College of Surgeons. To them was entrusted the care of John Hunter's great medical collection.

The two colleges could issue degrees and diplomas, the fees for which paid for the upkeep of the colleges. However, these were not the only bodies which issued degrees in medicine. Each university, as well as the Apothecaries' Hall, could issue similar degrees without interference or supervision from any higher authority. In this way there came to be many ports of entry to the medical profession and this strange multiplicity still obtains in England today. It was not until the Medical Act of 1858 was passed that the State began to exercise any real control over the profession.

This distinction between physicians and surgeons did not gain a foothold in the American colonies, although most of the medical practitioners in early colonial days were trained in the British Isles. It is of interest in passing to note that the first president of Harvard College, Charles Chauncey, had received his M.D. at Cambridge University, and that his successor, Leonard Hoare, had also studied medicine at Cambridge University.

The early efforts to regulate the practice of medicine in the colonies consisted of laws designed to put down quacks. The first statute of this kind was enacted in Massachusetts in 1649. The General Courts granted licenses to practice medicine to individuals upon presentation of their credentials. There were, however, many irregular healers of all sorts. Eventually, after the Revolution, the various states passed laws establishing the requirements for medical licensure. Thus it has come to pass that in the United States each state has its own licensing board which examines candidates according to its own standards. These standards vary considerably, even today. There is no national regulation of medical practice.

Just over a hundred years ago the British Medical Association was founded by Sir Charles Hastings at Worcester. This was a private organization of qualified doctors intended to represent the highest standards of the profession in England. Its aims included the advancement of both the learning and the social status of medical men. The Association has done much good work in pressing for reforms in matters of public health and can well claim to represent the opinion of the great majority of general practitioners in the country.

The American Medical Association, a similar private body of regularly qualified doctors in the United States, was founded in 1847. It likewise has been a powerful agent in bringing about public health reforms such as the Pure Food and Drug Act, in suppressing medical quackery of all sorts, and in elevating the standards of medicine and of medical education.

We have seen that in the 17th Century there were medical schools in different parts of Europe and that these were generally formed around some eminent teacher. In the 18th Century these centers of teaching began to expand and become more numerous. Anatomy was taught at Paris, Berlin, Strasbourg, and in Edinburgh, Cambridge, and Glasgow. Clinical instruction was more of a novelty. Professorships of clinical medicine were founded in Edinburgh in 1741.

It was largely at the voluntary hospitals that students in England gained experience and knowledge while they worked under the great physicians and surgeons of the time. From these beginnings, at Guy's, St. Thomas's, and St. Bartholomew's, for example, have grown up the great medical schools of today. A number of private medical schools which were run for profit by individual teachers constituted another important source of medical education. Among the more famous of these in London were William Smellie's school of obstetrics, William Cullen's for internal medicine, Joseph Black's for chemistry, and William Hunter's great school in Windmill Street, where some of the greatest surgeons of their day received instruction in anatomy, surgery and obstetrics. Such extra-academic schools were of immense importance elsewhere besides in London. It was largely due to these that Edinburgh attained its great reputation as a medical center. It is interesting to recall that the most celebrated anatomy school in that town was kept by the unfortunate Dr. Robert Knox, who suffered so much from his association with the "resurrectionists" Burke and Hare.

In the American colonies, on the other hand, the early medical schools developed within the academic organization. The first of these was set up at Philadelphia in 1765 as part of the College of Philadelphia (later the University of Pennsylvania). The Medical School of King's College in New York (which was eventually to become the College of Physicians and Surgeons of Columbia University) was the second in 1768. The Harvard Medical School, the third institution of its kind in the colonies, was opened in 1783, having developed from a lecture course in anatomy given to Harvard College students during the three previous years by the surgeon John Warren. All three of these schools were organized by the best qualified physicians of the respective communities; they set a high standard and had a strong influence on the subsequent development of American medicine.

At the time of which we write there was little specialization in medical teaching. The leading surgeons were also the teachers of anatomy, which they studied sedulously in such spare time as they could find. We read of Sir Astley Cooper rising at six o'clock to put in an hour or more in his private dissecting-room before starting the day's work. The private teachers who kept their own schools may have been more specialized.

The chief obstacle in the way of teaching anatomy lay in the great difficulty of obtaining corpses, or "subjects," as they are called, for dissection. The law on the matter of obtaining such corpses was not helpful in England. Under Henry VIII it was granted that the Company of Barbers and Surgeons should have the bodies of malefactors, and in 1752 it was ordered that the bodies of murderers executed in London and Middlesex "should be conveyed to the Hall of the Surgeons' Company to be dissected and anatomized." Since this was the only legal supply in the early 19th Century there was consequently a shortage of subjects, for the general public showed a natural reluctance to submit the bodies of their dead to suffer a murderer's fate.

A knowledge of anatomy was obviously essential, and indeed was insisted on by the Corporation of Surgeons for its member practitioners, who otherwise must experiment blindly on their patients. The result of the inadequacy of the law was that there grew up an illicit traffic in dead bodies, conducted by the notorious body-snatchers or "resurrection-men." This gruesome occupation was chiefly in the hands of a few "regulars," although outsiders also plied the same trade. The rivalry between different factions of the resurrectionists was so keen that there was no ingenuity or artifice to which they did not resort to obtain their prey or injure their rivals. Ordinarily they merely robbed newly filled graves, bribing the custodian if necessary. Sometimes, however, they would pose as relatives of the deceased and lay claim to the body from a hospital or workhouse. It was not uncommon for them to seize a body already on the dissecting table, and convey it elsewhere to be sold anew. Brawls in the very graveyards between rival gangs were far from rare.

The price paid for a subject rose at one time from two guineas up to fourteen or even sixteen, and besides this the teachers had to pay the men "opening money" at the beginning of each course to secure the monopoly of their services and a regular supply of bodies, as well as a retaining fee during the vacation, and compensation for any man who was unfortunate enough to get a spell of imprisonment. Some of the buyers formed an "Anatomy Club" in an attempt to regulate the prices and limit the extortion: but this was never very successful. Some teachers refused to pay the extra fees and of these men the resurrectionists made an example. A Mr. Joshua Brookes, of Great Marlborough Street, was rewarded by having decomposed bodies left on his doorstep and on one occasion was sold a live confederate of the resurrectionists done up in a sack.

As may be well imagined, popular feeling grew to a white-hot pitch of fury. Guards were instituted over recent graves and frequently came into conflict with the body-snatchers, whom they sometimes manhandled severely. The Government was reluctant to act. The need for subjects was imperative, but the popular outcry made it probable that any attempt at legislation might be fatal to the intended object.

Both the private teachers and the surgeons were hand in glove with the resurrection-men. Sometimes a surgeon would specially commission one of these miscreants to obtain for him the body of one of his patients who had been subjected to some interesting operation or who had suffered from some disease which made a post-mortem examination desirable. When giving evidence before the Select Committee on Anatomy (at which also some of the snatchers themselves were anonymous witnesses) Sir Astley Cooper said: "The law does not prevent our obtaining the body of an individual if we think proper: for there is no person, let his situation in life be what it may, whom, if I were disposed to dissect, I could not obtain. . . . The law only enhances the price and does not prevent the exhumation."

Some enlightened people saw the necessity for dissection and saw too how unwise it was to drive all the would-be doctors to Continental universities to learn anatomy. Jeremy Bentham went so far as to set the example of leaving his own body to be dissected. When he died in 1832 this was done by a friend in accordance with his instructions and his skeleton is still preserved in University College, London.

It was not until this same year, four years after the Select Committee had presented its report, that the Anatomy Act was passed. This was undoubtedly expedited by the still greater public feeling which was aroused when it came to light that certain malefactors, Bishop and Williams in London, and Burke and Hare in Edinburgh, had resorted to cold-blooded murder with the object of selling bodies for anatomy.

The Act abolished the dissection of the bodies of murderers, thereby removing the stigma attaching to being dissected. It provided that properly qualified practitioners, teachers and students should be given licenses to practice dissection. It insisted upon proper death certificates and a decent burial afterwards. It allowed executors or any persons having lawful possession of a body to give it up provided no relative objected. The Act was successful, for it secured a reasonable number of bodies and it also put the resurrectionists out of business.

In America, in the 18th Century, there were similar difficulties in procuring bodies for dissection. Because the amount of anatomical teaching was smaller and the demand for bodies correspondingly less, there were no such notorious resurrectionist scandals as those which occurred in London and Edinburgh. There were, however, so-called anatomical riots in which physicians were attacked by mobs in both Philadelphia and New York. Dr. William Shippen, Jr., the first Professor of Anatomy and Surgery in the new medical school in Philadelphia, was set upon several times and forced to go into hiding. In New York there was a serious riot in and around the New York Hospital where dissection was carried on. It began on Sunday, April 13, 1788, and lasted two days. The rioters broke into the dissecting rooms and got so out of hand that the militia was summoned, the medical students in the meanwhile having been placed in the city prison for their own protection. The mob was only dispersed when the militia fired upon it, killing and wounding several persons.

This episode resulted in the passage of a law in 1789 in New York permitting the bodies of executed criminals to be turned over to the surgeons for dissection. Massachusetts had enacted a somewhat similar law in 1784. These laws, as in England, failed to provide a sufficient number of bodies, and the bodies of paupers were exhumed by students and even, on occasions, by surgeons themselves. Massachusetts was the first state to meet the problem frankly, and in 1830 a law was enacted granting the bodies of unclaimed paupers for anatomical purposes. This law predated by two years the English Anatomy Act. Most of the other states in the union subsequently passed similar laws. Dissection still remains illegal in New Jersey, however, a fact which has hindered the establishment of a medical school in that state.

A notorious episode in the long story of the difficulties in enacting proper laws for providing anatomical material concerns the case of President Benjamin Harrison's father, who died on May 26, 1878. He was buried three days later in a cemetery in North Bend, Ohio. Several days later, his son went to the Ohio Medical College at Cincinnati to search for the remains of a friend. There he found the body of his father. This incident was one of the factors which led to a revision of the Ohio Anatomy Law in 1881, making proper anatomical material available to medical schools. It should be emphasized that such incidents no longer occur anywhere, now that bodies are obtainable by legal processes.

As the 18th Century ended, and the convulsions of the American and French revolutions shook the social and political world, medicine was still bound by its traditions and a lack of any fundamental understanding of the nature of disease. In the following century this obscurity was to be broken by a discovery as revolutionary to medicine as any readjustment that had occurred in the social sphere—namely, the cellular nature of disease.

PART TWO

Medical Science During the Last Hundred Years

10

THE NEW PATHOLOGY

THE 19TH Century brought a fundamental change of outlook, which has colored the whole of medical thought ever since. The decisive factor was the discovery of the animal cell, which led to the conception of the living body as a vast organization consisting of millions of tiny individual cells. It is difficult to give any adequate idea of the tremendously far-reaching results of this discovery or of the immensely fertile field which it was to lay open to medical science. Suffice it for the moment, before we go on to describe the development of the Cell Theory, that every doctor of today thinks of health and disease ultimately in terms of these cells.

In 1665 the initial discovery had been made by Robert Hooke, who found that if he cut a sufficiently thin slice of cork, he could see under the microscope that the whole substance of the cork was made up of little bladders of air with little wooden walls separating them from one another. The same was found to be true of green plants except that, as the great botanist Robert Brown showed more than a hundred and fifty years later, each little cell contained an essential structure called the "nucleus." Incidentally Brown was also the discoverer of the important fact that the pollen of the plant played the part of the male element in the process of fertilization.

Germany, however, was to have the distinction of elaborating the new biological theory. Mattias Jacob Schleiden of Hamburg, in 1838 demonstrated conclusively that every part of a plant was made of groups of cells and that the nucleus was the controlling influence inside each cell. Furthermore he believed that every part was developed from one or another group of cells.

Stimulated by these discoveries in the vegetable kingdom, Theodor Schwann began to look for cells in animal tissues, and he found them everywhere. He had received a sound biological training in the laboratories of Johannes Müller at Bonn and Berlin, and was already an experienced scientist when he began his study of the microscopical appearances of animal matter. Among other achievements he had disproved the theory of spontaneous generation which held that life might arise *de novo* from dead materials under suitable circumstances.

The stronghold of the supporters of that idea was the proved appearance of small organisms in material which was undergoing fermentation or putrefaction. Schwann was able to show that these processes were in fact the *effect* of the growth of the organisms and not by any means the *cause*. This will be seen to be of great significance when we come to discuss the work of Pasteur.

Schwann proved that all vegetable and animal tissues are composed of and developed from cells. The cells of each individual tissue are all alike. Different tissues have different kinds of cells, but any cell of a given tissue is like all the rest in the same tissue. He showed, too, that the ovum, the "seed" from which all plant and animal life developed, was itself a cell. He noticed also that the cells had some kind of internal substance besides the nucleus and pointed out the movements occurring in this stuff which today we call protoplasm. It is noteworthy that Schwann's religious convictions made him secure the approval of the Bishop of Malines before he gave to the world his remarkable work.

It was Rudolf Virchow, the most influential of all Germany's medical thinkers, who applied the discoveries of Hooke, Schleiden, and Schwann to the intimate study of disease. Virchow was above all a man of science and he believed that practical medicine must be based only upon the firm structure of applied theoretical medicine, which must in turn rest upon pure scientific physiology and pathology.

In 1839 Virchow arrived on the scene in Berlin just when the tremendous discovery of animal cells had been published from Müller's laboratory. To this he added the important truth that no cell ever arises except by direct formation from another cell. Life is continuous: *Omnis cellula e cellula*. Before this it had been assumed that in certain circumstances cells could develop from the "organization" of some more homogeneous animal substance, much as foam is formed from soap. This supposition had been found necessary to explain, for instance, how a homogeneous clot in a wound could be converted into a living scar composed of cells. Virchow showed quite definitely that these cells were not formed from the clot but grew out into the clot from the living cells of the surrounding tissues.

Virchow's academic career very nearly came to an untimely end owing to his left-wing political views. In 1848 there was an outbreak of relapsing fever in Upper Silesia and he was sent by the Prussian government as a member of a commission to investigate the cause. He quickly saw that famine and unwholesome conditions were the precipitating if not the ultimate cause of the pestilence. Accordingly his report, dealing largely with the villainous conditions which he found, had a political rather than a medical cast, and, in the storm of indignation which he aroused, Virchow was suspended from his post at Berlin.

Happily he was invited to take up a position at Würzburg where, as professor of pathology, he turned his attention to more purely scientific matters. He worked assiduously at the study of the animal cells in disease. In 1856 he was asked to return to Berlin as professor of pathology and two years later he gave to the world his greatest work, *die Cellular Pathologie*. In this he enunciated the doctrine that every diseased tissue consists of cells which arise only as the offspring of pre-existing cells. This may seem to us today suspiciously like a truism. But it was not so regarded in Virchow's day. Indeed the very fact that this truth seems so obvious goes to show how deeply the fundamental idea enters into our mental make-up.

In the 18th Century M.-F.-X. Bichat, the great French anatomist, had begun to study animal tissues under the microscope in an attempt to make some sort of systematic classification of them. He found, as was to be expected, that certain tissues recurred in different parts of the body. He counted as many as twenty-one distinct types of tissues or "membranes." He observed only the grosser features of each and that is why he supposed that there were so many.

Disease, he decided, must ultimately be some change in one or more kinds of tissue. Any tissue in any organ might be affected while the other kinds of tissue in the same organ might undergo no change. Indeed this is what often happens. This conception accounts for multiple changes all over the body in a generalized disease. Rickets, for example, affects the same kind of tissue everywhere. The fact that the disease attacks the tissue of the growing parts of bones accounts for the bony deformities which occur in every region of the body.

Bichat had carried pathology one step further than Morgagni. The latter considered *an organ* to be the seat of the disease while the former showed that it was a particular *tissue* that was at fault. Virchow thought, as we all do now, in terms of *cells*. Disease is simply abnormal cell life. In other words, sickness is the reaction of the cell to altered conditions. If the conditions become altogether too anomalous, the cell dies. Speaking prematurely in terms of the germ theory, we might add that the disease is not the germ but the behavior of the body cells towards the germ.

Virchow made many individual discoveries extending over a wide field, not only in pathology but also in anthropology and archaeology, but it is by his cellular pathology that his name will live. Upon this rests the whole edifice of the modern study of disease, and its influence extends to every branch of medical thought. Virchow's doctrine has been extraordinarily fertile. Because of it, the microscope has become a necessary part of the equipment of every doctor. In the diagnosis of cancer, of blood disease, and of kidney disease, to quote but three examples, the present-day pathologist is looking daily and hourly through the lenses of his microscope to observe the minutest variations from the normal appearance of cells. Here lies the key not only to diagnosis but to the discovery of the fundamental nature of disease.

Virchow became the Grand Old Man of German medicine. He was to medicine what Liebig was to chemistry, an acute thinker, an oracular figure-head, and an influence which is still felt in every corner of the civilized world.

In 1862 he returned to the political stage as a member of the Prussian lower house and later, in 1880, of the Reichstag, where he was among the most formidable of the opponents of Bismarck. Municipal affairs also claimed some of the attention of the indefatigable professor, and it is largely to him that Berlin owes its excellent water supply and drainage system. He died in 1902 at the age of eighty-one, but his work is being carried on in every pathological laboratory in the world—a supreme tribute to this remarkable man—while his name survives in the periodical which he founded and which is known to every doctor as Virchow's Archives.

NEW AIDS TO DIAGNOSIS

ONE OF the most striking changes in medical practice is the addition, during the last century, of various scientific weapons, physical and chemical, to the armament of the diagnostician. The important principle underlying many of these new inventions is that of accurate measurement, which replaces the mere qualitative observations of the signs and symptoms of disease.

Even before the invention of the modern thermometer, attempts had been made to estimate the temperature of the human body. In the 17th Century Santorio Santorio had used a bulb filled with air and opening into a tube. The other end of the tube opened under the surface of some water in a vessel. He placed the bulb inside a person's mouth and the air inside expanded as it became warm and issued in bubbles through the water. By counting these bubbles he could gain some idea of the "hotness" of the person in question. This was an extremely rough-and-ready method, but it was not until almost 200 years later that the researches of the physicists, notably Helmholtz and Sir William Thomson (Lord Kelvin), improved the thermometer and placed thermometry on a sound basis.

Although Boerhaave and others had certainly made some use of the thermometer, it remained for Carl August Wunderlich in Leipzig to show its real value to medicine. He began to collect careful records of the varying temperature of the human body in health and disease, and showed that in "fevers" the variations of temperature were an essential feature and indeed a guide to the precise nature and course of the disease. He published numbers of papers on this subject and followed them up in 1868 with his comprehensive work *Das Verhalten der Eigenwaerme in Krankheiten* (Body Temperature in Disease).

It is certainly due to Wunderlich that the thermometer has become an instrument for the everyday use of the bedside physician. The first instruments began to be used in the hospitals in England about 1866 and their use rapidly became universal. These early thermometers were quite unwieldy, being generally some ten inches long, and the quantity of mercury that they contained so large that five or more minutes were necessary if a reliable reading was to be obtained. Sir Clifford Albutt saw these grave disadvantages and it is to him that we owe the use of the accurate little pocket thermometers which everyone knows so well today.

During the 19th Century the science of chemistry as well as that of physics began to be the servant of the diagnostician. The first important contribution to chemical diagnosis was the discovery in 1838, by Apollinaire Bouchardat and Eugène-Melchior Peligot, that the sweet substance in diabetic urine was identical with grape-sugar (glucose or dextrose). Suitable chemical tests for such sugar were then devised. In 1848 Hermann von Fehling devised his famous method of testing for and estimating the quantity of sugar in urine by means of the alkaline copper solution that bears his name today. A more reliable sugar test has recently been developed by S. R. Benedict.

During the last fifty years advances in our knowledge of the chemical processes within the body have been so enormous that they have come to constitute a separate branch of learning called biological chemistry, which has an important place in the medical curriculum. This new science has given us a whole series of quantitative tests for substances present in the blood and urine, which are among the most valuable of all the aids to diagnosis that the modern clinician possesses. To a large extent these methods are the result of the ingenuity of the late Professor Otto Folin of Harvard Medical School.

Folin was born in Sweden in 1867 and emigrated to the United States when he was fifteen. He supported himself by working in the lumbering camps in Minnesota and got through high school. He then made his way through the Universities of Minnesota and Chicago, obtaining his doctor's degree in chemistry from the latter institution in 1898. After two years abroad spent at Marburg and at Upsala he returned to found a research laboratory to study the chemistry of the blood and urine at McLean Hospital in Boston. When he began his work at McLean there were no quick and simple methods for the quantitative analysis of the nitrogenous constituents of urine, and no methods at all for the determination of nitrogenous waste products in the blood. Folin devised methods for determining these substances by means of color reactions, and introduced the colorimeter, a simple but accurate optical instrument for comparing colors, into biochemistry. It thus became possible to measure with a high degree of accuracy the small amounts of non-protein nitrogen, urea, uric acid and creatinine in blood and urine. Folin's first paper, *Laws Governing the Composition of Normal Urine,* published in 1905, gained him immediate recognition. In 1907 a professorship in biological chemistry was created for him at Harvard Medical School. It was the first chair of its kind in an American medical school. From this laboratory came a long series of important contributions.

These chemical methods of analysis of the blood quickly proved their great value in clinical medicine. They have been so refined and improved that they can now be carried out with only minute amounts of blood. For example, a method is available for determining sugar in blood which requires only one-tenth of a cubic centimeter. These so-called micro-chemical methods of quantitative analysis have come to play an indispensable practical role in the practice of medicine. They indicate the progress and guide the diet of those suffering from renal disease; they make surgery, particularly prostatic surgery, far safer; they guide the use of insulin in diabetes; they are of crucial importance in the diagnosis of tumors of the parathyroid glands, of pancreatitis, adrenal disease, and biliary obstruction; they enable us to restore the fluid and salt balance of the body when it has been disturbed by shock. Their usefulness is constantly increasing as our knowledge of biochemistry grows.

Of all the new physical aids to diagnosis there was none that was so unexpected, unhoped for, and consequently unlooked for, as the roentgen rays. This discovery, like so many others, had its beginning in an accident. In saying this we have no wish to detract from the genius of the inventor, for had not Wilhelm Conrad Röntgen been a physicist of exceptional ability, the new rays might easily have been overlooked. Indeed it is certain that the rays had been produced previously in many physical laboratories all over the world but their existence remained unrecognized.

Towards the close of the last century almost every well-equipped physical laboratory possessed, in what is known as a Crookes tube, a potential means of producing the rays. These tubes were of glass and contained various gases at very low pressures. By means of wires sealed into the glass, high-voltage electrical discharges could be passed from an induction coil through the gas in the tube and the extraordinary phenomena which occurred could be studied. Heinrich Hertz and P. Lenard had made brilliant experiments with a new kind of ray which, under certain conditions, they found emanating from the negative wire inside the tube. It was while experimenting with these so-called cathode rays that Röntgen, professor of physics at Würzburg, made his startling observations on November 8th, 1895.

Working in the dark, with the Crookes tube completely enclosed, he noticed that a small piece of paper covered with a coating of barium platinocyanide shone brightly while the electrical discharge was taking place. This may not seem a very striking observation, but it was to have far-reaching effects. Röntgen told no one of his discovery, but with incredible energy set out along truly scientific lines to investigate the phenomenon.

Some weeks passed before he convinced himself that the astonishing results which he had obtained were indeed facts. He had worked out pretty completely the fundamental character of the new rays when, on December 28th, with some hesitation, he presented his astonishing communication *On a New Kind of Rays* to the Physical Medical Society of Würzburg. "Now there will be the devil to pay," he observed.

The paper showed at once how thorough Röntgen had been. He proved that the rays emanated from the point where the cathode rays struck the glass wall of the tube. The most surprising objects, a book for example, seemed transparent to the rays, and objects varied in their degree of transparency according to their thickness and their density. Other substances besides barium platinocyanide fluoresced in the path of the rays. A photographic plate was sensitive to the rays, but the human eye was not. The behavior of the new rays differed in many ways from that of light-rays, in that the former could not be reflected by any substance nor deviated by a prism; nor could he produce "interference" effects nor polarize the rays by any of the ordinary methods. Yet the rays seemed to travel in straight lines, for the shadows cast by a dense object were sharp. They differed, too, from cathode-rays in that the new rays traveled much farther through the air and other substances, and, unlike the cathode-rays, could not be deflected by a magnet.

Röntgen illustrated his communication with some photographic shadow-pictures including one of a human hand showing the shadow of the bones. Since the inventor admitted that he was unaware of the true nature of the rays, he proposed to call them the x-rays and he put forward the suggestion, which was subsequently disproved, that they differed from light in being longitudinal (as opposed to transverse) vibrations in the ether. After a demonstration before the Physical Medical Society it was de-

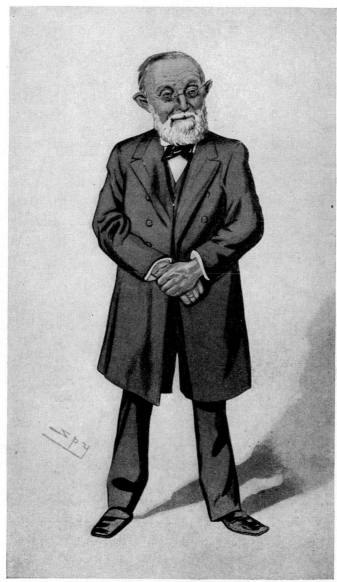

(From *Vanity Fair* for May 23, 1893)

Spy's Caricature of Virchow

Virchow was a typical German professor of his time, with a liberal social point of view but a conservative and critical attitude toward the innovations of some of his medical juniors. He disapproved, for instance, of Koch's work.

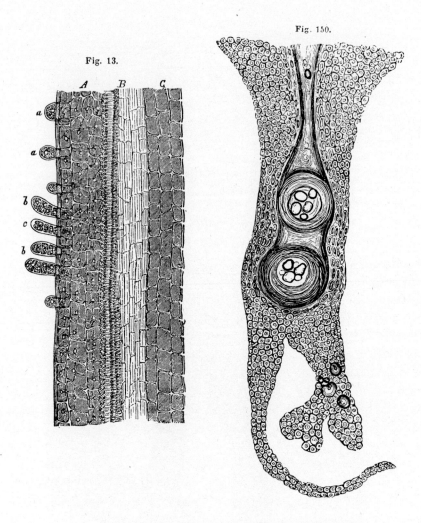

Fig. 13.

Fig. 150.

Illustrations from *The Cellular Pathology*

As an example of the biological law that cells always develop from pre-existing cells Virchow showed a longitudinal section of a lilac bud (Figure 13). The club-shaped outgrowths begin as single cells and grow by continual subdivision. Applying this principle to explain disease Virchow showed a cancer of the lip (Figure 150) in which the epithelial cells are seen multiplying abnormally and growing down into the substance of the lip.

cided that the rays should be called "roentgen's rays." However, they are more commonly known as x-rays today.

Unlike so many great men who have had to fight desperately for the recognition of their discoveries, Röntgen became famous at once (although it should be added that, scientifically, he would have been considered a great physicist even if he had not discovered his rays). When the news became known there was great excitement all over the world and, since almost every laboratory possessed or could obtain a Crookes tube, the existence of the x-rays was soon confirmed everywhere.

The immense value of the new discovery to medical diagnosis was quickly seen and it was not long before surgeons began to take shadow-pictures of fractures and dislocations. Shot or other foreign bodies showed up well on the plates, and photographs were also taken of teeth and stones in the kidney. The bony changes which occur in gout, rickets and other diseases began to be examined by the same method, while the heart and lungs, though not so dense as the bones, could also be photographed with a suitable length of exposure.

The new discovery was fortunately given active encouragement by educated opinion and was patronized by many persons in high places. The German Emperor, for instance, before whom Röntgen demonstrated his rays as early as January, 1896, was sufficiently impressed to have a picture taken of his crippled left arm with the object of determining the nature of the deformity. Queen Amelia of Portugal is said to have "had x-ray pictures made of several of her court ladies in order to demonstrate to them the evils of tight lacing." So Röntgen's fame spread and messages of congratulation began to reach him from all over the world. In 1901 he was awarded a Nobel prize.

The newspapers seized upon the imaginative aspects of the discovery, and whipped up a public interest which had its humorous aspects. A London firm offered x-ray-proof underwear to that section of the public that feared being seen by the new penetrating rays. In February, 1896, Assemblyman Reed of New Jersey

introduced a bill in the state legislature to prohibit the use of
x-rays in opera glasses in theaters! In New York in May, 1896,
Thomas Edison provided a public demonstration of x-rays that
delighted crowds of people. The subject of the new rays was a
favorite one for contemporary cartoonists.

Attempts were made to discredit Röntgen, including the alle-
gation that his discovery was really that of a junior assistant.
There were also many claims to priority in the discovery. But all
these have been carefully scrutinized and not one can be substantiated. Such recriminations seem to have embittered the discoverer, who was a modest and retiring man. He was wounded
by the vituperation of a few and, retiring into private life, he died
in 1922, lonely and neglected.

The uses of roentgen rays in medicine and surgery have steadily increased during the half-century that has elapsed since their
discovery. It was at once realized that if certain hollow organs in
the body, not ordinarily seen in an x-ray picture, were filled up
with some substance which was opaque to the rays, then a picture could be taken showing the shape of the inside of the organ
in question.

A beginning was made in 1896 when W. Becher of Berlin photographed the stomach of a dead guinea pig after filling it up
with a solution containing lead. Lead is very poisonous, so that in
order to apply the same process to human beings it was necessary
to find something that would be at the same time both opaque
and non-toxic. Walter B. Cannon, the distinguished professor of
physiology at Harvard, solved this problem while he was a medical student there. In December, 1896, he began to feed bismuth
subnitrate to various small animals and to follow the course of
this x-ray-opaque material down the gastro-intestinal tract by
means of a fluorescent screen. During the following six years, employing cats for the most part, Cannon used this method to describe for the first time the normal movements of the stomach
and intestine during the process of digestion.

Soon afterward several independent investigators studied the alimentary tract in man in this way, and within a few years the great importance of x-ray examination in diseases of the stomach and intestine was generally recognized. Today these examinations form a large part of the work in the modern x-ray laboratory. The patient drinks a glassful of barium sulphate mixture (which, by the way, was also introduced by Cannon as a substitute for the more dangerous bismuth), and this material is photographed during its passage through the whole of the gastro-intestinal tract. In this manner a variety of diseases of the tract can be diagnosed and their response to treatment followed. By this means also tumors can be detected while they are yet early enough to be cured by surgical removal. Thus countless lives have been saved.

Other opaque substances have been used to study various other organs. Much of our knowledge of disease in the bladder, ureters, and kidney is based on x-ray photographs taken following the retrograde injection of sodium iodide into the urinary tract. Such photographs are called pyelograms, and accurately reveal abnormalities of the contour of the cavities within these organs. Indeed, a method of studying the kidneys by means of injecting an opaque material into the bloodstream has recently been developed. The material is an organic compound of urea and iodine which is eliminated through the kidneys in a sufficient concentration to make x-ray photographs of the kidney possible.

An ingenious method of obtaining an x-ray picture of the gall bladder was devised by Evarts A. Graham and Warren Henry Cole of St. Louis in 1924. They discovered an opaque compound containing iodine, which, when ingested, appears later in the bile that is stored in the gall bladder. An x-ray picture may then show little holes, as it were, in the shadow of the gall bladder if there are gallstones present, for these stones are often more transparent to the rays than is the iodine compound. By this method one can clearly detect gallstones which might not be seen at all in the ordinary x-ray picture.

Great advances in our knowledge of diseases of the lungs have also been made by means of roentgen rays. In addition to the ordinary x-ray photographs, a method of revealing the structure of the lung by injecting opaque substances into the bronchial tree has been developed. The non-irritating oily substance used for this purpose is called lipidol.

Much work has been done with the object of improving the quality of x-ray photography. In the early days very long exposures were necessary to secure a good picture. Soon better and better tubes were devised. A target of platinum was found to be a better source of the rays than the glass wall of the tube. The American physicist, William A. Coolidge, in 1913 perfected the modern x-ray tube, which has since been known by his name. Photographic plates, too, were improved very much in quality and sensitivity. Nowadays films have superseded glass plates in x-ray work. The superiority of the films lies not only in convenience of storage, but also in the fact that they are sufficiently thin to allow a sensitive coating to be applied on both sides without too much blurring of the picture. In this way the time of exposure can be halved, and, by placing on each side of the film sheets of paper coated with material that shines in the path of the x-rays, the speed is still further increased. With this arrangement the actual picture is taken partly by the fluorescence of the coated paper as well as by the direct effect of the rays on the plate.

Apart from considerations of convenience, it was found highly important to reduce the exposure-time to the minimum because of the dangerous effects of the rays. Unfortunately, roentgen rays were not an unmixed blessing, for gradually among the pioneers of roentgenology appeared the distressing and disastrous effects of x-ray burns. Redness and brown pigmentation of the skin, dropping out of the hair, superficial ulceration, and skin cancer—all these followed insidiously and relentlessly in the wake of prolonged exposure to rays. There were many workers who lost limbs and lives in this horrible way. Twenty-eight American martyrs to roentgen rays have been listed by P. Brown in his book on the subject.

Now happily the danger is recognized and every worker with

x-rays protects himself, his neighbors, and his photographic plates with aprons, gloves, walls, and screens heavily impregnated with lead. Professor Röntgen himself escaped without harm because, although he never anticipated the evil effects which the rays have on the skin, for the sake of convenience he worked almost entirely inside an enclosed and metal-lined cabinet with only one window through which the rays were admitted from the Crookes tube outside.

Once it was known that x-rays had a direct effect on the skin it was natural that empirical attempts should be made to cure skin diseases with them. The rays were turned from diagnostic to therapeutic use. They have proved to be useful in controlling certain forms of cancer, as we shall point out in a later chapter. But they have also been used in the treatment of a wide variety of benign skin conditions, from athlete's foot to superfluous hair. For all of these benign conditions, x-rays are a dangerous method of treatment, for the margin between a proper therapeutic dose and one that will cause permanent and irreparable damage to the skin is very small.

One of the difficult economic problems of modern medicine lies in the fact that certain of these modern diagnostic methods which we have just described, particularly blood chemistry and x-ray examination, have added considerably to the cost of medical care. The charge to a private patient for x-ray study of the gastro-intestinal tract alone, for instance, may amount to as much as $75.00. This is a large sum in terms of the annual budget of the average man. Some way will have to be found of reducing the cost of these laboratory aids, for if we accept the humanitarian principle that human life is worth more than money, we cannot deny them to our patients. These laboratory aids are as necessary to the physician as modern instruments of navigation like the radio-compass to the sea captain. They guide him in diagnosis and therapy where the unaided eye and ear can but suspect lurking danger.

THE GERM THEORY:

INFECTIVE ORGANISMS

WHILE VIRCHOW and his pupils in Germany, through their discoveries regarding the cellular changes in disease, were laying a new foundation for medical science, another great advance was being made across the Rhine. There Pasteur, an equally fertile genius, was unravelling the mystery of the infective organisms responsible for many of the cellular changes just discovered by Virchow. Yet the work of these two men was quite separate. They knew but little of each other. Virchow began as an anatomist, Pasteur as a chemist. The former dealt with the cold reality of dead tissues, while the latter dealt with theory and living things.

From the remotest periods of history we find mention of plagues and pestilences, and it is scarcely surprising that mankind should have invented many different hypotheses to account for the undoubted fact that many diseases are epidemic. From antiquity to the Middle Ages these hypotheses postulated as the cause of disease factors which varied from cosmic influences (hence "lunacy" and "influenza") to witchcraft, and from the will or vengeance of the gods to the poisoning of wells by the Jews.

The doctrine of contagion is not a new one. The writer of "Leviticus" clearly recognizes this as the method of spreading leprosy and gonorrhea when he lays down the principle that persons who are suffering from these diseases should be restrained from mixing with their fellows. Thucydides, too, in his description of the plague at Athens, seems to have understood that the disease was conveyed directly from one person to another. More recently, in the 18th Century, the practice of inoculating smallpox from person to person was brought from the East, showing that contagion was recognized as the means of spread of this disease at least.

Another theory of epidemics that received wide recognition appears under a variety of forms and names. In general, it assumed that there was an "atmospheric influence" or "epidemic miasma" which might pass over a country, and that its progress might be shown by outbreaks in different localities where there was some determining factor or localizing condition. In other words, the air was to blame: there was a bad air, a *mal aria*. From this, of course, comes the name of the disease which, once common almost everywhere and known as ague, is now found chiefly in tropical and sub-tropical lands. This hypothesis of epidemic miasmata was by no means worthless, for it at least taught that filth was a predisposing cause of disease. It was believed pretty generally until the actual living germs of certain diseases were discovered, although it was fighting a losing battle against the theory of contagion. The latter theory was forced on medical opinion by the epidemics, quite obviously contagious, which swept over Europe from time to time. Notable among these was the Black Death (probably the bubonic plague) which entered Europe about 1348, killing over sixty millions there after it had ravaged Asia and Africa. The waves of syphilis in the 15th, smallpox in the 18th, and cholera in the 19th Centuries were likewise obviously contagious in origin.

Before the discovery of the living organisms that produce many diseases, attempts at the prevention of such diseases were for the most part unsuccessful. Isolation of the diseased, and quarantine for those who had been in contact with them, were the only available methods of control. There were successes, but more often there were failures. The greatest triumph claimed for the isolation method is the disappearance of leprosy from Western Europe. This disease, which was possibly introduced and

probably spread by the Crusaders, had been so far eradicated in
France, Italy, Spain, England, Denmark and Switzerland by the
middle of the 16th Century that we hear little, after this, of the
lazar houses. There had existed in England more than two hundred of these in the previous century. It must be added, however,
that modern experience in the East has shown that compulsory
isolation of lepers leads to endless concealment and consequently
is not very effective in preventing the spread of the disease. It
must have been even less useful in the past when no hope of cure
could be held out for the sufferers. Since the exact mode of transmission is yet uncertain, we cannot fairly assume that the isolation of the infected was the only cause of the disappearance of
leprosy from Europe.

More recently, by the method of muzzling all dogs, the
scourge of rabies was abolished in England. This was achieved
not only by the virtual isolation of dogs by muzzling them, but
by their further isolation from Continental infection by a very
strict quarantine. On the other hand, the quarantine method had
conspicuously failed to keep the plague from Venice in the 14th
Century and, in the light of our present knowledge of the means
of communication of this disease, this cannot be considered altogether astonishing.

Pasteur did not "discover" germs in the sense that he was the
first to see microbes through his microscope. In the latter half of
the 17th Century the great Dutch microscope maker, Antonj van
Leeuwenhoek, had described a variety of such minute organisms.
Bacteria, in fact, are found almost everywhere on the earth in
enormous numbers and countless species. Fortunately, only a very
few species are capable of producing diseases in human beings.
Pasteur's researches led him to the discovery that putrefaction is
a kind of fermentation, that both these processes are due to micro-
organisms and that putrescible material (such as blood, for example) can be kept indefinitely if care is taken to ensure the

absence of all living micro-organisms from it. These are, in fact, absolutely necessary to, and the cause of, putrefaction.

First of all, Pasteur began by trying to find what turns milk sour. He pointed to the little globules seen through the microscope, living globules that budded and multiplied, so that just a trace of these globules could sour the milk. Alcoholic fermentation he showed to be due also to self-reproducing globules, but these were different globules from the others: they could produce alcohol from sugar, but they could not turn the milk sour. Each fermentation had its own kind of organism and each organism its own kind of fermentation. This is the important principle of the specificity of organisms.

Pasteur showed that these ferments came from the atmosphere and multiplied in the putrefying or fermenting liquids. They were present in very different numbers in different places. They swarmed in towns and rooms, but were scarce in the high mountain air. He showed also that by heating air, by passing it through narrow curly tubes, or by filtering it through plugs of cotton wool, the germs could be excluded from sterile flasks. In his studies of the agent that produces butyric acid, which causes the smell of rancid butter, Pasteur discovered an astonishing phenomenon. Here was an organism which would only grow in the absence of air, or rather, of oxygen. This was the first germ of this kind discovered, the first of the *anaërobic* bacteria, as he called them.

All such fermentative changes he showed were due to these *living* microscopic beings and to them alone. The opposition which this idea roused was so enormous as to seem almost incredible to us now. Pasteur had against him the full crushing weight of the terrific Baron von Liebig, the leading chemist of his day. Liebig's dicta were looked up to by an enormous following; but since, while denying Pasteur's ideas, he absolutely refused to look through a microscope, the matter could not very well be argued to a conclusion.

This kind of controversy took much of Pasteur's time. He spent a long time demolishing Liebig's theory that fermentation and putrefaction were processes akin to slow chemical combustion and that the dead portion of the yeast alone was responsible for the production of alcohol. He spent even more time over his celebrated controversy with Félix-Archimède Pouchet concerning the "spontaneous generation" of life. Were the germs the cause or the effect of fermentation? After a bitter fight in which his experimental proofs were answered with flowery oratory and his arguments with rhetoric, he eventually, in 1862, succeeded in convincing the Academy of Sciences at Paris that "spontaneous generation is a chimera" and that all life comes from life and from life alone. Pasteur had a negative point to prove and that is not easy, but he convinced them all.

The wine industry in France was losing huge quantities of wine every year from a wine disease of unknown origin when Pasteur, whose every investigation seems to have been crowned with success, turned his discerning mind to the matter. As he had surmised, the disease of wine was due to an organized ferment, and he showed that by heating the wine for a short time to a temperature of between fifty and sixty degrees centigrade, the ferment could be destroyed while the wine remained unaltered and would keep indefinitely. The wine, as we would say, had been "pasteurized."

The wine industry was not the only one benefited by Pasteur. By showing how to breed silkworms which were free of two prevalent scourges—*pébrine* and *flacherie*—which had brought the silk industry almost to a standstill in his time, he earned the undying gratitude of all those engaged in the production of silk. He next gave his attention to the problems of brewers, and was able to demonstrate that the quality of every brew was determined by the nature of the micro-organisms present.

As early as 1863 we find him saying to the Emperor, to whom he had been presented by the great French chemist, Jean-Baptiste Dumas, that his "ambition was to arrive at the knowledge of putrid and contagious disease." He turned from diseases of wines and silkworms, to diseases of mankind.

Before Pasteur's time there had been isolated discoveries of microscopic beings which caused disease. The little rod-like organisms in the blood of animals dead of anthrax had been seen as early as 1838, but it was not until Casimir Davaine became acquainted with the work of Pasteur on fermentation that he began to inoculate rabbits with these organisms and to reproduce the disease. Beginning in 1863 Davaine carried out a long series of researches on anthrax which proved beyond doubt that the disease was due to the rod-shaped bodies to which he gave the name "bacteria." But it was Pasteur and his pupils who put the germ theory of disease upon a sound footing, and the whole structure of the science of bacteriology is built directly upon his work.

To a German, Robert Koch, however, we owe the beginnings of modern bacteriological technique. He it was who first laid bare the natural history or life story, of the anthrax bacillus, and showed how to grow the bacillus, and how to obtain it unmixed with other organisms in "pure culture."

From these first discoveries an enormously complicated technique has grown up, which enables the bacteriologist to separate and identify the different disease-producing agents. But even today the subject is far from being a complete and orderly one, and this is largely due to the fact that bacteriology has been an *applied* science and that "investigators have been more interested in what bacteria do than what they are, and much more interested in the ways in which they interfere with man's health or pursuits than in the ways in which they function as autonomous living beings," as Topley and Wilson have said. The general natural history of germs has been neglected for the study of the specialized behavior of a few species.

Pasteur had previously shown how to cultivate germs in his liquid media which he prepared synthetically in the laboratory. He had realized that different bacteria needed media which differed not only in the varying quality of the nutrient material, but also in the amount of oxygen or the degree of acidity. He had grown an organism in a tube and then sown one drop of the liquid into another tube, waited, then sown one drop from this into a third tube, and so on through a long sequence of tubes, so that any extraneous, non-living substances which might have been present in the first tube were inconceivably dilute in the last tube. But the organisms remained alive, reproduced themselves, and were as numerous and had the same disease-producing properties in the last as in the first tube. It was the organisms and they alone which produced the disease.

Koch showed how to grow the organisms on solid media. He showed also that different organisms took up different dyes from a solution, so that they could be distinguished one from another by observing what color they took on when dyed with different chemicals.

Following the work of these two leaders came the discovery of a large number of the bacteria responsible for many different diseases. Some were discovered by the masters, and more by the many pupils. Before the close of the 19th Century there had been discovered the causative organisms of leprosy, gonorrhea, suppuration, typhoid, malaria, tuberculosis, cholera, diphtheria, pneumonia, cerebro-spinal meningitis, Malta fever, tetanus (lockjaw), plague, botulism and dysentery; while more recently, in the present century, observers have found the organisms of sleeping sickness, syphilis, whooping cough, infective jaundice and scarlet fever. This list is far from complete and there are numbers of organisms which are almost certainly the cause of different diseases, but the absolute proof is sometimes lacking. Until it can be shown that the organism is always present in every case of the disease, that it can be cultivated through several generations and that the last generations can reproduce the disease with certainty, it cannot be asserted that this organism is the cause of the disease beyond any shadow of doubt.

The bacteriologists have invented a large number of clever expedients for studying germs and for distinguishing one kind from others. The first method is an obvious one, to see what the organism looks like, or, as they prefer to say, to study its morphology. The germs are of different sizes and shapes, they may have granules in them, or they may be surrounded with a kind of capsule. They may have one or more little thread-like appendages called flagellae, or they may be grouped together in certain definite formations such as clumps or long chains. Furthermore, a group or "colony" of bacteria which is large enough to be seen with the naked eye, has characteristics which often vary according to the species of the bacteria. The colonies are of different colors, different sizes, different shapes, and have different surface textures. Certain bacteria, when stained with certain aniline dyes and then washed in a solution of iodine, are easily decolorized by washing again in alcohol; other kinds of bacteria retain their color under this process. There are some kinds which remain colored when acted upon by strong mineral acids. By these and other microchemical means many bacteria can be distinguished from one another, although at first sight they may seem very much alike.

Other methods depend upon the behavior of growing cultures of the bacteria. Some will liquefy gelatin, others not. Some can set free the red blood-pigment of mammalian blood from the containing corpuscles, while others are unable to do this. Some can ferment different kinds of sugar with the production of carbonic-acid gas, while others cannot alter the sugars at all. There are some bacteria that need oxygen for their growth, some can do without it, while others still cannot grow at all except in the complete absence of free oxygen. There are many other delicate biological tests, too, but these we have not space to describe here.

It began to be assumed, then, that every infectious disease had its own particular organism which caused this disease alone. But today we know that the matter is not quite so simple as this. For example, the pneumococcus, though quite the commonest and most important, is by no means the only cause of pneumonia. As an antithesis to this we know that certain species of bacteria

can cause more than one disease. There seems little doubt that
the diseases scarlet fever, puerperal fever, infectious sore throat,
and erysipelas, besides some forms of wound infection, are all due
to streptococci. These are organisms which can be seen under the
microscope as minute rounded bodies arranged in chains. Controversy has raged between those who believe that these streptococci are all of one kind and those who think there is a separate kind for each of the diseases which we have mentioned. An
immense amount of work has been done during the last few years
and the view seems to be gaining ground that the organisms are
all of one kind and that varying factors, such as the different sus-
ceptibilities of individuals, may cause the disease to take on one
form or another. Certainly there is a relationship between these
diseases, and the bacteriologists have not succeeded in clearly
distinguishing different forms of streptococci. One fact remains
undisputed, that there has been a very great decline in the epidemics of these streptococcal diseases. Since puerperal fever,
when it does occur, still has an undiminished virulence, this decline seems to be more the result of hygiene than any decrease
in the virulence of the germs or increase in the cunning of the
physicians.

In their search for the microbes of disease, the bacteriologists
have met with one particularly great difficulty. There are a great
many diseases which are undoubtedly infectious, since they can
be produced by inoculation, but no one, search how he may, has
been able to see the organisms with the ordinary microscope.
The melancholy fact is that there is a limit to the power of the
ordinary microscope. When an object is much smaller than the
wavelength of the light used to view it, the light, because of its
wave nature, bends round the object so that the effect is as though
the light came uninterruptedly through the object: in other
words, the object is invisible, and this is true however powerful
the microscope may be.

If we use a microscope which throws a very bright beam of

light on to a small body and view the body sideways, that is, at right angles to the beam, we may be able to see the body by virtue of the light which is scattered. In theory the smallest bodies might be seen by this method, which is, indeed, an extension of the principle that the little motes, otherwise invisible, can be seen dancing in a sunbeam. In practice there are a number of difficulties which greatly limit the distinguishing power of such a microscope, although very small particles which cannot be properly distinguished can at least be made visible. The highest practical magnification obtainable with the ordinary microscope and well-stained biological material varies from x1,200 to x1,800.

We can, of course, use a light of shorter wavelength, and in fact this has been done. Barnard of New York has designed a microscope utilizing ultra-violet light, with which he has succeeded in photographing (for we cannot *see* such a "light") objects considerably smaller than those visible with the ordinary microscope. The difficulties of this method, however, are enormous. For example, the microscope lenses must be made of quartz, since glass is opaque to this kind of light.

The electron microscope is a more promising development. This instrument uses a beam of electrons instead of light, and a system of magnets instead of the usual lenses. This effect depends upon the wave nature of the electron. The experimental proof of electron diffraction was provided by C. J. Davisson and L. H. Germer of the Bell Telephone Laboratories in New York in 1927, and the electrostatic electron lens soon followed. The first electron microscopes were developed in Germany in 1932. In 1938 such a microscope was built in the physics laboratory of the University of Toronto under the supervision of its director, E. F. Burton, by two of his students, James Hillier and P. Prebus. Important advances in the design of the instrument have been made at Toronto and in American laboratories during the past few years. Electron microscopes are now available commercially, and are being installed in a number of American research laboratories.

The electron image can be photographed directly, and magnifications of x30,000 or more have been obtained. The tobacco mosaic, smallpox, and influenza viruses have been photographed by this method, and the possibilities of its usefulness in bacteriology are great.

Thus we have today photographic proof of the existence of disease-producing organisms which are too small to be seen with the ordinary microscope. The existence of these so-called viruses has been known for some time, however, owing to the demonstration that some diseases can be transmitted from man to man, from animal to animal, or between man and animal, by means of extracts prepared from the raw tissues of an infected victim, even when these extracts are filtered or shown to contain no visible organized cells whatsoever. The active principles in these extracts are known technically as the *filterable viruses*. Some of these viruses can be cultivated in the presence of living animal tissue. But in many instances the results obtained by different observers vary considerably. This is not surprising, since it is not possible to obtain the virus pure and unadulterated by extraneous organic matter. However, some viruses have definitely been shown to reproduce themselves through several generations of culture. This, of course, raises the question whether these viruses are themselves organized living beings or whether they are a kind of non-living ferment which becomes increased in quantity during its own action on the living cells. We cannot answer such a question yet. What we can state definitely is that they are self-reproducing and parasitic.

Filterable viruses have been found to be responsible for a number of diseases, to some of which human beings are susceptible. Others are diseases both of animals and men, others are confined to animals alone, and still others are found among plants. Among the most important of these diseases are smallpox, cowpox, infantile paralysis, rabies, foot-and-mouth disease, yellow fever, and encephalitis lethargica (the so-called sleepy sickness, a comparatively new disease first reported in Vienna in 1917, which caused 4,000 deaths in Japan in 1924). Distemper, which attacks

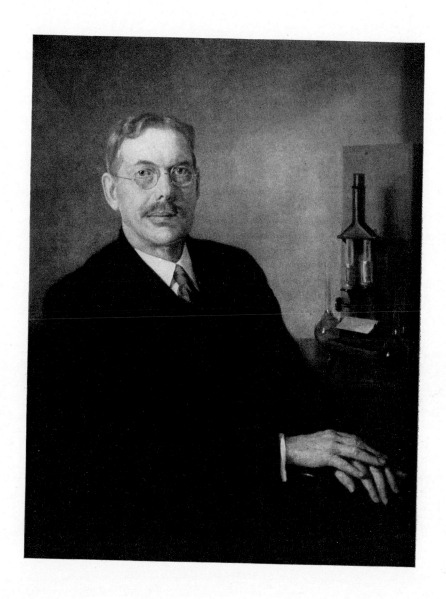

Otto Folin

In the background is Folin's colorimeter, the instrument that made blood chemistry determinations available for the clinician.

dogs and other carnivorous animals, is also a virus disease. There is an important group of virus diseases which chiefly attack the respiratory tract. This includes measles, influenza, the common cold, and psittacosis (the parrot disease which recently came into prominence). It seems likely that most of these are due to definite viruses, although many of the ordinary bacteria frequently found in the respiratory organs of men have been accused in turn of causing colds and influenza.

It is also of considerable interest that three forms of cancer in animals are due to viruses. These are the sarcoma of chickens discovered by Peyton Rous, the rabbit epithelioma discovered by Shope, and the renal carcinoma of the frog described by Lucké. It must be kept in mind, however, that the great majority of animal cancers, as well as those of human beings, cannot be transmitted by cell-free filtrates and are not contagious.

Hope ran high when the bacterial agents of contagious disease first began to be discovered. Here was something new and tangible. The mystery of contagion was laid bare. If these minute beings were the true cause of disease, it was thought, we had only to wage war on them, to exterminate them after they infected the body or prevent them from reaching the body, and there need be no more infectious disease.

Much has been discovered regarding infectious disease but many mysteries remain. In many instances, once the channel of infection, that is, the means of access of the germs to the body, has been found, it has been possible to prevent disease. But there have been many disappointments. In reviewing briefly the expedients to which experimenters have resorted in the war against disease-producing bacteria and the difficulties they have encountered, we shall abandon direct chronology and trace separately the two phases of the battle. First we shall describe the attack on germs outside the body, and then go on to all the various means, both natural and artificial, by which germs can be checked or slain inside the body.

THE GERM THEORY: THE ATTACK ON
THE GERM OUTSIDE THE BODY

I N O R D E R to prevent infectious disease the first important step is to determine the natural history of the causative organism, and this of course includes the means of access to the body. Some organisms are conveyed by food or drink, or through the air. Others enter the body as the result of direct contact of the skin with infective material, but generally, for this to occur, the skin must be broken. For example, hide-porters are frequently attacked with the malignant pustule of anthrax—primarily a disease of animals—which develops on the back of the neck where the infected hides are most liable to rub. The same disease sometimes attacks the faces of people who are unfortunate enough to have bought and used unsterilized and infected shaving brushes. Wool-sorters, on the other hand, are more likely to develop the disease in their lungs, since they are constantly inhaling quantities of dust which sometimes contains spores of the anthrax bacillus.

To develop certain other diseases, however, it is generally necessary to swallow the germs. Two striking instances of this mode of infection are seen in typhoid fever and cholera. From the fact that infection is through the alimentary tract, we would expect an epidemic of one of these diseases to follow the distribution of infected food or water. Such indeed has been the case, and we may take as an illustration the great cholera epidemics which recurred in England between 1831 and 1866.

It was John Snow who in 1855 first produced a mass of evidence to show that cholera was in general a water-borne disease. It had long been observed that the pestilence came out of the East along the great trade routes and proceeded from seaport to seaport, "never going faster than people travel." Snow definitely stated that some kind of material passes from the sick to the healthy "which has the property of increasing and multiplying in the systems of the persons it attacks. . . . As cholera commences with an affection of the alimentary canal . . . it follows that the morbid material producing cholera must be introduced into the alimentary canal . . . must, in fact, be swallowed accidentally." He went on to point out how the swallowing of "minute quantities of ejections and dejections" is favored by uncleanliness, and how the mining population suffered especially from the disease because they worked eight hours at a stretch and consequently took their food and drink, which they ate with unwashed hands, down with them into the pits, which were little better than "one huge privy."

In London the water-supplies were, in some districts, nothing more nor less than diluted sewage. The water was polluted by leaking sewers and overflowing cesspools. A fearful outbreak of cholera occurred in Broad Street, Golden Square, Soho, and caused 500 fatal attacks in ten days—and the mortality would have been worse had not the populace taken refuge in flight. Snow traced all these deaths, or nearly all, to the pump which stood in Broad Street, and endeavored to stay the pestilence by removing the pump-handle.

More convincing even than this was the information which he collected in the parts of London south of the river. This area was supplied with water by different companies whose services overlapped in certain areas. "It is extremely worthy of remark," wrote Snow, "that whilst only 563 deaths occurred in the whole metropolis, in the four weeks ending August 5th (1853), more than one-half of them took place amongst the customers of the Southwark and Vauxhall company and a great portion of the remaining deaths were those of mariners and persons employed in the shipping in the Thames, who almost invariably drew their drinking water directly from the river."

Snow's theories were hotly contested. Many adhered to the old theory of miasmata and epidemic influences. It was only reasonable to blame the air, since no one owned a vested interest in it, unlike the water supply, which had sturdy champions in the directors of the various companies.

Snow made excellent recommendations, including cleanliness about the sick and the sterilization of infected bed linen. He emphasized the importance of obtaining clean or, failing this, boiled water for drinking. He added that it was unwise to hide the fact that cholera was communicable from the people with the idea of preventing a panic. A true knowledge of the cause was likely to be far more helpful.

Cholera in epidemic form has not visited England since 1866 nor the United States since 1873. There is no doubt that this is due not only to quarantine measures but also to improved hygiene, particularly the excellent systems of sewage and water-supply which now exist. It was not, however, until 1884 that Koch was able to announce at the Berlin Conference that he had isolated the causative organism, the comma bacillus, which he had found in Egypt and in India.

Water, however, is not the only article of diet that can spread disease. Tuberculosis may, and often does, lurk in cow's milk. The diphtheria bacillus, too, can grow in milk without giving rise to any appreciable change in its appearance or taste. Undulant or Malta fever is also conveyed by milk. Dairy herds are now so generally infected with this disease that on this account alone it is unsafe to drink unpasteurized milk.

There is another important group of diseases spread by food which are generally known as "food poisoning." Everyone has heard of "ptomaine" poisoning, but contrary to general belief, it is not the most prevalent of the diseases in this group. The "ptomaines" are chemical products of putrefaction and any food containing enough ptomaine to do anyone a serious mischief would be likely to be extremely offensive both to the nose and the palate of the eater. Hence we cannot attribute more than a small fraction of all the cases of so-called "ptomaine" poisoning to the presence of these substances. The truth is that in many instances living germs are swallowed, while in others the trouble is caused by toxins produced by the germs.

We all have eaten shell fish or sausage meat at one time or another with the uneasy feeling that the result may be uncomfortable if not unexpected, but it may come as a surprise to learn that outbreaks of food poisoning have occurred also through eating canned fruits and cheese. In some cases it is possible to acquire the disease even though the food has been cooked or recooked before eating it, for it has been shown that the powerful poisons manufactured by some of these germs are not destroyed by boiling. These poisons can produce very severe internal derangements although, of course, the outlook is much more favorable than when the living germs are eaten and continue to brew their poisons in the intestinal tract of their unwilling host.

We occasionally read of sudden death from botulism following the eating of preserved meats. Fortunately meat containing this toxin almost always smells and looks peculiar, so that it is only rarely that it is eaten at all. The poison is one of the most powerful known and it is by no means necessary to swallow the living germs to develop a fatal attack.

Infection is not always communicated by ill persons. It has been shown that an unsuspected source of infection is from individuals who, though in perfect health themselves, carry about and distribute bacteria which spread disease among those who come in contact with them. These "carriers," as they are called, have sometimes suffered shortly before from the disease they carry. This is usually the case with those who carry typhoid fever. Diphtheria carriers, however, have often not had the disease themselves. The meningococcus, the organism of cerebro-spinal meningitis, is remarkable for the fact that the number of carriers enormously exceeds the number of persons who actually have the disease.

The importance of carriers in keeping diseases endemic among populations is very readily understood. Diphtheria persists in this manner although, as we shall see later, we now know quite enough about the habits of the diphtheria organism to abolish the disease if only the community would make up its mind to stomach the interference and inconvenience involved.

The enormous amount of harm that a single carrier can do is well illustrated by the remarkable story of Typhoid Mary. She was an Irish cook who was proved to be a carrier of typhoid by the clever detective work of Dr. George Soper of New York. In 1907, while studying an isolated outbreak of typhoid fever in a Long Island house, he came to suspect the cook, Mary Mallon, of being a carrier, because all of the other sanitary conditions of the house were beyond reproach. Mary had by this time left her employers and Dr. Soper set out to trace her. He found that in the previous six years she had caused seven household epidemics of typhoid. When he finally caught up with her she was cooking in a Park Avenue house in which the laundress and the only daughter of the family were ill with typhoid.

Mary violently resented the suggestion that she was a carrier. She had to be taken into custody by the police and confined in the Willard Parker Isolation Hospital before specimens of her feces could be obtained for examination. From these a pure culture of the *bacillus typhosus* was isolated. After being incarcerated for two years and eleven months, Mary was released on her pledge that she would never again cook or handle food for others. She promptly broke this pledge, and during the succeeding five years infected a long series of people. The complete story of her doings remains unknown, but she was finally caught again by Dr. Soper at the Sloan Hospital for Women in New York where, serving as a cook, she had caused more than twenty cases of typhoid among the patients. She was then arrested a second time, and was confined on North Brother Island for the remaining three years of her life. She died in 1938. A total of 53 cases of typhoid and three deaths were traced to her.

Mary refused to have her gall bladder removed. It is known that the focus of propagation of the *bacillus typhosus* in the intestinal tract of carriers is the gall bladder and the bile ducts. Removal of the gall bladder suffices, in the majority of cases, to cure the condition. It is unfortunate that this surgical means of control is not more frequently used. The magnitude of the problem of supervising the lives of these typhoid carriers in such a way as to render them harmless to the community is illustrated by the fact that the New York City Department of Health reported that 420 of them were listed in its registry at the end of 1939.

Man himself is by no means the sole offender who carries about with him diseases which may prove the undoing of his fellows. Everyone knows that the hopeless disease of hydrophobia or rabies may follow the bite of a mad dog. As we have seen, it has been possible to eradicate this disease in Great Britain by means of muzzling orders when necessary, and by the strictest possible quarantine for immigrant dogs. In Continental countries the matter is one of much greater difficulty since the methods which have been used in England cannot easily be applied on so enormous a scale. Another difficulty arises because dogs are not alone in spreading rabies. A number of other animals are susceptible to it, including cats, wolves, jackals, and ruminants. When infected they also can inoculate humans by biting. Recently, too, it has been suggested that the Sangre Grande daylight bat of Trinidad may also communicate the disease. Another example of an illness produced by animal bites is the so-called rat-bite fever of Japan, where the rats may inoculate man with a little spiral organism which has been known by the name of *Spirochaeta morsus muris*.

Insects, however, are responsible for far more widespread afflictions than animal carriers. The first discovery of the remarkable fact that insects can cause disease was made by Patrick

Manson. In 1879 he demonstrated that the embryos of the worm which causes a common tropical disease are taken from the blood of an infected human being by a female mosquito. These embryos then develop inside the mosquito, and are finally injected into another human being by the bite of the same insect. This discovery was of tremendous importance, although it was not so regarded at the time. It was, however, directly due to this theory of insect-borne disease that Ronald Ross was able, in 1898, to show that the parasite of malaria, which had been discovered eighteen years previously by Alphonse Laveran in Algeria, is conveyed from man to man in a similar manner. Ross demonstrated that the parasite has a double life-cycle. One set of changes occurs in the body of man at regular intervals, which accounts for the remarkable regularity of the recurring fevers of malaria. The other cycle of change takes place within a special kind of mosquito, until the insect's spit glands are heavily charged with the spores of malaria, ready to infect the next victim of the mosquito.

The cause found, the remedy becomes evident. Malaria is no longer a "bad air," an exhalation from the marshes, but a phase in the life-cycle of a known organism. To abolish the spread of malaria it is necessary to break the life-cycle at some point. The first and most obvious way is to avoid being bitten by the mosquito, and since the habits of the insect are nocturnal, the provision of fine-mesh screens in the windows of houses and nets under which to sleep has procured safety for those who stay indoors after dark.

This, of course, is not an ideal method. The next most feasible way to break the life-cycle of the malarial organism is to destroy the mosquito itself. The anti-mosquito campaign began in 1901 and has met with considerable success. Mosquitoes breed in stagnant water on the surface of which the eggs are laid. The eggs hatch into little wriggling larvae which swim about in the water, coming to the surface occasionally to breathe. The fullgrown mosquito emerges from the water after an interval of seven to ten days.

We have then four methods at our disposal for ridding ourselves of the insects. We can dry up the breeding places or convert the stagnant pools into running streams, we can poison the
larvae, we can asphyxiate them, or we can find some animal which
will eat them. All these methods are employed. The poisoning is
done with "paris green," a powder containing arsenic and copper,
while asphyxiation is accomplished by pouring on the surface of
the water some kind of oil—fuel oil, kerosene, or waste oil is commonly used—so that the larvae cannot breathe. Small predatory
fish will feed with avidity on "the wrigglers" and have proved invaluable. In spite of all these possible ways of killing off mosquitoes there are often considerable practical difficulties in getting
rid of them. For example, it is almost impossible to deal with
every collection of stagnant water, and any small quantity such
as might occur in the fork of a tree or a puddle is quite sufficient for the breeding of mosquitoes provided it remains in
existence for the few days required for the eggs to develop completely.

Furthermore, there is more than one species of "anopheles"
mosquito which can carry malaria, and the species often have
different habits. One kind may breed in small pools, puddles,
quarries, or wheel-ruts. Another may prefer large fresh-water
swamps, another brackish swamps. Sir Malcom Watson has
warned that "only about one species of anopheles in ten carries
malaria and care must be taken to do nothing that would increase the number of the dangerous species. Indeed, the unwary
medical officer may easily stir up a virulent outbreak of malaria
by the adoption of a method that would be 100 per cent successful in another type of land perhaps only a few miles away."

The methods outlined above have been employed with great
success in many parts of the world, although in some instances
success has been marred by the inhabitants' dislike of interference. To take a recent example, in the Shanghai area the oil was
voted too smelly, the "paris green" was mortal to the local ducks,
and the fish placed in the ponds to eat the mosquito larvae were

too well appreciated as a delicacy by the Chinese and the ducks. Fear of political difficulties slowed down the zeal of the municipal authorities. Consequently, the incidence of malaria among the British troops stationed in Shanghai rose from 26.9 per thousand in 1929 to 77.2 per thousand in 1930.

On the whole, however, energetic and skilled organizers have succeeded in making admirable reductions in the incidence of malaria in certain districts. It must also be realized that malaria not only kills directly, but also, by weakening the resistance of those who are attacked, it allows other diseases to gain entry to the damaged body. It is very noticeable that where the incidence of malaria has been greatly reduced by general sanitation and special anti-malarial measures, there also the number of deaths from other diseases is lessened. This has been particularly noticeable in Malaya and in Northern Rhodesia.

Malaria still flourishes over vast tracts of the earth's surface and will continue to do so in spite of an almost complete knowledge of the means of preventing it. The lack of sufficient money to carry out the known preventive measures is the greatest factor in its continued prevalence. The only hope of eradicating it seems to lie in the discovery of cheaper and more ingenious methods of attack.

It follows from what we have seen that human beings are also real carriers of malaria. The mosquitoes do not infect each other but must bite an infected person in order to become bearers of the disease. It will therefore be realized that an important factor in its control is to keep those who are suffering from it out of reach of the voracious anopheles mosquito. This could be done either by effective screening or, perhaps better, by sending the malarial patient to some district where the pestiferous insects do not dwell. The large numbers of the infected, however, make this impossible.

Yellow fever, or yellow jack, the appalling pestilence which has played such havoc in the tropics, has its chief seats in Central

America and the West Coast of Africa. It was formerly common in the United States, having appeared there every year with but two exceptions between 1800 and 1879. It developed among American troops in Cuba during the Spanish American war, and remained such a menace in Havana that in 1900 a commission of American army officers was sent there to study it. The chairman of the commission was Major Walter Reed, and his associates were James Carroll, Jesse W. Lazear, and Aristide Agramonte. As long ago as 1881 Dr. Carlos J. Finlay of Havana had suggested that the mosquito was the carrier of the disease, but had not brought forward any experimental proof. Reed and his associates adopted Finlay's hypothesis as being the right one and set to work to provide proof. The story of their experiments is one of the most dramatic in the whole history of public health work. It is well told in Howard Kelly's biography of Walter Reed, and in the recent play, "Yellow Jack," by Sidney Howard and Paul de Kruif.

Since lower animals were not known to develop yellow fever, human beings had to be used as subjects. The Commission reached the conclusion, after careful consideration, that the results of such an experiment, if positive, would be of sufficient service to humanity to justify it, provided that each individual subjected to the experiment was fully informed of the risks he ran, and gave his free consent. The members of the Commission all agreed that it was their duty to run the risk involved themselves before submitting anyone else to it.

Dr. Carroll, on August 27th, allowed himself to be bitten by a mosquito that had previously bitten four patients with yellow fever. Four days later he developed the disease, and was desperately sick. Fortunately he recovered, as did Private W. H. Dean, who was the second subject to develop the disease after being inoculated in this manner.

Dr. Lazear, however, got the disease shortly afterwards as the result of an accidental bite by one of the infected mosquitoes, and died after some days of delirium.

In order to test the matter thoroughly an experimental station, called Camp Lazear, was then established, and volunteers were called for from the American troops. More came forward than were needed, Private John R. Kissinger being the first to volunteer. The experiments that were carried out proved beyond all doubt that yellow fever was transmitted only by the bite of a variety of mosquito called *Aëdes aegypti*. No other form of contact transmitted the disease, as was proved by seven volunteers who lived for twenty days in a small screened but poorly ventilated room into which clothing, bedding, and the discharges from yellow fever patients were put. They all escaped infection.

Following these experiments a campaign was at once begun in Havana to screen the rooms occupied by yellow fever patients and to destroy all the mosquitoes in the neighborhood. As a result there were only six deaths from the disease in Havana during 1901, while there had been an average of 750 deaths from it per year during the preceding half century.

General William C. Gorgas applied these same methods of yellow fever control in Panama four years later. This region had formerly been a veritable pesthole. Gorgas transformed it into one of the healthiest of places. Without these sanitary measures the Panama Canal could not have been built.

The campaign against yellow fever has been continued in other parts of the world, and much progress has been made during recent years with the support of the International Health Board. There have been further tragedies in the story, however. Hideyo Noguchi, of the staff of the Rockefeller Institute, died of the disease in Africa, where he had gone to study it. Thus also died Adrian Stokes, whose great contribution to the pathology of the disease was the discovery that certain Asiatic monkeys could be successfully inoculated with yellow fever. This did away with the necessity for human experimental subjects.

The actual cause of yellow fever is now generally believed to be a filterable virus. Noguchi in 1918 found a spiral organism in the blood of a patient with yellow fever in Guayaquil, but no one has confirmed his work. It now seems probable that there was a mistake in his diagnosis and that his patient must have been suffering from hemorrhagic jaundice, because this disease is certainly caused by a spiral organism which is identical with the one Noguchi claimed as the germ of yellow fever.

In spite of the successful campaigns against yellow fever, the danger of its further spread is very real. The distribution of *Aëdes aegypti* has been widely studied and it has been found to extend over immense tracts of the earth in every continent, not excluding Europe, so that presumably it is only necessary for a few cases of yellow fever to travel to such areas to provoke explosive outbreaks. In addition to this there is reason to suppose that *Aëdes aegypti* is not the only carrier of the disease, for, in South America—in the emerald-mining village of Muzo, for example—epidemics have occurred *in spite of the absence of Aëdes aegypti.*

The bubonic plague in the western world is, at least in its epidemic form, almost a matter of past history. This history is gruesome enough when we recollect that the Black Death in the 14th Century accounted for one-half of the inhabitants of Great Britain and probably one-quarter of the population of the known earth. But plague has not been exterminated, and may yet come again out of the East where it remains widely but patchily endemic. Indeed, in the last seven years of the 19th Century, the old scourge threatened the whole world. From Hong Kong in 1894 it spread to India, Japan, Turkey and Russia. In 1897 it was at Madagascar and Mauritius. By 1899 it was in Europe again and had even reached Hawaii. In India alone, between 1898 and 1918, more than ten million deaths from plague were recorded. As may be imagined from this figure, the mortality in proportion to the numbers of persons attacked is enormous. When it assumes the bubonic form not less than sixty per cent perish, but when the plague is pneumonic not one escapes.

It was at the beginning of this last pandemic that the bacillus of the plague was found independently by Shibasaburo Kitasato

and Alexandre Yersin at Hong Kong. The means of spread of the
disease was unlike any other yet discovered. Early in the 20th
Century it was found that the plague is, in the first place, a disease of rodents and in particular of rats, and is conveyed from
rat to rat by the bites of fleas. These particular fleas generally live
upon rats, but when pressed by hunger will bite human beings.
The rat dies of the plague, the fleas leave the dead body for new
pastures, and so the pestilence is spread.

This discovery throws some light on various pestilences recorded in history. When the Philistines had carried the ark of God
to Gath, the Lord "smote the men of the city, both small and
great, and they had emerods [hemorrhoids] in their secret parts."
In order to appease the Lord the priests and diviners advised offerings of golden "images of your emerod and images of your
mice that mar the land." That the rodent and the bubo (or
emerod) should have been linked together indicates an awareness
by the ancient Hebrews of an association between the two.

The prevention of plague, then, consists in keeping down the
numbers of rats and avoiding human contact with them, in other
words, in good hygiene. In certain focal areas there is always
some plague among the rodents—for example, a district in the
South-west Himalayas. Other rodents which convey the infection besides rats are the ground squirrels of California and the
gerbilles in South Africa. It is, of course, highly important to
prevent the rats from migrating from one country to another.
The circular metal discs on the mooring ropes of ships in port are
designed to stop them from landing at will. If a ship arrives with
the plague on board the authorities at once set about the extermi-
nation of all the rats by chemical fumigation.

Recently yet another disease-bearing parasite has been shown
to have been responsible for endless mischief. The three fevers,
relapsing fever, trench fever and typhus fever, are all conveyed
by lice. In these instances it seems that it is not the bite that
causes the infection but that the lousy person scratches himself

and thus inoculates himself with the infective body fluids of the louse.

Relapsing fever, or famine fever, is a malady of which we hear little at the present time, although it still flourishes in Eastern Europe, Asia, and Central and South America. But during the last century this disease, together with typhus (gaol fever) and dysentery, caused frightful distress, especially in Ireland. These three furies came savagely upon the unfortunate people in the midst of the appalling potato famine of 1847. A correspondent writing from Dingle, said: "The state of the people of this locality is horrifying. Fever, famine and dysentery are daily increasing; deaths from hunger daily occurring, average weekly twenty—men, women and children thrown into the graves without a coffin—dead bodies in all parts of the country, being several days dead before discovered—no inquests to inquire how they came by their death, as hunger has hardened the hearts of the people."

The causative organism of relapsing fever is a *spirochaete* which was discovered by Otto Obermeier during the Berlin epidemic of 1867–68, and it has been shown that it is transferred by blood-sucking insects. In the Congo and in Central and South America it is transferred by a tick and thus earns its alternative name of "tick fever," while in Europe, Asia and North Africa it is carried by lice.

Typhus, or gaol fever, is uncommon where sanitation and hygiene have reached a high level, but this sickness also was widespread during the 19th Century. It is yet endemic in the Slav countries and indeed it follows closely the geography and the history of dilapidation and dirt, wretchedness and war. Typhus used always to occur not only in gaols but also among armed forces. It has been suggested that this fever in the English Navy was for long recruited directly from the prisons through the press-gangs who forcibly enlisted newly discharged convicts.

The organism which is generally believed to be responsible for typhus was named by da Rocha-Lima in 1916 *Rickettsia prowa-*

zeki, to commemorate Howard T. Ricketts and Stanislaus von Prowazek, who had both fallen martyrs to the study of this disease. The *Rickettsiae* are minute organisms which form a class by themselves. They are not only much smaller than ordinary bacteria, but they vary in size and shape and are difficult to stain. They were first described in 1909 by Ricketts in the blood of patients ill with Rocky Mountain spotted fever, a disease closely related to typhus. In 1910 Ricketts and Wilder found similar organisms in typhus blood smears, and in smears from lice who had fed on typhus patients. Von Prowazek made the same observation in Serbia in 1916, and da Rocha-Lima, Wolbach and others subsequently confirmed the discovery.

The prevention of these louse-borne diseases is simple in principle and consists essentially in preventing the louse from changing his host. This is most easily done by preventing overcrowding, and "delousing" the inhabitants as far as possible.

There is another important channel by which disease germs may enter the human body and which we must now consider. This is the respiratory tract. How do germs actually get in through the nose, larynx, windpipe and lungs?

Pasteur himself had shown that the air in inhabited places was swarming with micro-organisms, but most of these are harmless. However, harmful germs certainly do get loose about the air. When a person coughs or sneezes a fine spray consisting of innumerable droplets of moisture is thrown into the air. The patient may be suffering from some disease in his respiratory system, or he may be a carrier of some respiratory disease. He may be coughing diphtheria germs or scarlet fever germs into the air. When a person who has consumption spits into the street, the sputum dries and forms a fine powder which may be carried to others in dust stirred up by wind. There is very little doubt that many common infectious diseases, ranging from the common cold to the pneumonic plague, are spread in this way.

There has been much dispute about whether pulmonary tu-

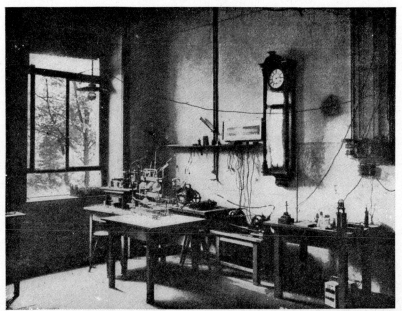

Röntgen's Laboratory

*The Laboratory in the Würzburg Physical Institute
in which Röntgen discovered x-rays.*

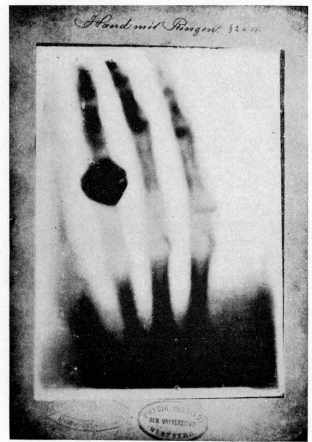

(From Otto Glasser's biography *Wilhelm Conrad Röntgen*)

The First X-ray Photograph

*Made by Röntgen of his wife's hand on Dec. 22, 1895,
and now in the Deutsches Museum.*

berculosis (consumption) gains entry by the air or by the food. Now there are at least two kinds of tubercle bacilli which may infect human beings. The one is called the *human* and the other the *bovine* type. These can be distinguished from one another by the fact that the bovine bacillus is much more virulent in certain lower animals such as the rabbit than the human bacillus. It has been found that 99 per cent of tuberculous infections of the lungs and 95 per cent of tuberculous infections of the glands in the neighborhood of the air passages are caused by the human type of tubercle bacillus. It therefore seems not unlikely that most of this kind of tuberculosis is inhaled, for bovine tuberculosis is only likely to come from drinking milk.

The air, as we have seen from the miasm theory, has been suspect from time immemorial. The great prison reformer, John Howard, believed that the poisonous effluvia of the nauseous dungeons which he inspected were the cause of gaol fever. Florence Nightingale, too, declared her belief that fevers arose *de novo* from bad air and filth. The diseases were seen to spread rapidly and mysteriously and it is, therefore, scarcely surprising that the air was blamed. In 1750 the prisoners of the Old Bailey conveyed their typhus fever (surely through the air, it was thought) even to the Bar and the Bench, so that many died, including the Lord Mayor and other notables.

A hundred years ago Maidstone gaol was rid of gaol fever by the energetic use of soap, water, quicklime, clean clothes, sulphur and nourishing food. The same methods are now used with fuller knowledge of the rationale. Thus we see that gradually the number of diseases for which the air can be blamed is declining; but it seems very probable that certain respiratory diseases, at least, will remain in this category. Certainly no one will deny the beneficial effects of fresh air, yet we send our children and go ourselves into the foul air of moving picture theaters and schoolrooms where, as Leonard Hill has pointed out, the air is usually much more laden with germs than the comparatively healthy atmosphere of a well-conducted sewer!

In some instances the remarkable rapidity with which a disease will spread, especially in a population unused to the disease, almost forces us to conclude that the spread is by means of the air. For example, it is stated that in the island of Wharekauri, 480 miles east of New Zealand, the visit of a ship to the island is followed by a four-day illness (called murri-murri) of both whites and colored. "The mere appearance of murri-murri is proof to the inhabitants *even at distant parts* of the island, which is thirty miles long, that a ship is in port."

In many of these influenza-like diseases, it is fairly certain that the air is the channel of infection, but it is very difficult to prove the matter if we cannot see the microbes. In consumption and diphtheria, it can be readily demonstrated that morbid germs are coughed into the air. Can germs travel long distances in the air and appear spontaneously at some distant site? Considering the fact that disease almost always can be kept out by strict quarantine, we must admit that this appears unlikely. However, it has recently been shown by the United States Bureau of Plant Industry that the spores of the black stem rust, the dreaded pestilence of American wheat, can be collected on glass microscope slides, by means of an aeroplane, at the astonishing height of ten thousand feet above the earth. These spores fall so slowly that it has been calculated it would be possible that regions a thousand miles and more to the leeward of the original source *might* become infected. We must, therefore, not be too sure about how far germs may travel in the air. It should, however, be stated that the viruses which are known are essentially parasitic and are found in association with living matter, so that it does not seem probable that they will be found borne passively by themselves on the wind.

Bacteria are not possessed of any organs that enable them to fly and in general any movement they make is a passive one. We may note, however, that certain germs—such, for instance, as those which cause typhoid fever—are able to move about in liquids. Other organisms such as the ameba of dysentery and the various disease-producing spirochaetes are very active while swimming, but they definitely cannot fly. We must not, then, conclude that because a disease seems to appear independently at a fresh geographical focus isolated from the source, it has propagated itself through the air. We must, for example, consider that common pests like the domestic house-fly can, and often do, act in the odious role of disease carriers and may infect our food with their germ-laden feet as they fly from the dunghill to the dinner-table.

THE GERM THEORY: THE ATTACK ON
THE GERM INSIDE THE BODY

IT MUST surely have been noticed at a very early stage in the history of man that certain diseases rarely, if ever, attack the same person twice. Thucydides categorically states that no one was ever attacked a second time, at least with a fatal result, by the plague at Athens, and this belief was so strong in those who had had the malady and recovered that they even entertained the innocent fancy that they could not die of any other sickness.

The practice of inoculation of smallpox with the idea of "getting it over" and in the hope of inducing a mild attack came first from the east of Europe. It is supposed that this practice originally contained no idea of engendering in the body antidotes to the contagion, but was intended by magical symbolism to rid the patient of the disease by passing it on either to another person or to an animal. It is said that there is the germ of this idea in the scapegoat of the Israelites and the miracle of the swine of Gadara. This kind of belief exists today. For example, the writer has heard the opinion expressed among the Riffs in North Africa that a certain distressing and very prevalent contagious disease can be cured most easily by passing it on in the same manner in which it was acquired to a negress, or, failing this, to a donkey. According to this point of view disease is an entity, a sort of possessive devil, as it were, that goes from one person to another. Our modern concept, however, is that contagious disease is due to infecting or-

104

ganisms, and that any immunity which develops is due to the building up by the body of specific substances which either destroy the germs in the body or neutralize the poisons given out by them.

Inoculation of smallpox matter from a mild case was certainly almost always successful, if it produced an artificial attack, in preventing a subsequent natural attack. The method was widely used in the latter part of the 18th Century, but unfortunately it was not always possible to gauge the virulence of the inoculated matter, so that the results were sometimes fatal and often disfiguring. Moreover there was considerable risk of infecting the patient with other diseases. Nevertheless numbers of people were successfully protected from smallpox by this means, and without too much disfigurement, if we may judge from the remark of Mrs. Hardcastle in Goldsmith's *She Stoops to Conquer*: "I vow, since inoculation began, there is no such thing to be seen as a plain woman." The story of Jenner's substitution of vaccination (the inoculation of cowpox) for the more dangerous procedure has already been told. This was the beginning of the science of immunology.

No further progress at all was made until Pasteur published his brilliant discoveries of the microbic nature of infectious disease. Pasteur's discovery of preventive inoculation was a kind of accident, but an accident of which a less acute mind might easily have overlooked the importance. He had been studying the disease of fowls which is vulgarly called "chicken cholera" and of which the microbe had already been found. One evening he attempted to inoculate a bird with a stale culture of chicken cholera germs some weeks old. The bird sickened slightly and then recovered. Using the same bird and a fresh tube of virulent germs he was delighted to find that the bird was resistant to the infection although the germs were quite virulent to any normal chicken. He was quick to notice the prime importance of this discovery. The oxygen of the air was responsible for the attenuation of the germs. He could now cultivate germs to any lessened virulence that he desired and with these produce an immunity to future infection.

These studies led him to an attempt to provide a preventive inoculation for sheep and cattle against anthrax (splenic fever). With the discovery of the principle that the virulence of germs can be attenuated or reinforced by passing the germs through suitable animals—that is, by inoculating the animals and recovering the germs later in a fresh culture from the animal—he brought this line of research in 1881 to a triumphant conclusion. In 1882 he completely annihilated the opposition of those who constantly contradicted his opinions and impugned his scientific honesty, by the world-famous and classical experiment on the farm of Pouilly-le-Fort near Melun. Here he had three groups of sheep. The first group, consisting of ten sheep, were control animals. Of the remaining fifty, twenty-five had been previously inoculated with an attenuated culture of living anthrax germs and twenty-five had not. In the presence of an interested audience of friends and sceptics, Pasteur publicly injected all but his control group with a virulent culture of anthrax germs. To the confusion of his enemies and the jubilation of his friends, all of the unprotected sheep died, just as he had predicted, while the inoculated ones remained alive and well.

Hydrophobia was the first human disease which Pasteur tried to prevent by inoculation. He started with the assumption that the rabid virus was in the spittle of the mad dog. He was unable at first to transmit the disease to animals by inoculating them with human saliva from a patient with hydrophobia. It then occurred to him that, from the nature of the symptoms of the disease, the virus surely attacked the central nervous system. He found that he could convey the disease to animals by trephining them. Thus he came to use the central nervous system of rabbits as a culture medium for growing the virus, which of course he was unable to see in a microscope since it belongs to the class of filterable viruses. By drying the infected spinal cord from rabbits for varying lengths of time, he could produce samples which had their virulence attenuated to any degree he required.

Pasteur saw clearly that it would be impossible to inoculate all French dogs against rabies since there were some hundred thousand in Paris and two and a half million in the provinces, and each dog would require several inoculations. He came to the reluctant conclusion, therefore, that the method must be one which could be applied to human beings *after* they had been bitten by mad dogs. This opportunity came to him in 1885. Courageously, but with some mistrust of a treatment which up to then he had used only on dogs, he began by inoculating with gradually increasing strengths of virus a little Alsatian boy, nine years old, who had been bitten in fourteen places by a rabid dog. There was no doubt that the dog was mad and Pasteur adopted the method in the one hope of saving the boy's life. The result was successful, and as all the world soon knew, the boy remained well.

This was the beginning of the justly celebrated Pasteur treatment for the prevention of hydrophobia. It was followed shortly afterwards, in 1888, by the inauguration of the Pasteur Institute in Paris. At the present time there are Pasteur institutes scattered throughout the world where persons bitten by rabid animals are given one or another modification of the original methods of Pasteur.

The discovery that the virulence of bacteria can vary under different conditions is extremely significant in the study of epidemics. It may, in fact, account for the disappearance or sudden virulent outbreak of an epidemic in the history of nations. Pasteur looked upon these inoculations as preventive and not curative. His hope was that every infectious disease could be combated in a similar way, but unfortunately his success was limited.

IMMUNE SERA

In order to trace the further development of methods of fighting infectious disease within the body, particularly as regards the use of immune sera, it will be convenient to study the history of diphtheria.

Diphtheria used to be a mysterious sickness. Before the middle of the last century it was little known. The older epidemics of "throat-distemper" cannot be definitely differentiated as diphtheria or scarlet fever. Quite suddenly, between the years 1856 and 1859 diphtheria, as we now know it, became common. The reason for this can only be surmised, but it seems not to be due entirely to improved diagnosis. Friedrich Löffler's masterly researches on the diphtheria bacillus, which had actually been observed before by Edwin Klebs, marked the beginning of the bacteriology of the disease in 1884. The important point about this bacillus is that it is found in the body only at the site where it first takes root. It does not spread throughout the body like anthrax and most other disease germs. Four years after Löffler's discoveries it was shown that there is a potent poison given out by the bacillus. This toxin circulates in the system and is responsible for the mortality from diphtheria. The bacillus itself multiplies only in the throat or wherever it was first implanted.

By inoculating a horse with gradually increasing doses of this powerful toxin it has been found possible to make the horse immune to further large doses. This is a modification of the method used by the great Mithridates IV, King of Pontus, to protect himself from death by poison. The blood of the horse then possesses antitoxic properties. The horse is bled from the jugular vein, the blood is allowed to clot, and the serum is filtered off. The strength of this is carefully standardized by measuring its protective action in guinea-pigs against a standard dose of toxin. This serum is used in the *treatment* of diphtheria. It is sold under the name of diphtheria antitoxin, although of course it is really a very diluted solution of the antitoxin in the blood-serum of the horse. The importance of this method is so great that it is rarely necessary to provide any other specific treatment for diphtheria. The serum must be administered without delay and in large amounts. The statistics show clearly that the case mortality is considerably reduced by this procedure.

It must be emphasized at this point that the principles involved in vaccines and sera are quite different. A vaccine is a poisonous product consisting either of living, or, as we shall see later, dead germs, which provokes the formation of resistance in the body. An antitoxic serum, on the other hand, is an animal's blood-serum containing substances which can neutralize bacterial poisons.

We have also learned from statistical surveys that diphtheria is more prevalent in certain classes of society and in certain age-groups. This has been explained by the demonstration that some people are immune in a greater or less degree because they have some antitoxin in their blood. This is called natural immunity. In 1913 Bela Schick developed the technique of the famous "Schick test," which enables us to determine whether individuals possess any natural immunity to diphtheria. A minute and measured quantity of a standardized solution of toxin is injected into (not under) the skin of the forearm. A positive reaction is said to occur when a red flush appears at the site of the injection within twenty-four or thirty-six hours. It reaches its maximum on the fourth day. This means that the patient has little or no antitoxin in his blood and is therefore susceptible to diphtheria. Those who show a negative reaction are immune.

We have seen how the antitoxin can be used for the treatment of diphtheria. It has also been used in epidemics in order to immunize those who have been in contact with persons suffering from the disease. Such an injection of antitoxin rapidly brings about immunity, but unhappily it is not a lasting one. Within a few days or weeks the antitoxin disappears again and the immunity goes too. A fresh exposure may then result in an attack of the disease. Such "passive" immunity is therefore of limited use, since it is clearly of value only when there is a risk for a limited time.

A serum is also effective against the disease known as tetanus (lockjaw). In this disease the organisms gain entry by means of a wound, and grow in it and elaborate poisons, without themselves being disseminated all over the body. It has been found that the injection of anti-tetanic serum, prepared in a similar manner to the anti-diphtheritic serum, has had a remarkable effect in lowering the incidence of tetanus. Here is an ideal situation for the use of passive immunity. The risk is only for a short time, while the wound is infected. Anti-tetanic serum is now given as a routine measure in all cases where there are dirty wounds, especially those contaminated with mud or manure.

Its use on a large scale in war casualties was begun during the First World War, in the middle of October, 1914. The figures regarding the incidence of tetanus among wounded British soldiers before and after its introduction are remarkable. In September, 1914, 15.9 out of every thousand developed tetanus. In October the figure had risen to the horrible rate of 31.8, but the following month saw an immediate drop to 1.7. It is impossible not to ascribe this magnificent result to the general preventive use of the serum.

Can we not produce some lasting immunity to infectious disease? If the horse can produce antitoxin when injected with toxin, cannot the same process be applied to man? It is obviously unwise to inject unaltered toxin into human beings, but it has been found that the human body will produce antitoxin when we inject a suitable mixture of toxin and antitoxin. For example, this method produces a lasting immunity from diphtheria. The Schick test is very useful in this connection, since we can determine those who are susceptible and then proceed to immunize these alone without the necessity of having to do it to everyone. Further, we can see if the immunization has been successful, for if it has, the Schick reaction should become negative.

Wholesale immunization of children against diphtheria has been carried out in many American communities with striking success. In New York City, for instance, there was an average of 14,282 cases of diphtheria with 1,290 deaths per year during the years 1910 to 1919. The intensive campaign to immunize all school children was begun in 1929. The decrease in the disease has been phenomenal. In 1940 there were only 408 cases with only 10 deaths in a population of 7,392,000. This represented a fall in the diphtheria death rate from 83 per 100,000 children under 15 years of age during the 1910–1919 period, to 0.7 per 100,000 in 1940.

Diphtheria is spread by contact with those suffering from the disease, by human carriers and by cows. The latter develop diphtheria lesions on their teats which may discharge highly virulent bacteria into the milk. All of these sources of diphtheria, once known, can be stopped and if this were done and all Schick-positive persons could be immunized, there seems every possibility that we could extinguish the malady entirely.

In scarlet fever a test similar to the Schick test has been devised to detect those who are susceptible. This was worked out by George F. and Gladys H. Dick in 1924. It consists in the intradermal injection of a toxin prepared by filtration from a bacterial culture. The culture used is of streptococci which are almost certainly the cause of scarlet fever. The test is positive at the beginning of the illness but negative in 80 per cent of the cases after the attack. A serum has also been prepared from the blood of animals who have been inoculated with increasing doses of the same streptococcal toxin. This anti-streptococcal serum is now used in the treatment and sometimes in the prevention of scarlet fever, though it produces only a temporary (passive) immunity.

There is also available a method of producing artificially a permanent immunity to scarlet fever. As with diphtheria, this is done by injecting gradually increasing doses of toxin, and it is claimed that this procedure will effectively protect the majority of susceptible persons.

We have also ground for hoping that in the not far distant future there may be some kind of serum treatment for influenza. Before 1933 experiments with the alleged filterable virus of this highly infectious disease had been difficult because no animal had been found to be susceptible to the infection. At that time it was shown by Wilson Smith and his associates, that ferrets could be infected with filtered throat washings from patients ill with influenza. Furthermore, the infection could be readily transferred from ferret to ferret. If the virus is mixed with serum from a ferret which has been infected and recovered, it becomes harmless. Ferrets that have recovered are not susceptible to a further infection for at least some weeks. Most important, too, is the fact that neutralizing antibodies have been found in serum from human beings who have recovered from this disease. In 1934 it was further discovered that mice also can be infected. This will probably expedite the research. It is unlikely, however, that any really good method of inducing an active immunity will be found because one attack of influenza does not protect against another.

VACCINES

We have seen how immunity can be artificially produced first by inoculation with an attenuated *living virus,* and second by the use of *toxin-antitoxin* mixtures. There is now available a third method which, in certain instances, has proved invaluable. This is the injection of emulsions of *dead* germs. These emulsions also have regrettably been christened "vaccines" although they have nothing whatever to do with cows. The original anti-smallpox vaccine of Jenner was prepared directly from infected cows and in this instance only does the name seem justified.

Pasteur believed that immunity could be acquired only by infection with living bacteria. In certain diseases where it has been impossible to grow the organisms in pure culture, unmixed with other substances, we continue to use the living virus. This is still done in rabies and in smallpox. More recently efforts have been made to deal with tuberculosis by wholesale immunization with living germs of lowered virulence. Dr. Albert Calmette of Paris in 1924 produced a strain of weakened tubercle bacilli generally known as B.C.G. (Bacillus Calmette-Guérin) which is lineally descended, through successive sub-cultures made at fourteen to twenty-five day intervals over a period of many years, from bacilli originally isolated in 1901.

The results of prolonged investigation go to confirm Dr. Calmette's view that B.C.G. can be used as a vaccine without any danger of causing progressive tuberculosis. Obviously, however, we should feel happier if some method could be found by which dead germs could secure effective immunity. This is clearly the safer course. In this connection it may be wise to bear in mind the ghastly affair at Lübeck in Germany. In the winter of 1930–31 some two hundred and fifty infants were given by mouth (*not* by injection) this B.C.G. vaccine, which was prepared by subculturing the organisms received from Paris. Within three months sixty-eight of them were dead of acute tuberculosis. The question at issue was whether the B.C.G., for some unexplained reason, had become suddenly virulent, or whether there had been some blunder whereby another virulent strain of organisms had been given in error. The court of inquiry took the latter view, and punished those whom it held responsible, so that Calmette's vaccine was vindicated; but it may be observed that legal and scientific proof are not always the same. It is certainly true that many thousands of infants have been treated with B.C.G. without untoward results except at Lübeck. How far this treatment attains its object cannot be calculated with any scientific accuracy. It is too early to judge the results.

Robert Koch, the founder of modern bacteriological technique, and discoverer of the tubercle bacillus, hoped that his work would be the key to a definite cure for tuberculosis. Koch had prepared a non-living toxic substance from cultures of tubercle bacilli which he named tuberculin. If a very small quantity of this is injected into a new-born infant who has not been infected, there is very little reaction. With a healthy adult who is not clinically tuberculous, but who has at one time been infected, there is more reaction. Any animal that has once been infected is, in fact, very sensitive to the toxin. It has been found that ninety per cent of persons in cities react positively to tuberculin. It would seem, then, that most people are, at one time or another, the victims of a slight infection with tuberculosis, that they recover and have some degree of resistance to the disease. This accounts for the fact that, in spite of the widespread possibility of infection, only a relatively small number of people seem to develop obvious signs of the disease. This is corroborated by the fact that in post-mortem examinations old and healed tuberculous foci are often found in people who have no history of having suffered from tuberculosis.

Tuberculin is of great value in diagnosis both in man and in animals. Thus it has been possible to test cattle and to collect herds of tested cows that are guaranteed to give milk free from all tubercle bacilli. In the United States, public health laws requiring periodical tuberculin tests of dairy herds have to a large extent eliminated the spread of tuberculosis from milk. In Britain such laws have not been enacted, and more than two thousand children die every year in England and Wales from bovine tuberculosis, which probably comes from drinking tuberculous milk.

In some diseases other than tuberculosis, however, vaccines made from dead organisms have given gratifying results. The classic example of this is the anti-typhoid inoculation, for the successful exploitation of which we are indebted to Sir Almroth Wright and his co-workers. Typhoid and paratyphoid fever are in general conveyed by sewage—polluted water—either directly or through some agency such as oysters which have been grown in contaminated water. Consequently any community which builds an efficient system of sanitation can reduce the incidence of these diseases almost to the vanishing point. There is always likely to be some difficulty in dealing adequately with chronic typhoid carriers. War, of course, produces conditions under which sanitation is often inadequate and typhoid is apt to appear. In former wars it has caused great numbers of deaths among the troops. As recently as 1898 the disease reached epidemic proportions in some American army camps. At Camp Chickamauga, in August, 1898, for instance, there were at one time more than 500 cases of typhoid. Today all American troops are inoculated against typhoid and the disease is no longer seen in the army.

A method of producing active immunity against typhus by means of vaccination has recently been worked out. Several types of vaccine have been devised, but the one generally favored is prepared from the growth of rickettsias in the yolk sac of the developing chick embryo. The suspension of typhus organisms thus obtained is inactivated by the addition of phenol or formaldehyde. The vaccine is given subcutaneously in three doses at weekly intervals. Although the value of the vaccine has not been extensively tested, the United States War Department has enough confidence in it to administer it to all American troops going abroad. Reports indicate that typhus is already rampant in the Balkans and on the Russo-German front, and it is hoped that this new vaccine will protect our troops from this great scourge of army life.

ONE DISEASE USED TO ATTACK ANOTHER

The idea of using one infectious disease to attack another can be traced to an interesting experiment conducted by Pasteur. Pasteur had been unable to infect birds with anthrax. Léon Colin had claimed that nothing was easier, but he never produced the chicken, dead of anthrax, which he had promised to Pasteur. However, Pasteur turned the tables on Colin by finally producing the infected bird himself. Now chickens, and other birds too, have a much higher temperature than mammals. The normal temperature of a chicken is about 107 degrees Fahrenheit, as compared with 98.4 degrees Fahrenheit in human beings. Pasteur wondered if the immunity of chickens to anthrax lay in this difference of temperature. He took a chicken and gave it a prolonged cold bath. Its temperature was lowered, and sure enough, the bird came down with the disease and died.

This impressive demonstration led other men to wonder whether the fever which accompanies many infections might not be a reaction hostile to the invading parasite. The hypothesis was first put to a test in general paralysis of the insane, which is an occasional late manifestation of syphilis. Its truly syphilitic nature, long suspected, was proved by Noguchi, the Japanese bacteriologist, who, after a long and unwearied search, found the spirochetes in the brain of a man dead of general paralysis. The disease is progressive and results, as its name implies, in both paralysis and insanity. Its march is slow but unrelenting. To the untreated comes almost certain death when the brain is gradually destroyed, leaving the body speechless, paralysed and insane.

The story of Wagner-Jauregg's fifty year battle with the disease and his eventual relative success is one of the most stimulating in modern medicine. Julius Wagner-Jauregg was an Austrian who took his medical degree in Vienna in 1880. During the next six years he worked in pathology there and finally obtained a post as an assistant in psychiatry. It was at this time that he was deeply impressed by seeing an insane patient cured following an attack of erysipelas. In 1890, following Koch's discovery of tuberculin, Wagner-Jauregg began to use it to produce fever in the insane with the hope that such artificially induced fever might have the same effect as the fever of erysipelas.

His results at first were thoroughly discouraging. Nevertheless he kept at it. In 1901 he gave up trying to influence miscellaneous forms of insanity and concentrated his efforts on general paralysis. Now for the first time he began to get suggestive results. In 1914 he was able to report that among 86 paretics he had treated between 1907 and 1909, 21 were still alive and seven were actually working. He then screwed up his courage to the point of inoculating paretics with malaria, an experiment he had had in mind for thirty years but had not dared to try, for malaria, of course, is sometimes fatal. The results of this heroic therapy were indeed miraculous—about one-third of those who were given malaria were cured of their insanity, and their disabilities relieved to the point where they could return to society. Wagner-Jauregg carried his therapy one step further, namely, he gave the malaria treatment to syphilitics who had not yet become insane but who

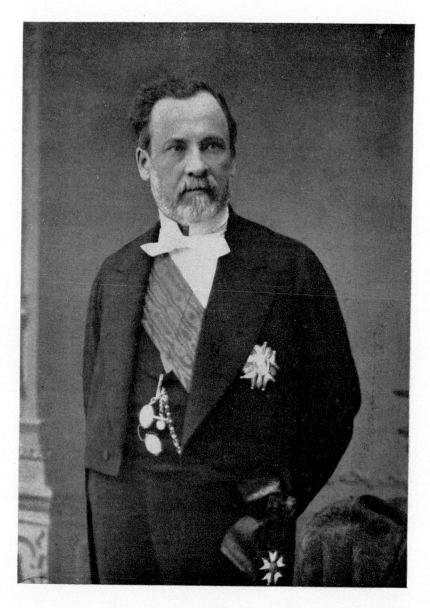

Pasteur

One of the remarkable things about Pasteur was the manner in which he triumphed over a great physical handicap. In 1868 when he was 46 years old, just after he had completed his studies on wine, he was struck down with a cerebral hemorrhage. Although his mind was not affected he was left with a partial paralysis of his left side which persisted for the remainder of his life. This photograph, taken after he was awarded the Grand Cross of the Legion of Honor in 1881, gives no hint of his infirmity.

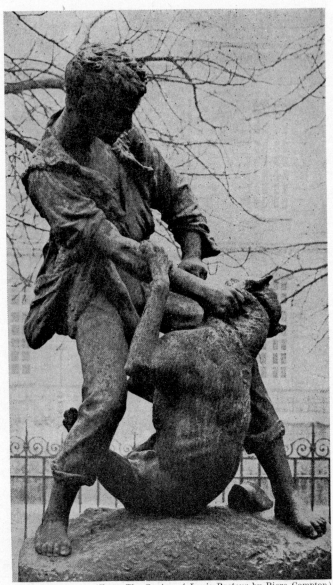

(From *The Genius of Louis Pasteur* by Piers Compton)

The Shepherd Boy Jupille Subduing the Mad Dog

Jupille volunteered to be inoculated by Pasteur and became the second person to be saved from rabies. In his honor this statue was raised in Paris.

were doomed to develop general paralysis because of the known presence of the spirochetes in their central nervous system. In a large proportion of these patients the disease was arrested and the development of insanity prevented. Thus after forty years of the most discouraging effort, Wagner-Jauregg attained a degree of control over one of the worst afflictions of mankind. He was awarded the Nobel Prize in 1927, and lived to see his work generally accepted. He died in 1940.

Recently more simple and less dangerous methods of producing artificial fever have been discovered and substituted for the malaria therapy. Willis R. Whitney, a physicist in the General Electric Company Research Laboratory at Schenectady discovered that a powerful high frequency electric oscillator would raise the temperature of those working near it. This discovery was tested upon animals by Carpenter at the Albany Medical College, and finally put into use upon patients at the Psychiatric Institute of the Columbia-Presbyterian Medical Center in New York. Other methods of raising the temperature of the body by electrical devices have since been developed. It is yet too soon to know whether malarial fever or machine made fever is the more effective in the treatment of general paralysis.

STOREHOUSES OF INFECTION

There is yet another method of doing away with the ill effects of microbes in the human body. This is by removing them *en masse* where this is possible, that is to say, when they are all collected in some localized situation which is accessible to the surgeon's knife.

The opening of abscesses, with subsequent drainage by means of tubes or other types of drains, is ancient history. More recently it has come to be realized that there are certain organs in the body which frequently become infected and act as a kind of reservoir, from which germs and their toxins are disseminated. The tonsils, appendix, gall bladder, and nasal sinuses—all can, and frequently do act in this way. Pyorrhea or abscesses around the roots of the teeth sometimes form such a focus of infection.

A patient with such a hidden focus of infection may be ill in some rather indefinite way, while at other times there may be symptoms which definitely point to one or another of these organs as the source of the trouble. Chronic rheumatism, for example, may be exacerbated if not actually caused by a localized infection. In all diseases where the general health is at fault it is now considered important to examine a patient with the thought of these foci of infection in mind.

CHEMOTHERAPY—THE MAGIC BULLETS OF MEDICAL SCIENCE

WE ARE living today in an epoch of medical progress which will certainly be known to our descendants as the *chemotherapeutic epoch,* and which certainly marks the most important conquest over disease that man has yet achieved. This epoch began with the discovery of the anti-streptococcic power of a sulfonamide compound by Gerhard Domagk in 1932, and as we write these words in 1942, the list of bacterial diseases successfully attacked by the sulfonamide compounds continues to grow.

But the history of chemotherapy of course goes farther back. Indeed, one of the most ancient methods of combating sickness has been by the use of chemicals or drugs. Many people seem to think that there must be a drug appropriate to every disease and that once the disease is diagnosed it is only necessary to find the right physic. Unhappily there are very few drugs which have a direct action in curing the diseases for which they are administered. Most of the drugs in the pharmacopoeia are useful only in removing some unpleasant symptom, or in treating some aspect of the disease. For example, we give aspirin for a headache. This often removes the headache but not the cause of it. If the cause is a trifling one, it may have vanished before the aspirin loses its effect, but this is not always so, for headache may be due to a serious disease.

Among the drugs which do have a definite specific effect on

the causal organism of a sickness is quinine. The crude Cinchona bark (Peruvian or Jesuit's bark) was first imported into Europe from South America in the 17th Century. The purified drug quinine was isolated in the early 19th Century. Cinchona is now grown chiefly in the Far East, in Java. The bark was formerly used for the ague without any understanding of why or how it was effective. It has since been discovered that quinine exerts a definitely hostile action on certain phases of the life-cycle of the malarial parasite in the blood of the patient. Unfortunately, it has little or no action on other phases of the parasite. More recently certain synthetic products have been found to attack the parasite in its other phases. Some of these products are too poisonous to be used regularly in preventing infection with malaria. The results of trial with various drugs have not always been consistent, and this may be due to the fact that there are different breeds, so to speak, of malarial parasite which are more or less resistant to the effects of these drugs.

Since quinine acts only at one period in the life-cycle of the parasite, it has certain grave disadvantages. First, it does not prevent infection even when taken in huge doses. Second, it does not always prevent relapses. Finally, it does not prevent mosquitoes from becoming infected from the blood of human beings. Plasmochine and atebrin, two synthetic drugs, will attack the parasite at other stages and in certain cases will prevent the infection of human beings from a mosquito bite. Plasmochine will also keep the parasite under control during the phase when the mosquito is liable to become infected. Thus these two drugs are valuable not as substitutes for but as auxiliaries to quinine.

The search still goes on for some product which may be at the same time lethal to the parasite, less harmful to the patient and, what is of very great importance, cheap enough and abundant enough to be used on a large scale. It will be recognized how necessary is this last condition when it is known that the British Empire, within which the bulk of the three and a half million deaths from malaria recorded annually occur, spends about £450,000 each year on quinine alone.

Another chemical product which has proved of very great value is emetine, used in treating certain forms of dysentery. There are two main forms of this disease, namely, that caused by certain bacilli, and that which is due to a species of ameba called *entamoeba histolytica*. Emetine, which has a lethal action on the entamoeba, is of value only in amebic dysentery. The entamoeba has the power of burrowing, or rather digesting, its way into the tissues of the patient's bowel, and may form abcesses in more distant sites. These require surgery. Bacillary dysentery can be treated with a specific serum.

But it was in connection with syphilis that chemotherapy scored its greatest triumph of the last generation. The chemical was Paul Ehrlich's "magic bullet," salvarsan. Born in Silesia in 1854, Ehrlich was one of the brilliant young men who were attracted to Koch's laboratory in Berlin in the eighties. He won a place for himself in the laboratory by discovering a method for staining the tubercle bacillus with a dye in order to make it visible under the microscope. Thus a practical diagnostic test for tubercle bacilli in the sputum became available. Ehrlich contracted tuberculosis himself in the process of making this discovery. He went to Egypt to rest and was cured.

Returning to Germany and to his work, he eventually became, in 1896, director of a state laboratory for testing serum, near Berlin. His next move was to a bigger and better laboratory that the government built for him at Frankfort on the Main, and it was there that, in 1901, he became interested in some research done by Alphonse Laveran with a trypanosome which is the cause of a disease in horses. Laveran had inoculated mice with the organism and tried to cure them with arsenic, but the mice always died under the treatment. Ehrlich took up the task of trying to cure this mouse trypanosome disease because the microbe was a good one to work with. He did not begin his work with the cure of syphilis in mind, for he did not then know that the *spirochaeta pallida* was the cause of syphilis. This was only established by Shaudinn in 1905.

With incredible tenacity Ehrlich kept at the discouraging task of testing arsenic compounds against the mouse spirochetal infection. Finally, in 1909, the 606th compound tested, dioxy-diamido-arsenobenzol-dihydro-chloride, cured the mice. By now fully aware of the possible significance for the treatment of syphilis of any chemical that destroyed any kind of a spirochete, Ehrlich tested 606 upon syphilitic rabbits. They were cured! Human beings with advanced syphilis treated with the chemical also showed miraculous improvement.

Unfortunately, 606 proved to have certain disadvantages. Since it is a poison both to the *spirochaeta pallida* and its host, the patient, great care must be exercised in administering it. It has to be given in dilute solutions, in small doses at a time, into the veins of the patient, so that it is rapidly diluted by the patient's blood and as rapidly disseminated throughout the system. Formerly the doses had to be given at lengthy intervals of time, in order to allow the patient's system to recover from the poisonous effects of the drug.

Recently, however, a new so-called "massive dose" method of treating syphilis with neoarsphenamine has been worked out by Drs. H. T. Hyman and L. Chagrin of the New York City Department of Health. The drug is diluted with dextrose solution and run into the veins very slowly, along with considerable amounts of fluid. The intravenous treatment is kept up continuously over a period of four or five days, by the end of which time a large total dose of the neoarsphenamine has been administered. The results of this new method of treatment give promise of being better than those obtained with the old method.

By the end of the third decade of the present century, synthetic chemical remedies had been found for most of the protozoal diseases, as we have described above, but no chemical had been found that would destroy bacteria within the body. Bacteria are ordinarily classified as belonging to the vegetable kingdom, while the parasites of malaria, amebic dysentery, and syphilis are members of the single celled and primitive animal group called protozoa. Many chemicals had been found that would destroy bacteria in a test tube, but when injected into the body they proved useless. Research workers in general all over the world had given up the problem as insoluble.

But in the laboratories of the *I. G. Farbenindustrie,* the great German dye trust, the routine testing of the bactericidal power of new chemicals continued. The director of the trust's Institute for Experimental Pathology at Elberfeld was Dr. Gerhard Domagk. He was born in Lagow, Germany, in 1895, and trained as a pathologist. After teaching in Griefswald and Münster Universities he took charge of the dye firm's laboratory in 1927. When he made his great discovery he had been working for some years with the azo dyes. He had been led to concentrate his attention on them because they had proved so valuable in the treatment of various protozoal diseases. He was in a way continuing the hunt for the magic bullet that Ehrlich had begun in a previous generation. At the great chemical laboratories of the *I. G. Farbenindustrie* there were elaborate facilities for working with azo dyes, for these are among the best known for dying cloth in fast colors. The corporation employed a large staff of chemists who were continually trying to find new and better ones.

Domagk used as a test object for his dyes a strain of hemolytic streptococci which, when inoculated intraperitoneally in mice, always proved fatal. This was a method of testing the efficacy of chemotherapeutic agents generally used in research laboratories.

It is interesting to interpolate that in 1915 two American investigators, Michael Heidelberger and Walter A. Jacobs, at the Rockefeller Institute, had studied the bactericidal properties of a large series of azo dyes, including several sulfonamide compounds. Their method of testing them, however, was limited to observing the action of the dyes upon bacteria in the test tube. We know now that had they used animals as test objects as Domagk did, they would have anticipated his great discovery by many years.

The first hint that Domagk had hit upon something was a patent issued to his company, dated Christmas Day, 1932, for a compound given the trade name of Prontosil. This was a dark red dye, the hydrochloride 4-sulfonamido-2,4-diamino-azobenzene, synthesized by Domagk's chemists, Fritz Mietzsch and Joseph Klarer. There was no public notice of this patent at the time it was granted; it was not published until January 2, 1935. Then there was a burst of publicity. In the last months of 1934 two German clinicians had reported favorable results with the compound in streptococcus infections in human beings, and in the *Deutsche medizinische Wochenschrift* for February 15, 1935, Domagk presented the astounding fact that Prontosil would cure streptococcus infected mice. Domagk's paper was accompanied by three clinical reports from as many different German clinics claiming that Prontosil cured a variety of streptococcal infections in human beings. Domagk's mouse experiment bore the date of December 20, 1932, and the clinicians wrote that they had been using the compound for two years. The *I. G. Farbenindustrie* had apparently withheld knowledge of the therapeutic value of Prontosil so that its chemists could have time to prepare and test a large number of chemically related compounds. This they did during 1933 and 1934, taking care to patent the compounds that seemed valuable.

But the German effort to control the discovery failed. It failed because of the keenness of French chemists who had heard rumors of what was going on across the Rhine and promptly went to work to find out for themselves which of the several components of the complex compound patented by Domagk was really responsible for its surprising power of killing streptococci. A group of able workers including M. and Mme. J. Tréfouël, F. Nitti, and D. Bovet in the laboratory of Ernest Forneau at the Pasteur

Institute in Paris soon discovered that azo-compounds which did not contain a sulfonamide group attached to one benzene nucleus were inactive, whereas para-amino-benzenesulfonamide, which lacked an azo-group, was just as effective as Prontosil, and unlike Prontosil, was effective in the test tube as well as in animals. Para-amino-benzenesulfonamide (sulfanilamide for short) was a comparatively simple white organic substance that had been known to chemists since 1908, and was not patentable. The French concluded that this substance was the miracle-working factor in Domagk's Prontosil, and subsequent events have proved them right.

This was a stroke of genius on the part of the French chemists. In a few months they solved the chemical riddle and identified the essential component of Domagk's new drug. They deserve an equal share with Domagk in the credit for the discovery of the value of the sulfonamides. After the French showed that simple and inexpensive sulfanilamide protected mice against streptococci just as well as Prontosil, the latter compound was soon forgotten and the German patents brought but little profit.

The third and final act in the drama took place in London in January, 1936. The value of the drug in protecting mice against streptococci had now been corroborated in several laboratories. But there was as yet no definite proof that it cured human beings. About a dozen reports had appeared from German clinics regarding its use in human infections. They were all favorable. But, as Dr. Leonard Colebrook, the distinguished English bacteriologist, said about these reports, "their evidential value must be regarded as small, since in most cases the recovery of the patients is unhesitatingly ascribed to the treatment, and too little allowance is made for the tendency to spontaneous cure of these infections. The bacteriological and clinical data supplied are nearly always very scanty. . . ." In a word, the German clinical reports were unscientific and unconvincing.

Fortunately Dr. Colebrook had at his disposal in London an organization in which the value of a method of therapy for streptococcal infections could be tested in a genuinely scientific way. This was the Isolation Block, or ward, of Queen Charlotte's, a large obstetrical hospital. To this Isolation Block were sent not only the cases of puerperal sepsis (childbirth fever) that developed in its own wards, but about one-half of all the cases of puerperal sepsis from other hospitals in Metropolitan London. This disease, the great hazard of child bearing, which still persists to some extent despite the most rigorous aseptic precautions, is usually due to the streptococcus. These patients therefore formed an ideal group in which to test the value of the new drug under carefully controlled conditions. Colebrook obtained a supply of Prontosil from the *I. G. Farbenindustrie* and began to give it to patients with proved streptococcus infections in January, 1936. By June he had treated a total of 38, and only three, or 8 per cent, had died. He then began to use sulfanilamide instead of Prontosil, and by December, 26 more patients had been treated without a single death. The death rate in the whole series of 64 cases was thus only 4.7 per cent, whereas during the preceding five years it had varied from 16.6 per cent to 31.6 per cent. Colebrook had proved for the first time that sulfanilamide cured an infectious disease in human beings. Of great significance was an associated demonstration by Colebrook and his associates, that the blood of normal or infected individuals receiving sulfonamide compounds by mouth rapidly became endowed with the capacity to kill large numbers of hemolytic streptococci. This provided a rational explanation of the successful clinical results.

It is worthwhile to pause for a moment in our story and define this accomplishment. The disease, puerperal sepsis, that Colebrook was dealing with was one of the most intractable known to man. No specific method had ever been found of influencing it once it developed. Yet here was an inexpensive and relatively simple chemical agent, which could be taken by mouth and which had little or no toxic effect, that cured it. Truly, this is the miracle come true that such pioneers as Koch and Ehrlich had dreamt of so long ago. Nothing like it has ever been achieved before in the struggle with infectious disease.

The next important step in the story of the sulfonamides also took place in England. Colebrook had established the value of sulfanilamide in combating streptococcal infection, but he discouraged attempts to treat other infections with it. Nevertheless, three of his collaborators, Buttle, Gray and Stephenson, tried it in cases of cerebrospinal meningitis, an inflammation of the lining membranes of the brain caused by the meningococcus, and found that this disease, too, subsided miraculously. This observation was quickly confirmed in the United States, where extensive studies with sulfanilamide had begun.

The next disease to be conquered by the magic bullet, sulfanilamide, was gonorrhea. No really effective method of treating this great social scourge was known, and its toll of women sterilized and made invalids by inflammation of the pelvic organs, of limbs crippled by arthritis, and of social distress, surpasses imagination. Sulfanilamide at once cured a considerable proportion of the cases.

A new phase in the story next developed. High hopes were raised that sulfanilamide would be of value in combating other infectious diseases caused by bacteria belonging to the streptococcus family, such as pneumonia. It was indeed found to have a slight effect upon pneumococci, but was not potent enough to be of clinical value. In many laboratories chemists were at work trying to combine sulfanilamide with other compounds in the hope of finding a substance that would be more effective. In this search the English chemists, A. J. Ewins and M. A. Phillips, were the first to succeed, in 1938. They recalled that back in 1914 two Russian chemists had claimed that pyridine was useful in infections, so they combined it with sulfanilamide to form the compound 2-sulfanilylaminopyridine—called sulfapyridine for short. It was tested against various organisms in experimental animals by L. E. H. Whitby, and found to have a far wider range of bacteriostatic action than simple sulfanilamide. It was effective against pneumococci as well as hemolytic streptococci. Administered to human beings ill with lobar pneumonia, sulfapyridine has reduced the mortality of the disease from about 25 per cent to 5 per cent. All the tediously produced and costly pneumonia antisera were superseded overnight. Not only lobar pneumonia itself but the other forms of infection due to pneumococci are favorably influenced by sulfapyridine, including pneumococcal meningitis and pneumococcal peritonitis. Empyema, a common complication of pneumonia in which pus collects between the lung and the chest wall, has almost disappeared since the discovery of this drug. Sulfapyridine, furthermore, was found to be more effective than sulfanilamide against the gonococcus. Whereas the latter cured from 40 to 50 per cent of the cases, sulfapyridine cures almost 70 per cent.

These miraculous accomplishments have naturally led to an intense study of the mode of action, the manner of excretion, and the chemical relationships of sulfonamide compounds in hospital and commercial laboratories. The greatest part of this work has been done in England and in America. These drugs are not without danger, and must be administered with care. Reliable methods have been worked out for measuring their concentration in the bloodstream. New sulfonamide compounds are being developed so rapidly that it is difficult to evaluate them.

In 1939 another important magic bullet called sulfathiazole (2-sulfanilylaminothiazole) was synthesized. This compound attacks all the bacteria that sulfanilamide and sulfapyridine kill, and others besides. Perhaps its most important advantage is its effect upon the deadly and ubiquitous staphlococcus. This is the organism that causes boils, carbuncles, abscesses in bones, and many other infections. Sulfathiazole does not cure them all but it is a powerful remedy in many cases.

In 1941 a new and even more promising sulfonamide compound appeared—sulfadiazene (2-sulfanilamidopyrimidine). It has been shown to be just as effective against bacteria as the other sulfonamides, and it is tolerated by the patient a great deal better than they are. It is absorbed more slowly, but this is not necessarily a disadvantage. Because of its lesser toxicity sulfadiazene is rapidly superseding the other sulfonamides.

Two new sulfonamide compounds have recently appeared that possess the special property of not being absorbed to any great extent from the gastro-intestinal tract. These are sulfaguanidine (2-sulfanilaminoguanidine) and sulfasuccidine (succinyl 2-sulfanilaminothiazole). Other sulfonamides, when taken by mouth, are absorbed and taken up into the blood stream, and they therefore have little or no effect upon the contents of the intestine. But enough sulfaguanidine and sulfasuccidine remain in the intestine and have a considerable effect upon the bacteria in the bowel contents. Both of these drugs are so new that their usefulness in infections of the gastro-intestinal tract, or as prophylactics when the bowel has to be opened surgically, is as yet unknown, but they may prove to be of great value.

As time has gone on evidence has accumulated that sulfanilamide itself, as well as its newer derivatives, is a valuable agent in combating a frequent cause of infection which was originally thought to be resistant to them—the colon bacillus. This organism is a normal inhabitant of the gastro-intestinal tract, and in association with other organisms is commonly the cause of peritonitis which may follow appendicitis or other disease within the abdomen. Ravdin, Rhoads and Lockwood, at the University of Pennsylvania, have been able to reduce the mortality from appendicitis and peritonitis strikingly by means of sulfanilamide. Sulfanilamide has also been found to be of value in infections of the urinary tract due to the colon bacillus.

The sulfonamides are being rapidly introduced into other phases of surgery with astonishing results. Traumatic wounds of the type that previously gave bad results are now treated by placing several grams of sulfonamide powder in them after the usual cleaning and debridement has been carried out. Serious infections appear to be much less frequent with this method. In burns, unfortunately so common in modern warfare, the sulfonamides give promise of being a very important means of controlling infection. It is the secondary infection that is responsible for a large part of the crippling contractures from burns, and if this can be kept down the eventual results of burns will be much improved. Indeed the saving of life and limb through the use of sulfonamides in war wounds surpasses the imagination. At Pearl Harbor the drug was used with much wisdom, and the fact that not a single patient with a gunshot wound of the abdomen who reached the operating table alive, and in whom the visceral wounds could be repaired, subsequently died, can be attributed largely to the sulfonamide that was used. There never has been such a record in military surgery before.

No one can foretell the further triumphs of the sulfonamide magic bullets. We can, however, sum up the infectious diseases that have been brought under control by them in the eight years that have elapsed since Domagk discovered Prontosil. They are:

Hemolytic streptococcal infections: bloodstream infections, puerperal sepsis, peritonitis, lymph node infections, acute tonsilitis, mastoid infections, erysipelas, and meningitis.
Meningococcal infections: cerebrospinal fever and bloodstream infections.
Gonococcal infections: male and female gonorrhoea, gonococcal arthritis, bloodstream infections, ophthalmia neonatorum, and vaginitis in children.
Pneumococcal infections: lobar pneumonia, peritonitis, meningitis, and mastoid infections.
Staphylococcal infections: osteomyelitis.
Colon bacillus infections: peritonitis and urinary tract infections.
Virus infections: trachoma and lymphogranuloma venereum.

One may ask why sulfonamides have succeeded where the stronger antiseptics had consistently failed to influence infections? Lockwood has pointed out that the explanation is to be found in the fact that the sulfonamides do not produce a *direct* destructive action on bacterial protoplasm which would necessarily be accompanied by a similar destructive action on the cells of the host.

Carbolic acid, for instance, will kill bacteria in large numbers but it is much too poisonous to the host to be used internally. The sulfonamides, on the other hand, attack bacteria through *blockade* of their food supply, and thus subtly induce a cessation of multiplication and a corresponding weakening of the bacteria so that they fall an easy prey to the defending cells of the host. Since this blockade does not interfere with the nutrition of the host's cells the action of the sulfonamides becomes a selective one on the parasite. It is an extraordinary fact that a saturated solution of sulfanilamide, approximately 1 to 60, is not injurious to body tissues, while a concentration of the drug as low as 1 to 1,000,000 will definitely retard bacterial growth.

One of the curious features of this story is the fact that since Domagk's original discovery of Prontosil nothing of real value has been contributed by German workers. All of the subsequent advances have been made elsewhere, at first in France, and later in England and America where new discoveries in chemotherapy are now being made in an ever increasing tempo. Has this German apathy been due to limitation of research by the Nazi regime? We know of course that Domagk, when awarded the Nobel Prize in 1939 for his discovery, was forced, or chose, to refuse it. Perhaps it was an ironic Malthusian adjustment which led the German scientist to his great discovery, a discovery which will no doubt save more lives than all the barbaric fury of his Nazi masters will destroy before they are checked.

TUBERCULOSIS

Among all the infectious diseases that we have described in the preceding chapters tuberculosis particularly merits special consideration. Throughout the history of mankind it has been one of the most ubiquitous and persistent scourges. The bones of the ancient Egyptians show that it was common among them, and modern surveys, by means of x-ray films, of the chests of supposedly well inhabitants of our great cities reveal a shocking prevalence of the disease. Yet it is a disease in which modern medicine has made great advances. We probably know enough today to eradicate tuberculosis if we had the will and the money to do it.[1]

We must go back to Laennec to begin the story, because his stethoscope made the diagnosis of tuberculosis possible. Laennec was a thin, tense, dynamic little Breton who came to Paris when he was twenty to complete his medical education. He had a keen mind and unbounded curiosity about disease. Following the example of his master, Corvisart, at the Hôpital de la Charité, he followed every patient that died to the autopsy room and he shortly became a master pathologist.

It was in 1816 that he got the idea for his stethoscope. He was examining a young woman with heart trouble. Her age and sex made him hesitate to apply his ear to her chest, as was the cus-

[1] The story of how all this has come about has been superbly told in a recent book by a leading American authority on the disease, Lawrason Brown, the late Director of the Trudeau Sanitarium. Much of what we have to say here has come from this book.

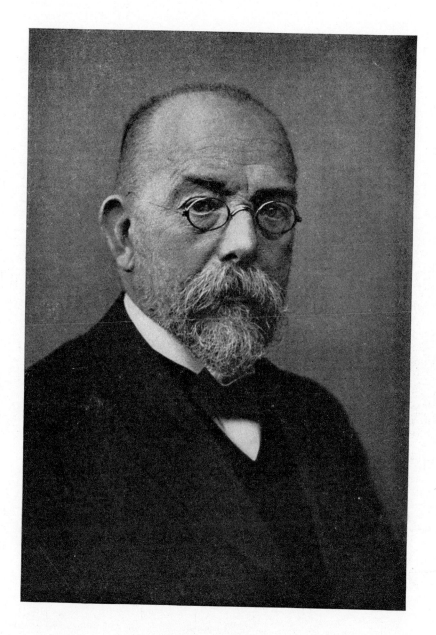

Robert Koch

His career in research began in 1872 when his wife gave him a birthday present of a microscope. He was then 28 years of age, doing general practice in a small town in Silesia. This was an agricultureal region where anthrax was common among sheep and cattle, and it was in the microscopical study of this disease in rabbits that Koch made his first great discovery.

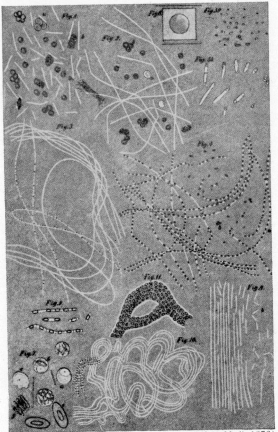

(From Koch's *Ätiologie der Milzbrandkrankheit,* 1876)

Koch's Illustration of Anthrax Bacilli

In his epoch-making work on anthrax Koch included a single illustrative plate, which we have reproduced. He isolated the anthrax bacilli from the spleens of guinea pigs infected with the disease. The rod-shaped organisms mingled with red blood cells are seen in the upper left corner of the plate. He cultured them on blood serum and watched them grow as long chains, which are seen in the middle of the plate. As the cultures grew older rounded spores formed in the ends of the bacilli. These are pictured in the upper right corner of the plate. This was the first description of spore formation.

tom of the day. He recalled the acoustic phenomenon in which the ear placed against one end of a beam of wood hears a pin scratch against the other end. He took a sheaf of paper, rolled it tightly, and placed one end against the patient's chest over the heart and placed his ear against the other. He was surprised to find that he heard the heart sounds more clearly than he had ever heard them before.

He attempted to improve his device by taking three paper copy books, rolling them up tightly, and gluing a cover of paper around them. These were not permanent, however, so Laennec, who had always been fond of wood-turning, himself made a copy of the device out of wood. It was simply a cylinder of light wood about twelve inches long and an inch and a half in diameter. At first the baton, as Laennec first called his instrument, was solid, but he soon found that he could hear better through it if he bored a hole some three-eighths of an inch in diameter through its length. Subsequently he found that if he widened the thoracic end of the instrument into a funnel shape, he heard râles and breath sounds more clearly.

Laennec was so impressed with the diagnostic possibilities of his instrument that he resolved to devote his life to studying them. He had at this time but ten short years of it left, for he was to die himself in 1826 of the disease to the knowledge of which he contributed so much. But in these ten years he accomplished a prodigious amount of work. He had a service of a hundred beds at the Necker Hospital, and he threw himself into the task of making careful observations of what he heard in his patients' chests, and correlating his interpretations with the autopsy findings. By 1819 he got out the first edition of his book on auscultation, but his health was so broken that he had to give up work and retire to Brittany. Two years later, somewhat restored, he returned to Paris and again plunged into clinical work. His strength was just sufficient to enable him to complete the second edition of his book. He had returned all the proof to the printer, and printing had begun, when he died in Brittany on August 13, 1826.

In this great work of Laennec, the fundamental features of a whole series of diseases of the lungs, never before clearly differentiated, are described. He differentiated between pulmonary tuberculosis, pulmonary abscess, gangrene of the lung, bronchiectasis, pulmonary emphysema, pulmonary infarction, and pneumothorax. He described râles, bronchial breathing, bronchophony, and a number of other auscultatory signs, upon which his diagnoses were based. As Lawrason Brown, the historian of the disease, says, Laennec found pulmonary tuberculosis a conglomeration of disease, pulmonary and general, and he left it a clear-cut entity.

Laennec had focussed his attention at the advanced and terminal stages of pulmonary tuberculosis. He was not interested in early tuberculosis—or to put it another way, he did not live long enough to have time to attack this phase of the problem. It was left to his successors and their pupils. A number of these, Frenchmen, Englishmen, and Americans, saw the necessity of detecting the disease in its early stages if cure was to be hoped for, and during the succeeding generations worked out the clinical picture of early pulmonary tuberculosis. In Paris in the early years of the 19th Century, there were unequalled opportunities for clinical research. All hospitals had been taken over by the government during the Revolution, and were now administered with great efficiency by a general board of governors. New patients were examined at the central office of the board and assigned to be cared for on the services of those attending physicians in the various hospitals who were specially interested in special diseases. Autopsies were almost always done. This system had enabled Laennec to study a great number of cases of chest disease in a relatively short time.

Among his successors who made important contributions under this system, Pierre-C.-A. Louis was outstanding. By painstaking recording of the early symptoms and physical signs in patients that he suspected of having pulmonary tuberculosis, Louis learned a good many of the important signs of the early stages of this disease. A persistent dry cough, shortness of breath, pain in the chest, loss of weight, if accompanied by hemoptysis, were strong indications of the presence of the disease. If percussion showed dullness below one of the clavicles and auscultation revealed feeble breath sounds accompanied by râles at one apex, Louis was convinced.

Louis was exceedingly popular with American students. Brown states that a total of 36 of them studied with him between 1830 and 1840. Included in this group were three brilliant young Bostonians, Oliver Wendell Holmes, James Jackson, Jr., and Henry I. Bowditch. These three young men had fateful fortunes. Holmes became a leading teacher of medicine, a distinguished essayist, and the father of the late Justice Holmes. James Jackson, who went to Paris in the spring of 1831, when he was just 21, became an expert stethoscopist. He wrote a series of letters describing the Paris medical scene which his father published, together with a series of case reports which the son had written, in a memoir of his son in 1835. The boy died suddenly in 1835 just as he was about to begin practice in Boston. These letters give the best picture available in English of this heroic age of Parisian medicine, and medical students would profit by reading them.

Henry Ingersoll Bowditch graduated in medicine from Harvard in 1832 and went to Paris to study with Louis. He, too, became interested in the diagnosis of chest diseases, and particularly in tuberculosis. Returning to Boston he became a distinguished clinician, and professor of medicine in Harvard Medical School. He was a man of strong character and took an active part in the attempts of his fellow Bostonians to circumvent the carrying out of the Fugitive Slave Law in the early 1850's. In 1846 he wrote a book, *The Young Stethoscopist, or the Students' Aid to Auscultation,* which had a strong influence on the practice of medicine and particularly on the diagnosis of pulmonary tuberculosis in the United States. Lawrason Brown states that it contains the best and most detailed description of early pulmonary tuberculosis that had appeared in America or any other country up to the

time—indeed, so good a description that it is better than those
contained in many modern text books. Bowditch emphasized one
diagnostic procedure which in the course of time has come to be
generally recognized as one of the most important methods of revealing early pulmonary tuberculosis, namely, making the patient
cough during the stethoscopic examination. This brings out râles
which may otherwise escape detection.

Bowditch's book brought the knowledge of the clinical diag
nosis of pulmonary tuberculosis to the point where it enabled the
general practitioner to diagnose the disease with some accuracy
The therapeutic attack against the disease could then, for the firs
time, begin to make progress. Certain it is that nothing could be
worse for the tuberculosis patient than the treatment in vogue
during the period we have been discussing. Laennec himself
when he was sick unto death, was bled. Blisters and liniment
were popular forms of local treatment. Emetics were used fo
hemoptysis. If he had money the patient was advised to take up
horse-back riding or go off for a long sea voyage. A change o
climate, in any case, was desirable: Madeira and Italy were popu
lar. Few patients with well marked signs of the disease recovered

It was not long after Laennec's death that the first step to
ward the modern treatment of tuberculosis was taken in England
Dr. George Bodington, a graduate of Oxford and St. Bartholo
mew's Hospital, London, passed his life as a general practitione
in Warwickshire. There he saw a great deal of tuberculosis. H
estimated that one-fifth of the annual deaths in England wer
caused by it, cure being scarcely ever heard of. Bodington becam
convinced that the prevailing method of treating consumptives b
shutting them up in a close room and excluding fresh air, an
plying them with antimony and digitalis, blisters, leeches, an
plasters, was not only useless but harmful. He advised his patient
"to live in and breathe freely the open air." He pointed out tha
those who lived in the open, farmers and shepherds, rarely go
tuberculosis, while those who lived in towns and were confined i
close rooms were often affected. He advocated the creation o

special sanitaria for tuberculous patients in the vicinity of large towns, and the training of specialists in tuberculosis.

Bodington presented these surprisingly modern ideas in an essay written in 1840. It was viciously attacked by an editorial in *The Lancet*. There was still a tax on windows in England, and fresh air was generally abhorred. Nevertheless, Bodington put his ideas into practice in a small way at Sutton-Coldfield, and reported some remarkable cures. But he failed so completely to convince his fellow practitioners that he turned his attention a few years later to the care of the insane. Yet Bodington deserves credit for discovering and emphasizing one of the fundamental features of the modern tuberculosis regime—the value of the out-of-door life. To be sure he failed to perceive that rest was also essential, for he followed the custom of his contemporaries in advising exercise by walking or riding.

The importance of rest in the treatment of tuberculosis was first put forward in Germany by Peter Dettweiler, a generation later. It is interesting that Dettweiler's contribution stemmed from the fresh air sanitarium idea which had, it so happened, been put into successful operation in Silesia by another German, Hermann Brehmer. Brehmer wrote his graduation thesis in 1853 on the subject, *The Laws Concerning the Beginning and Progress of Tuberculosis of the Lung.* He contended that the disease was curable when treated in separate institutions with an abundant diet, fresh air, hydrotherapy, and graded exercise. All this sounds much like Bodington, but we have no way of knowing whether Brehmer's ideas were arrived at independently or were copied after his English contemporary. Brehmer took over an unsuccessful hydrotherapeutic institute at Goerbersdorf, Silesia, and put his regime into active operation, wrote a book which went through several editions, and eventually put the idea of sanitarium treatment for tuberculosis across to the medical profession in Germany.

Dettweiler was himself a patient of Brehmer's at Goerbersdorf and subsequently became his assistant. During his own "cure" Dettweiler found that he was not strong enough to be up and about out-of-doors as much as he wished. He therefore adopted the expedient of resting in the open air in a hammock. When he founded his own sanitarium in Falkenstein in 1876 he made this idea of out-of-door rest an essential part of his plan of treatment. He had his patients spend many hours of the day in all seasons of the year resting in open air pavilions, whereas at Goerbersdorf they spent much time in their rooms, particularly in the winter. Dettweiler devised a special bamboo chaise-longue in which patients could sit well wrapped up and be comfortable out-of-doors even in cold weather. Dettweiler not only advocated rest: he emphasized the danger of exercise. Thus he discovered the foundation stone of our modern tuberculosis treatment. It should not be assumed that the value of the sanitarium rest cure was at once recognized. Quite the contrary. Its acceptance came only in the following generation, with the turn of the century.

In America the idea was carried out with striking success by one of the most heroic and beloved figures in modern medicine, Edward Livingston Trudeau. He was born in New York City in 1848 into a medical family of French extraction. In his youth he was greatly attracted by out-of-door sport, sculling on the Hudson and hunting in the Adirondacks. He acquired this interest from his father, who had accompanied Fremont on his expedition to the Rocky Mountains in 1841.

Edward Trudeau entered the College of Physicians and Surgeons in 1868 and graduated three years later. When his six months' internship was finished, he married, and after a summer spent in Europe, settled down to practice in New York. Just as he was getting well started he began to have attacks of unexplained fever, and on being examined by Dr. Edward G. Janeway, found that he had advanced pulmonary tuberculosis.

It is significant to note the treatment that Janeway, the leading expert on diseases of the chest in his day, advised Trudeau to follow: he was to go South, live out-of-doors and ride horseback. The winter spent in Aiken in this manner left Trudeau no better.

In desperation he thought of the Adirondacks. He had learned to love this great wilderness forest and its wild life on a previous hunting trip. In May, 1873, he said goodby to his wife and two babies and set out for Paul Smith's hunting camp, forty-two miles from the end of the railroad. And in the Adirondacks he lived for the rest of his long and useful life.

Soon after his arrival he lost his fever, began to eat and sleep well, and gained in weight and strength. At that time he knew nothing of the essential value of rest, but he unconsciously kept at rest much of the time, lying in his boat and fishing, or watching for foxes or deer in the forest runways. The following spring his wife and children came to the Adirondacks to be with him. Thereafter the Trudeaus lived in Saranac Lake in the winter and at Paul Smith's camp in the summer.

During his first few years in the Adirondacks Trudeau almost forgot that he was a physician. He was convinced that he could live but a short time, and he made no plans for the future. But as time went on and he got no worse, although he still continued to have periods of fever, he began to practice medicine a little among the natives and to care for a few consumptives who were sent to winter at Saranac Lake. In 1880 he began to read medical journals and to take an active interest in medicine again. It was in this way that in 1882 he came across an article describing Dettweiler's sanitarium and rest cure. He decided to try out this new method of treatment on some of his patients and conceived the idea of developing a sanitarium at Saranac Lake made up of a number of small cottages. It was to be a sanitarium for patients of limited means supported by voluntary contributions. He went to New York and raised $3,000. His friends, the Saranac Lake guides, bought and gave him the site which he coveted. In 1884 the main building was begun, and in February, 1885, the first cottage was completed. This was the beginning of one of America's most important medical institutions.

Meanwhile Trudeau had begun to work on the laboratory aspect of tuberculosis, which just at this time had come into prominence. In 1882 Koch announced his discovery of the tubercle bacillus as the cause of tuberculosis. This was a great step forward in the understanding of the disease, and of great practical value in the diagnosis, and in controlling the spread of tuberculosis. Trudeau's imagination was fired by the discovery. He went down to New York and learned how to stain the new bacilli from Dr. T. Mitchell Prudden, professor of pathology at the College of Physicians and Surgeons. Armed with the new method, he soon proved to some of his doubting medical colleagues that the demonstration of the little red rod-shaped bacilli in the sputum was conclusive proof of the presence of pulmonary tuberculosis.

This kind of work was important at the time, for although many pathologists had been convinced for some years of the infectious nature of tuberculosis, most practicing physicians were still doubtful about it. As far back as 1869, Jean-Antoine Villemin, a professor at the French army medical school at Val de Grace, had demonstrated conclusively in a series of careful experiments that tuberculosis is a specific infection transmissible by inoculation from animal to animal and from man to animal. He inferred that the tissue of the tubercles with which he inoculated his rabbits contained some foreign agent or virus which was responsible for the disease, but he could not identify this agent. The microscopical structure of the tubercle, the characteristic cell formation that developes in tuberculosis in all parts of the body, was first described in 1868 by Theodor Langhans, the Marburg pathologist. The central giant cells surrounded by zones of epithelioid cells and lymphocytes made the tubercle a relatively easily recognizable microscopical structure.

Villemin's claim was soon confirmed. Edwin Klebs, the brilliant itinerant German pathologist, transmitted human tuberculosis to animals by inoculating them with human sputum, among other materials. And the Neapolitan pathologist, Luciano Armanni, produced characteristic tubercles in the guinea-pig's eye by inoculating the cornea with a needle dipped in a suspension of tuberculous tissue in water. There could now no longer be any doubt about the infectious character of the disease, and many were ready for Koch's demonstration of the tubercle bacillus as the causative agent when it was announced. It required some time, however, for the adoption of the simple and obvious precautions against the transmission of tuberculosis. The careful disposal of the sputum of tuberculous patients in small containers that can be burned is of course fundamental. Trudeau made this a part of the sanitarium routine at Saranac. Public health regulations against spitting in any public place came later, but unfortunately these regulations are even today poorly enforced.

In 1890 Koch discovered tuberculin, a boiled glycerin extract from cultures of tubercle bacilli growing in artificial media. Tuberculin has the property of producing a specific reaction when injected into patients with tuberculosis. Koch, whose career had been a brilliant one up to this point, made the tragic mistake of concluding that tuberculin was a cure for tuberculosis. He began to treat patients on a large scale with it before he finally learned that it only made them worse. With desperate hope they rushed to Berlin from all over the world. Many lives were lost as a consequence. Indeed, Koch's tuberculin fiasco remains one of the best examples in modern medicine of how pernicious it is to raise the hopes of sufferers from a common disease like tuberculosis or cancer by unsound therapeutic claims. Modern newspaper publicity has done, and continues to do, a great deal of harm in this way.

Like others working with tuberculosis all over the world, Trudeau, in the early 1890's, attempted to verify Koch's claims for tuberculin by cautiously trying it out on some of his patients at Saranac. But he soon found that it was of no value therapeutically. The local reaction at the site of injection of tuberculin into the skin, however, has proved to be a helpful diagnostic test.

Although the Trudeau sanitarium served the poor and those of limited means, many famous people came to Saranac Lake to be under Dr. Trudeau's care. Among these Robert Louis Stevenson was probably the best known. He spent the winter of 1887–88 there, and wrote several essays and parts of *The Master of Ballantrae* there. When he left he inscribed a copy of *Dr. Jekyll and Mr. Hyde* to Trudeau with the following couplet:

> Trudeau was all winter at my side;
> I never spied the nose of Mr. Hyde.

Trudeau's sanitarium grew steadily in size, and its influence reached all parts of America. The fundamental value of the out-of-door rest cure was proven beyond all doubt. Physicians and nurses trained at Saranac staffed the new sanitaria that were springing up everywhere. At the present time there are over 600 sanitaria in this country, with a total of over 95,000 beds.

Trudeau lived to see the triumph of his ideas, and wrote the story in a moving autobiography which he completed just before his death in 1915. It is a book which every student of tuberculosis should read. He succumbed finally to his old enemy, tuberculosis, which during the last years of his life made him almost a complete invalid. Yet it is fair to say that Trudeau won the battle even when his life is considered from the purely physical point of view. He learned to adjust himself to the limitations which the disease imposed upon him, and nevertheless succeeded over a period of many years in doing a good deal of medical work himself; and he raised the $30,000 yearly deficit of the sanitarium entirely by his personal efforts, going down to New York for a couple of weeks in the spring and fall of each year to solicit for it.

Two technical procedures developed during the present century have been of great value in the control of tuberculosis. The first of these is roentgen-ray examination of the chest. Dr. Francis H. Williams of Boston, whose story we recount elsewhere, was one of the first to realize the possibilities of the new rays in the diagnosis of tuberculosis. He began studying the lungs fluoroscopically in 1896, and in May, 1897, was able to report the results of this kind of examination in 400 patients. He claimed that by means of the x-ray it was possible in some cases to diagnose pulmonary tuberculosis which was otherwise not detectable. Most of the clinicians remained unconvinced, but in 1898, Dr. Edward R. Baldwin, Trudeau's assistant at Saranac Lake, went to Boston to observe Williams' work, and introduced x-ray examination at the Trudeau sanitarium on his return. The Trudeau sanitarium was one of the first to examine all patients with x-rays.

Slowly the technique of this new method of examination and the interpretation of the findings improved. By 1910 a number of the leading roentgenologists had found x-ray films superior to the fluoroscopic method of examination. By 1916 a group of them suggested that the x-ray findings might well be used as a basis for the classification of the extent and type of pulmonary tuberculosis, because they are the most accurate guide to the condition of the lungs. In 1924 the National Tuberculosis Association actually adopted a classification of this kind.

Today it is generally agreed that the x-ray is a better means of diagnosis of pulmonary tuberculosis, and provides more information regarding its course and prognosis, than any of the older methods of examination. The method is inexpensive enough so that x-ray films could be taken of all the members of a community. This has recently been done on a small scale in certain sections of Detroit and Chicago. In this way the hidden carriers of active tuberculosis who are responsible for its continued spread can be detected and rendered harmless, and the public welfare enormously benefited. Unhappily, most public authorities have not as yet found the money with which to undertake so worthy a project, and they probably never will until the public itself becomes aware of the advantages that it would gain from it and forces its adoption.

The second event of great importance in the control of tuberculosis since the turn of the century was the introduction of pneumothorax. In this procedure air is injected into the chest cavity, compressing and collapsing the lung, stopping its expansion, and providing the rest which favors healing in all body tissues. In 1819 a Scot, James Carson, who practised in Liverpool, reported a series of experiments on rabbits before the Royal Society, in which he demonstrated that one lung could be collapsed with safety, and suggested pneumothorax for tuberculosis. His understanding of the basic principles involved was astonishingly clear, viewed from our modern perspective. Carson actually tried out this method on two patients but it was not successful. During the next generation a few isolated attempts at pneumothorax for tuberculosis were made in the British Isles, Germany and America, but without any convincing success.

Then about 1880 a number of careful students of pulmonary tuberculosis called attention to the fact that patients in whom pneumothorax developed spontaneously were sometimes strikingly benefited. Effusion into the pleural cavity on occasion has a similar favorable influence. Carlo Forlanini, an internist in Milan, wrote a provocative paper on the question in 1882, in which he suggested the use of pneumothorax. He waited ten years more, however, before he dared attempt it. He then found that the pleural cavity tolerated this kind of treatment very well, and that many patients were helped. He used nitrogen, injecting it slowly in small quantities each day until the absorption capacity of the pleura lessened. The treatment then needed to be repeated only at long intervals.

Forlanini's method of treatment was at first ridiculed, but he persisted with it and finally in 1906 published in the *Deutsche medizinische Wochenschrift* his results during fourteen years of work. The method was then quickly recognized as having merit and tuberculosis specialists all over the world began to use it.

In the United States, in the meantime, the dynamic Chicago surgeon, John Benjamin Murphy, quite independently got the same idea that Forlanini had had. There had been tuberculosis in his own family and he was deeply interested in the disease. To put the lung at rest he began, in 1895, to produce artificial pneumothorax with a single injection of a large quantity (700–3,000 cc.) of air into the pleural cavity. By 1902 over 400 patients had been treated in America by Murphy's method.

As time went on, however, the superiority of Forlanini's technique of multiple small injections of air became apparent, and when pneumothorax treatment was widely adopted in America during the succeeding decade it was Forlanini's method that was used. In a certain proportion of cases in which pneumothorax is attempted, the lung is prevented from collapsing by bands and sheath-shaped adhesions to the chest wall. In 1910, Hans Christian Jacobaeus, an internist at the University of Stockholm, worked out a method of cutting these adhesions, employing an instrument similar to a cystoscope inserted through the chest wall. The instrument, called the thoroscope, has since been improved, and the technique of its use developed to the point where it is a valuable aid to the tuberculosis expert.

During the last hundred years, while our knowledge of tuberculosis has steadily grown, a remarkable change has taken place in the incidence and character of the disease, a change so startling that we can scarcely ascribe it to improved therapy alone. Tuberculosis reached its peak incidence at the beginning of the industrial revolution. The concentration of the population in cities, the poverty, confined work, and poor hygiene, all favored it. In England in 1780 the recorded mortality rate for "consumption" was 1,120 per 100,000 population. To realize the magnitude of this figure we need only point out that in 1930 the total mortality for all disease was only 1,140 per 100,000 in England.

In American cities tuberculosis was similarly prevalent during the early part of the last century. In the decade 1820–1830, for instance, the proportion of tuberculosis deaths to the total mortality was 1:5.2 in New York City. It was overwhelmingly the most frequent cause of death. By 1900 a great reduction in its frequency had occurred. In the United States registration area in 1900 the mortality for all forms of tuberculosis was 201.9 per 100,-000. The proportion of tuberculosis deaths to the total mortality was 1:20.8. At this date the modern sanitarium facilities for the disease were just being organized, and we can not, therefore, credit them with this decrease in the incidence of the disease.

During the present century this downward trend in the mortality from tuberculosis has continued. In 1937 the mortality from all forms of the disease in the United States was only 53.6 per 100,000. This gave tuberculosis sixth place in rank as a cause of death. During this period, of course, our modern methods of treatment played an important part in curbing the disease. But there are several facts which indicate that the main reasons for the decrease have been better living conditions on the one hand, and a gradual development of a natural immunity by the white race on the other hand. History has repeatedly shown that when tuberculosis is newly introduced into an isolated population its ravages are frightful. Thus tuberculosis decimated the Polynesian peoples, the African Negroes, and our own American Indians, after the white man brought it to them. The nomad Indians of the Canadian northwest were the last to face this scourge. Crowded together in reservations, they were an easy prey. In 1882 the mortality from tuberculosis reached a peak of 9,000 per 100,000 among them.

Another fact indicating the development of a relative immunity to tuberculosis is the change in the character of the disease that has occurred during the last century. Acute generalized tuberculosis, which was common a hundred years ago in Europeans, is today rarely seen in this stock. Tuberculosis of the lymph nodes of the neck, known as scrofula, was in olden times exceedingly common, being a manifestation of the generalized disease. It was known as the King's Evil, and the royal touch was supposed to cure it. To illustrate its prevalence, Charles II is said to have "touched" 92,000 persons with scrofula between 1662 and 1682, in a time when transportation was rudimentary and patients must have had a difficult time to reach the king. Esmond R. Long has estimated that today non-pulmonary tuberculosis, including scrofula, constitutes less than one-twentieth of all cases of tuberculosis. The disease tends more and more, as its incidence decreases, to be chronic in character and to affect the lungs exclusively.

These facts should not, of course, cause us to lessen our ef-

forts to wipe out tuberculosis. On the contrary, they should en-
courage our anti-tuberculosis campaign, because today we can
begin to visualize the possibility of actually stamping out the
disease. This means the detection, chiefly by means of x-ray examination, of all of the tuberculous in the whole population, their
proper care in sanitaria or under home supervision, and the eradi-
cation of the bad hygienic conditions which favor the disease in
our crowded cities.

THE VITAMINS

No SCIENTIFIC subject has caught the public fancy today as the vitamins have. Drugstore windows are filled with vitamin preparations which the public buys and swallows in ever increasing quantities, quite without any real knowledge of whether or not they are needed, or of the possible harm that may come from overdosage. Our newspapers and magazines are filled with advertisements featuring vitamin-containing foods. All this has come about through the publicity given scientific experiments today. But our knowledge of the so-called vitamins is very recent and certainly incomplete. The word *vitamine* was coined in 1911 by the Polish physiologist, Casimir Funk, who wrongly believed at the time that the unknown substances necessary to life which he was naming were *amines,* that is nitrogen-containing compounds.

After the discoveries of the great 19th Century chemists and physiologists, it appeared that the knowledge of the necessary constituents of food was fairly complete. Yet it soon became evident that an adequate diet could not be built up from chemically pure substances. This striking fact was discovered in 1880 by a Russian chemist, Nikolaj Lunin. Working in the Department of Physiology at the University of Basel, he fed mice on a synthetic diet of casein, fat, and cane sugar and found that they did not survive beyond three weeks. He subsequently found that mice survived even after two and a half months when fed on milk powder alone, and he concluded that *milk contained besides the*

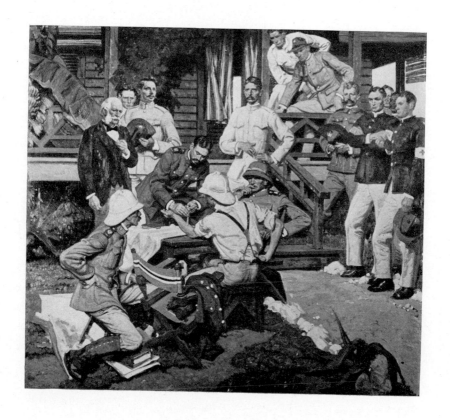

"The Conquerors of Yellow Fever"

Dean Cornwell's recent painting of the scene in which Dr. James Carroll (seated with his arm bared) was inoculated with yellow fever. Dr. Lazear is applying the mosquito in a test tube to the arm. Dr. Reed stands on the stairway with his hand on his hip. The white-haired man in civilian clothes at the left is Dr. Carlos Finlay, who had believed for many years that the mosquito was the carrier. The two privates with red cross arm bands at the right are Kissinger and Moran, who were the first volunteers for the inoculation experiment.

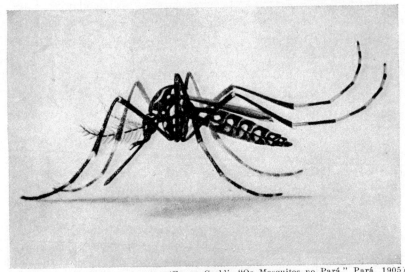

(From: Goeldi, "Os Mosquitos no Pará," Pará, 1905)

The Yellow Fever Mosquito

Aëdes aegypti. Female. Usual view when resting.

known elements, other unknown substances essential to life. This important conclusion, although reiterated in the textbook *Physiological and Pathological Chemistry* written by his chief at Basel, Gustav Bunge, received little attention at the time.

Ten years later another pupil of Bunge's, and also Bunge himself, repeated and confirmed the experiment. Similar and more exact feeding experiments were done during the next few years in several German, Italian, and English laboratories, utilizing rats, chickens, pigeons and other animals. They all confirmed the fact that synthetic diets lacked certain essential substances necessary for good nutrition.

This was the simple beginning of the experimental attack on the problem of the vitamins. The next step was to find which natural foods possessed these substances and which lacked them. It had been known of course for a long time that certain human diets were deficient. English seamen had known since the 17th Century that scurvy was due to a lack of fresh fruits and vegetables. But the task of identifying these missing substances chemically did not really begin until the first years of the 20th Century. A considerable part of these discoveries was made in the laboratories of the University of Wisconsin, in research inspired by that dean of American chemists, Stephen Moulton Babcock. With a sound training in American and German laboratories, Babcock came to the University of Wisconsin in 1888. Early in his career there he devised the famous Babcock test for the fat content of milk, which has been of greater benefit to the dairy industry than anything else science has done for it. In 1907 Babcock and his associates, the chemist E. B. Hart, and the professor of animal husbandry, G. C. Humphrey, showed by the simple experiment of feeding one group of cows exclusively on oats, another group on corn, a third group on wheat, and a fourth group on a mixture of oats, corn, and wheat, that corn contained an unknown factor which made it, alone among the three foods studied, adequate to sustain good nutrition in cows.

VITAMIN A

Vitamin A, the growth-promoting vitamin, was the first of the vitamins to be identified. Several investigators found it independently, but the outstanding work was that of Elmer Verner McCollum and his associates at the University of Wisconsin. McCollum had been brought there by Babcock and Hart to attack the riddle of the corn fed cows.

In 1912 the English chemist, Frederick Gardner Hopkins, had done the first experiment calling attention to a growth vitamin. He fed groups of rats upon a synthetic milk diet consisting of pure casein and certain carbohydrates and salts. At the same time other groups of rats were fed with exactly similar food with the addition of a minute ration of fresh milk. If the constituents were pure the rats who had no fresh milk failed to grow although they ate just as much as the others. Later their appetites failed, but the important part was that they ceased to grow before they ceased to eat. The synthetic milk diet was evidently wanting in some factor which is found in fresh milk and which is essential for growth.

In Wisconsin, McCollum turned his attention from cows to rats, and soon made an important discovery. He found that young rats, fed on a carefully prepared artificial diet, grew normally for about three months. They then ceased to grow although their general health remained good. In 1913 McCollum and his associates proved that the missing growth-promoting vitamin was contained in certain fats, particularly butter fat and egg-yolk. Almost simultaneously, McCollum's former teachers at Yale, the distinguished chemists, Thomas Burr Osborne and Lafayette Benedict Mendel, published a paper confirming McCollum's work. They found cod liver oil to be a rich source of the vitamin. Osborne and Mendel also made the important observation that an eye condition called xerophthalmia, in which the conjunctiva becomes dry, the glands of the eye atrophy, and the cornea degenerates, which developed in their rats fed on an artificial diet, was cured by feeding purified butter fat.

The discovery of Vitamin A has also thrown new light on an old clinical observation that a deficient diet results in loss of visual acuity in dim light, or so-called night blindness. Such night blindness has commonly developed among prisoners and among sailors on long voyages. It occurs with xerophthalmia. In the same year that Osborne and Mendel found that they could cure the sore eyes of their rats by feeding them butter fat, the Japanese investigator Kikutaro Ishiwara cured night-blindness in human beings by feeding them cod liver oil.

It was not until recently, however, that an explanation has been found for the development of night blindness in Vitamin-A-deficient states. Visual adaptation in dim light is a function of the visual purple of the retina. Visual purple is a pigment that forms in the retina when light is excluded from the eye. In 1935, the American biologist George Wald showed that in mammals, birds, amphibians, and certain marine fish, Vitamin A unites in the retina with a protein to form visual purple. This process goes on continuously and depends upon a sufficient supply of Vitamin A. If the diet is deficient in this vitamin, night blindness eventually results. Tests for night blindness carried out recently among school children in midwestern states suggest that about 25 per cent of rural children and about 50 per cent of city children have subnormal power of visual adaptation to darkness. Administration of Vitamin A brings recovery to normal in about six weeks. These studies, and clinical reports from many sources, suggest that night blindness due to Vitamin A deficiency may be somewhat more prevalent than has been suspected. It is possible that some automobile drivers have dangerously poor vision at night on this account.

The next step in the story of Vitamin A was the discovery that its chief source is the yellow-red plant pigment carotene. Harry

Steenbock at Wisconsin, in 1919, extracted Vitamin A in the form of a yellow pigment from alfalfa, sweet potatoes, yellow corn, carrots and other vegetables. His extract was a concentrated and potent one. But he was unable to explain how this yellow carotene was related to the colorless Vitamin A of liver oil. It was not until 1928 that Thomas Moore in the Nutritional Laboratory at Cambridge University solved the riddle by showing that carotene is converted in the body into Vitamin A. We now know that this transformation goes on in the liver. The chief sources of carotene in our diet are the green and yellow plants, fruits, seeds, and vegetables. A green color is an indicator of potential Vitamin A because carotene always accompanies chlorophyl, the green pigment of plants. The outer green leaves of iceberg lettuce, for instance, contain more carotene than the inner whiter leaves. Peas, beans, corn, squash, spinach, peppers, tomatoes, asparagus, sweet potatoes, pumpkin, carrots, apricots, yellow peaches, and bananas are rich sources.

Among the animal foods, liver, animal fats, eggs, whole milk and milk products are the most important sources of Vitamin A. The cow normally derives her Vitamin A from the carotene in the plants she eats, but she does not convert all of the carotene into Vitamin A, excreting some of both substances in her milk.

Cooks who worry about vitamins may take comfort in the fact that cooking does not destroy Vitamin A to any appreciable extent. It is fairly stable when heated and does not dissolve in water. Canned and frozen foods also retain it.

Important advances in the chemistry of Vitamin A have recently been made by the Swiss chemist, Paul Karrer and his associates at the University of Zurich. In 1930 and 1931 these investigators worked out the chemical structure of carotene and Vitamin A. They proved to be nitrogen-free hydrocarbons. The exact structure of Vitamin A being known, it was not long before its synthesis in the test tube was accomplished. The American chemists, Reynold C. Fuson and Robert E. Christ achieved it in 1936 at the University of Illinois.

VITAMIN B

The story of Vitamin B is bound up with that of the disease beri-beri, which has been prevalent for centuries among the eastern peoples who live largely on polished rice. Beri-beri is characterized by degenerative changes in the nervous system which cause pain, weakness and paralysis of the limbs, by edema, and by hypertrophy of the heart, which causes shortness of breath and other cardiac symptoms, and frequently ends in heart failure and death. This disease used to be common in the Japanese Navy, and it was a Japanese who, in 1882, proved that it was due to a dietary insufficiency. He changed the navy diet of rice to one in which meat, bread, fruit, and vegetables were included, and beri-beri disappeared.

A decade later a group of Dutch medical officers in the Dutch East Indies carried out studies of fundamental importance to our knowledge of Vitamin B. One of them, Christiaan Eijkman, discovered the cause of beri-beri through a curious circumstance. His stock of chicken feed for his laboratory chickens ran out and he had to feed them the table scraps from his hospital, where beri-beri was prevalent. The scraps consisted mostly of remnants of polished rice and the chickens got beri-beri! He found that the addition of the skin of the rice kernel, or even rice bran, to polished rice prevented the disease in chickens. A study of Javanese prison diets confirmed the discovery. It was found that beri-beri was vastly more frequent in those to whom polished rice was fed than in those who ate unpolished rice regularly. Eijkman's method of producing the disease experimentally was of great value to those who subsequently worked on the identification of Vitamin B in the laboratory. This anti-beri-beri vitamin became generally known among research workers as the antineuritic vitamin because of the degenerative changes in the nervous system caused by the lack of it. In 1916 McCollum distinguished it from the growth vitamin that he had discovered, on the basis of the difference in solubility between the two, calling the growth vitamin "fat soluble Vitamin A" and the antineuritic vitamin "water soluble Vitamin B."

Already, however, one of the most direct and original research workers of his time, Joseph Goldberger, was at work proving that another component of Vitamin B was responsible for the important disease, pellagra. In 1914 Goldberger was sent down south by the U. S. Public Health Service to study this chronic disease of the rural south which had been endemic there for a long time. Characterized by soreness of the mouth and tongue, a red rash on the backs of the hands, face, and neck, and ultimately by the development of signs of degeneration of the nervous system, pellagra has been known for hundreds of years to occur among the peoples who live largely on corn. During 1915 there were 10,663 fatal cases in the United States, of which 1,535 occurred in Mississippi alone. Although some keen observers had long attributed pellagra to an inadequate diet, the theory that it was infectious had recently become popular.

Goldberger looked into the homes of those who had pellagra and saw that it was a disease of the rural poor who lived almost exclusively on corn meal, white flour, and fat hog meat. He found it rampant in poor orphanages and insane asylums where the diet was also limited. His first experiment was done in two Mississippi orphanages in 1914. With government funds he arranged to provide two cups of milk and one egg each day, and meat four times a week, for these children. Under this regime pellagra soon disappeared in the two institutions where the year before there had been over 200 cases of it. Goldberger then persuaded the Governor of Mississippi to allow him to attempt to induce pellagra in a group of 12 convicts (all volunteers) at the state prison farm. He placed them on a strict corn meal, white flour, and white hog meat diet. Seven months later six of the eleven who completed the experiment showed signs of pellagra, and as a reward all eleven were freed. Paul de Kruif has told the story dramatically in his book, *Hunger Fighters*. It was some years later, in 1923 to be exact, that Goldberger hit upon yeast as a rich and inexpensive source of the anti-pellagra vitamin. He had been studying a pellagra-like disease in dogs, the so-called black tongue, when it occurred to him to attempt to prevent its development by adding ordinary brewers yeast to the dogs' diet. It worked in the dogs and has since proved highly effective in human beings.

From Goldberger's work, and from chemical studies carried on contemporaneously in several laboratories, it was now apparent that the water-soluble vitamin hitherto called Vitamin B was a complex substance containing a number of different components. How these components have been identified and subdivided again and again in the intervening years is best shown by Figure I.

The Vitamin B complex today includes the following main components: Vitamin B-1, anti-beri-beri or antineuritic vitamin; Vitamin B-2, also called Vitamin G or riboflavin; nicotinic acid, the pellagra-preventive factor; Vitamin B-6, pyridoxine; and pantothenic acid.

An American chemist, Robert R. Williams, director of the chemistry laboratory of the Bell Telephone Laboratories in New York, deserves most of the credit for our knowledge of the chemical nature of Vitamin B-1. He began his efforts to extract the vitamin from rice polishings while employed as a chemist in Manila in 1910. He worked at it intermittently in his spare time and at his own expense. When his work took him back to Washington and eventually to New York he intensified his vitamin studies. By 1933 his procedure was perfected to the point where he was able to prepare some twelve grams of the vitamin in pure crystalline form from two and one-half tons of rice polishings. With this amount of crystalline material to work with he was shortly able to determine the structural formula of the vitamin. In 1935 he succeeded in making the vitamin synthetically. He gave it the name *thiamine,* and it is now available commercially in quantity at a comparatively low price as thiamine hydrochloride.

Vitamin B-1 has been used with striking success in beri-beri and in the neuritis that develops in chronic alcoholism as the result of vitamin insufficiency. This vitamin occurs naturally in a wide variety of foods, but few of them contain much of it. In the ordinary well balanced diet we take small quantities of it from several foods. Vegetables, including potatoes, nuts and grains, eggs, meats, liver, and milk are the most important sources. Bread is more important than the others, because, on account of its cheapness, it is the largest single source of calories in the diet of western peoples. In the United States it has been estimated that bread provides about one-fourth of the total calories in the average diet. In wheat, Vitamin B-1 is found in the wheat germ. Unfortunately, modern milling processes ordinarily remove the wheat germ in making white flour. It is discarded and sold for cattle food as so-called bran or shorts. The practice has developed because flour in which the wheat germ is retained does not keep well. The result is that our ordinary bread does not contain the Vitamin B-1 which we need so much. The public over a period of years has been led to accept, and indeed prefer, the soft white bread, so much resembling cake, that contains almost no Vitamin B-1. Bread made with flour from the whole of the wheat kernel is coarser and is brown in color. It contains the full vitamin content of the wheat, however, which makes it much preferable to white bread as nourishment. An amusing incident occurred recently at a scientific meeting at which the advantages of whole wheat bread were being discussed. One speaker pointed out that the storage of whole wheat flour was difficult because it is attacked by weevils, while refined white flour escapes the pest. One of the authorities on deficiency diseases who is an enthusiastic advocate of whole wheat bread replied, "Of course—even the humble weevil has enough sense to prefer whole wheat flour."

Vitamins have so caught the public fancy that bread manufacturers have now begun to "reinforce" their white and brown breads by adding some thiamine and riboflavin to them. It is improbable, however, considering the incompleteness of our present knowledge of vitamins, that bread of this kind equals genuine whole wheat bread.

Vitamin B-1 is destroyed to some extent by cooking processes. Its greatest loss occurs in boiling, for it is soluble in water. Cooks should therefore boil their vegetables in as small an amount of water as possible, and save this liquid to serve in sauces or soups, for it contains valuable vitamins. The addition of soda, which many cooks use to keep their vegetables green when they boil them, more than doubles the amount of Vitamin B-1 destroyed. Freezing and canning do not destroy this vitamin to any extent.

The chemists had known for many years of the water-soluble yellow-green fluorescent pigment, lactoflavin, found in whey and widely distributed in plant and animal tissues, but they attached no special dietary significance to it. In 1933, simultaneously in several different laboratories, it was discovered that lactoflavin was identical with a new vitamin which had been discovered in 1926 by Goldberger and his associate, R. D. Lillie, and which had been called Vitamin B-2, or Vitamin G, by American biochemists in honor of its discoverer. Goldberger discovered this vitamin while working with rats in the course of his pellagra studies. The rats developed sore eyes and a dermatitis which caused their hair to fall out about the ears, neck, chest, and paws. This deficiency disease was not pellagra for it could be cured by Vitamin G, which, on the other hand, would not prevent human pellagra.

Following the isolation of this new vitamin (now called *riboflavin* instead of lactoflavin) from a variety of foods in 1933, the riddle of its chemical structure was attacked vigorously in several German laboratories. In 1935 Richard Kuhn and his associates at Heidelberg were able to announce the synthesis of riboflavin, and it shortly became available commercially.

It has since been shown that riboflavin deficiency in human beings is indicated by the occurrence of fissures at the corners of the mouth, erosions around the eyes, and itching and redness of the eyes themselves. This syndrome has been found most often in rural areas of the southern states where the diet consists chiefly of biscuits, corn bread, gravy and syrup. Small doses of riboflavin have cured the syndrome.

Riboflavin is widely distributed in plant and animal tissues, but it is less abundant in the plant seeds which form a large part of the human diet, than Vitamin B-1. In order to obtain a sufficient amount of it, the diet should include lean meat, milk, the green leaves of actively growing plants such as spinach or broccoli, or the particularly rich sources of Vitamin B-2, liver or brewers yeast.

Vitamin B-2 is not destroyed to any great extent by heat, or by the canning or freezing processes. It is, however, like Vitamin B-1, soluble in water and cooks should therefore take care not to dissolve it out and throw it away with the water in which they boil their vegetables or meats.

Nicotinic acid was identified and synthesized 75 years ago, but it was not until 1937 that C. A. Elvehjem and his associates at the University of Wisconsin discovered that this acid or its amide were marvelously effective in curing the pellagra-like disease of dogs, black tongue. In human pellagra nicotinic acid has been found to be equally effective. The red lesions of the skin and mucous membrane, the gastro-intestinal symptoms, and the mental changes characteristic of this disease promptly disappear, and the patients feel well and strong again. Already this miraculous remedy has been widely used in the pellagra-ridden rural south, and it promises to be a great help in controlling this disease. Like other components of the Vitamin B complex, nicotinic acid is found in greatest abundance in liver, yeast, lean meats.

In 1939 another component of the Vitamin B complex was isolated, its chemical structure determined, and its synthesis accomplished. The American chemists Stanton A. Harris and Harry Folkers completed this last stage of the study of this new vitamin, called Vitamin B-6 or *pyridoxine*.

Little is as yet known regarding its role in the human diet. It has, however, been found to be of value in the treatment of some cases of pellagra, and it seems to be helpful in relieving certain forms of muscular weakness and rigidity.

Recently, still another component of the Vitamin B complex has been identified. It has been called *pantothenic* acid (from the Greek root meaning universal) by its discoverer Roger J. Williams, because of its wide occurrence in living matter and its presumably fundamental importance in diet.

Williams began his studies of pantothenic acid while professor of chemistry at the University of Oregon, and completed them at the University of Texas where he now teaches. During 1939 and '40 he succeeded in determining the structure of the new vitamin and in preparing it synthetically. For this achievement he was awarded the Chandler Medal by the American Chemical Society in 1941. At the same time, his brother, Robert R. Williams, whose work with thiamine we have described above, was also given the Chandler medal.

As yet little is known of the role of pantothenic acid in the human diet, although it has been shown that the content of the vitamin in blood and urine from human beings with severe dietary deficiencies is abnormally low. Pantothenic acid will cure a special kind of dermatitis in chicks, which develops when it is lacking in their diet.

Roger J. Williams is now working with still another component of the Vitamin B complex. He calls it *folic acid* because of its abundance in the leaves of trees.

Several other substances, believed to be parts of the vitamin B complex, have also been identified recently.

VITAMIN C

The story of Vitamin C is the story of scurvy, "the plague of the sea and the spoyle of mariners." As soon as the 15th Century navigators began to make long voyages, their sailors, crowded together in damp quarters, and subsisting for months mainly on salt meat and mouldy bread, developed scurvy in appalling numbers. The great English sea hero of the 16th Century, Sir Richard Hawkins, estimated that it had killed 10,000 men during his twenty years at sea. An excellent description of the symptoms of scurvy is to be found in Hakluyt's account of Cartier's voyage to Newfoundland in 1535—"Some did lose all their strength, and could not stand on their feete, then did their legges swel, their sinnowes shrinke as black as any cole. Others also had all their skins spotted with spots of blood of a purple color; then did it ascend up to their ankels, thighes, shoulders, armes and necke; their mouth become stincking, their gummes so rotten that all flesh did fall off, even to the rootes of the teeth which did almost all fall out." In Anson's famous voyage around the world in 1740 he lost four-fifths of those aboard his ships from scurvy.

Scurvy has not, of course, occurred only among seamen. It has regularly followed in the wake of wars and famine. Joinville, the biographer of St. Louis, gave an exact account of its ravages among the crusaders as they besieged Egypt in 1249. Hirsch, the authority on the history of epidemic disease, tabulated 143 land epidemics of scurvy between 1566 and 1877. No war was omitted from his list.

It was not until 1753 that James Lind, a Scottish naval surgeon, proved by clinical experiment that orange and lemon juice were a miraculous cure for scurvy. He worked out a practical method of concentrating and preserving orange and lemon juice, as well as the juice of various vegetables and berries. But it was not until 1795, after a devastating outbreak of scurvy in the fleet, that a regulation issue to every seaman of one ounce of lemon juice daily was ordered. Scurvy at once disappeared. It is of historical interest to add that it is improbable that the blockade of France would have succeeded, and Napoleon's naval power crushed, if scurvy had not been controlled in the English fleet.

One of the important steps in the modern understanding of scurvy was the identification of the disease as it occurred in infants. In 1883, Thomas Barlow, a London pediatrician, described the clinical picture and the pathological changes characterizing the disease in infants. Once recognized, it was found to be relatively common in England and America where infants were bottle-fed. Further progress had to wait for the development of a method of studying scurvy in the laboratory. This was found in 1907 by the Norwegians, Axel Holst and Theodor Froelich, while studying deficiency diseases among sailors of the Norwegian Navy. They put guinea pigs on a diet of oats, hay, and water and produced in them a disease syndrome which was in almost every respect identical with the scurvy of human beings.

Although it was now easy to attack the problem of scurvy experimentally, attempts to isolate the scurvy vitamin chemically progressed very slowly because of the ease with which the vitamin is destroyed by oxidation. It became known as Vitamin C. In 1932 Charles Glen King of the University of Pittsburgh, after years of systematic effort to concentrate and identify this vitamin, succeeded in isolating it in pure crystalline form from lemon juice. He identified it as "hexuronic acid." The following year the Swiss chemist Tadeus Reichstein and his associates at the University of Zurich succeeded in synthesizing the vitamin, which has been given the name *cevitamic acid* by the American Medical Association.

A great deal of chemical study of the Vitamin C content of various foods, and of the metabolism of this vitamin, has been carried on in recent years. Much remains to be learned. The following table (quoted from Sherman's *Essentials of Nutrition*) shows clearly the high concentration of Vitamin C in citrus fruits, but the thrifty housewife will readily see from it that much less expensive sources are also available.

Vitamin C in the Edible Portion of Certain
Raw Foods—Milligrams per 100 Grams

Lemon 56
Orange 54
Grapefruit 39.3
Cabbage 35
Strawberries 34.4
Cantaloupe 29.2
Turnip 26.2
Tomato 22.7
Peas 22.4
Beans 15.4
Lettuce 13.5
Potatoes 12.6
Corn 9.4
Bananas 7.6
Apples 7
Carrots 4
Milk 2.1

Care must be used in cooking vegetables or a considerable portion of their Vitamin C may be destroyed by oxidation. Prolonged cooking, exposure to the air, and particularly cooking in water made alkaline by the addition of soda, all increase the percentage of the vitamin lost. About two-thirds of the Vitamin C content of some vegetables passes into the water in which they are boiled, so that it is desirable to use as little water as possible, and to serve this as a sauce or in soup.

VITAMIN D

The story of Vitamin D is the story of another long known deficiency disease, rickets. Rickets was accurately described by the great English clinician and anatomist, Francis Glisson, in 1650. The name comes from the old English verb, *wrickken*, to twist. And twisted indeed have been the bones of the little children of the poor in the slums of the great cities who have suffered from it. A disturbance of the deposition of calcium in the bones keeps them soft after the time that they should be hardened, and when the child begins to walk a twisted spine, deformities of the ribs and pelvic bones, knock-knees, and bow-legs result. As high as 50 to 80 per cent of the children of Vienna and London had rickets a generation ago, according to Osler. In 1917, in New York, Hess found that 90 per cent of the children in a Negro quarter had rickets.

The experimental attack on the disease, which has led to its conquest, was begun in 1918 by an English physician, Edward (later Sir Edward) Mellanby. It was long known to dog breeders that puppies under certain conditions developed rickets. Mellanby found that a diet consisting chiefly of white bread and skimmed milk would result regularly in characteristic rickets after six weeks. He proved that the disease could be prevented by the addition to the diet of a variety of substances rich in Vitamin A, particularly butter, cod liver oil, certain animal fats, meat and meat extracts, and by increase in the milk ration. Four years later McCollum carried the solution of the problem one step further by proving that the anti-rachitic vitamin was different from Vitamin A. He destroyed the Vitamin A in cod liver oil by bubbling oxygen through it while boiling it, and found that the oil still retained its power to prevent rickets in rats. From that time on the rickets vitamin has been called Vitamin D.

These experiments seemed to indicate that the cause of rickets was a lack of a sterol found in high concentration in fish oil. But another etiological factor that had been brought to light a generation earlier had to be integrated with this fish oil effect. It had been known for a long time that rickets was rare in the tropics and common in the north temperate zone. As long ago as 1822 a Polish physician, Jedrzij Śniadecki, had written that exposure of the body to sunlight would prevent and cure rickets. In 1890 an English medical missionary, Theobald T. Palm, who had practiced and traveled widely in eastern countries, published a classical paper on rickets in which he pointed out that the one factor common to all countries where rickets was unknown was an abundance of sunlight. He noted also the frequency of the disease in thickly populated districts, and its rarity in rural areas. He did his best to emphasize the value of "sunshine as a means of health." But his prophetic message was ignored. It was not until 1919 that a German pediatrician, Kurt Huldschinsky, proved by a clinical experiment that ultra-violet rays would cure rickets. Huldschinsky was working in a pediatric hospital outside of Berlin, after the last World War. He knew that cod liver oil prevented rickets but he had no way of obtaining it for his impoverished patients. Recalling that rickets was rare in children who got a lot of sun, and having available a quartz lamp that would produce ultra-violet rays equivalent to the sun's rays, he treated his rachitic children intensively with it, and saw to his amazement the rickets miraculously disappear.

Harry Steenbock at the University of Wisconsin, who had been studying the effects of vitamin-deficient diets on rats for some sixteen years, read of Huldschinsky's success and went to work with his rats to solve the riddle of how ultra-violet rays could accomplish the same thing that cod liver oil did. Steenbock is a man of extraordinary patience and ability to master detail, otherwise he would never have succeeded. But he did and the story is a fascinating one. He began giving ultra-violet light treatment to young rats fed a purified diet that did not contain enough butter fat to make them grow. The ultra-violet light treatments did make them grow for a while, but what attracted Steenbock's attention was the fact that when the rayed rats were put, after their treatment, into the same cage as their unrayed brother controls, these unrayed rats also began to grow. It was as if in some magic way the growth-stimulating power of the rays had been transferred from one rat to another. This gave Steenbock the idea of raying the rats' food instead of the rats themselves, and to his astonishment he found that ten minutes of exposure of the food under ultra-violet light was as effective in promoting growth as raying the rats themselves. He then repeated his experiment with rats made rachitic by being fed a Vitamin-D-deficient diet. Exposure

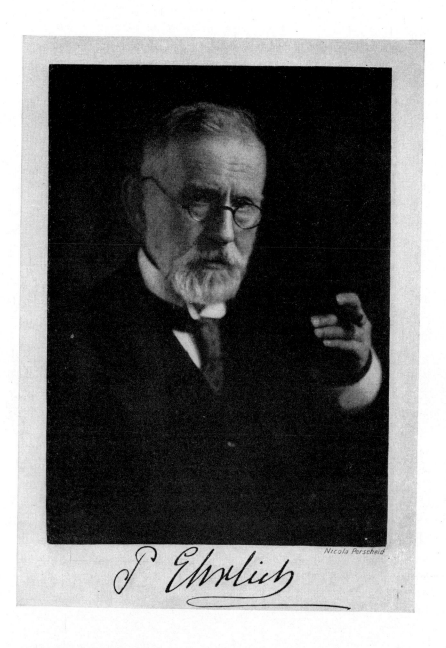

Nicola Perscheid

P Ehrlich

Ehrlich had a "one-track" mind which he applied with intense concentration during most of his waking hours to the chemical problems which were his chief interest. Strong cigars, which he smoked constantly, reading detective stories, and listening to his wife play light opera on the piano in the evening were his diversions. He claimed that he got his best ideas while pacing the floor and listening to his wife's playing.

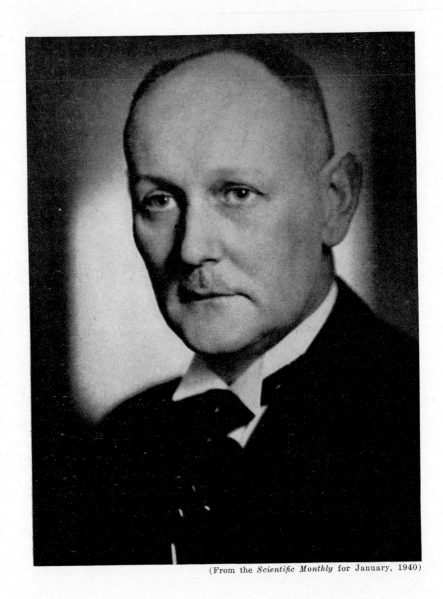

(From the *Scientific Monthly* for January, 1940)

Gerhard Domagk

of the food to ultra-violet light for a few minutes cured their rickets just as effectively as treating the rats themselves with ultra-violet light.

Steenbock found that a variety of foods could be given anti-rachitic powers in this way. Corn, oats, wheat, and milk, that normally had no anti-rachitic action, became, after radiation, as effective as cod liver oil. Steenbock now knew why the unrayed rats had caught, so to speak, the growth factor from their rayed cage-mates in his earlier experiment. The rayed rats had had enough food particles and refuse on their paws and other parts of their bodies while they were being rayed so that this minute amount of radiated material carried back to, and eaten by their unrayed cage-mates, supplied the lacking vitamin.

Steenbock's superiors at the University of Wisconsin were slow to realize the magnitude of his discovery and its commercial possibilities. Finally a group of Wisconsin alumni underwrote the patent rights and formed the Wisconsin Alumni Research Foundation. Steenbock turned over his rights to this corporation, asking nothing for himself. The foundation has since made large sums of money available for research at Wisconsin.

From this point onward the story of Vitamin D is a chemical one, concerned with the isolation, identification and synthesis of the various forms of this vitamin. For there are today no less than ten forms of Vitamin D known to the chemists. Only two of these are of practical importance, however. These are *activated ergosterol* and *activated 7-dehydrocholesterol*.

At first it was thought by Steenbock, and by others who had become interested in the problem, that it was the cholesterol in the food stuffs that was activated and converted into an anti-rachitic vitamin by the radiation. In 1926, however, it was proven simultaneously in three different laboratories that the activatable substance, or provitamin, as it is called, was not cholesterol but a persistent impurity. The next year it was announced by Adolf Windaus and his associates in the chemistry laboratory at the University of Göttingen, that this substance was ergosterol, the characteristic sterol of plants. Ergosterol has been known for over a century. It was so named after the ergot from which it was originally extracted. Yeast is a particularly rich source of it. Professor Windaus and his associates succeeded in isolating activated ergosterol in pure crystalline form. They shortly determined its chemical composition and eventually its structural formula. Vitamin D, made commercially by activating ergosterol with ultra-violet rays and dissolving it in oil, is called *viosterol* in America, or *calciferol* or Vitamin D in Germany.

The other important source of Vitamin D, activated 7-dehydrocholesterol, is derived from animal fats. It is the form of Vitamin D developed in the skin of living animals as the result of the action of the sun's rays. For several years after the identification of activated ergosterol in plants, it was thought that this sterol was also the one that was activated by ultra-violet rays in animal tissues. In 1934, however, an American chemist, James Waddell, proved that irradiated ergosterol was nowhere near as effective in curing the rickets of chicks as irradiated cholesterol. The following year Windaus and his associates identified this highly potent provitamin D of animal tissues as 7-dehydrocholesterol. In 1937 they actually isolated it in pure form from hog skin. Known as Vitamin D-3 it is the anti-rachitic vitamin found in cod liver oil, irradiated milk, and in irradiated animal products generally.

The natural dietary sources of Vitamin D are few. Most important are the fish liver oils, and to a lesser extent the flesh of oily fish such as salmon, sardines, herring. Halibut liver oil is richer in the vitamin than cod liver oil. The liver of beef, lamb and hog contain a varying amount of vitamin D. Eggs contain it. Finally, the so-called Vitamin D milk, that is milk which has been enriched in its Vitamin D content by the addition of a purified concentrate of the natural animal vitamin, is a common source. Vitamin D is not destroyed by the temperatures used in ordinary cooking, and since it is not soluble in water, it is one of the most stable vitamins from the cook's point of view.

There is clear evidence that in animals over-dosage with vitamin D causes excessive and harmful calcification in the kidneys, blood vessels, heart, lungs and muscles. The Germans, H. Kreitmair and T. Moll of Darmstadt in 1930 first showed these changes occurring in rats, mice, guinea pigs, rabbits, cats and dogs.

VITAMIN E

The discovery of Vitamin E, the so-called fertility vitamin, was made at the Institute of Experimental Biology at Berkeley, California, where for many years Herbert McLean Evans and his associates have been studying the fundamental aspects of the reproductive process. In 1921 they noted that rats fed on what was then thought to be an adequate diet, sometimes remained sterile. By trial and error they found that the addition of a small amount of wheat germ made the animals fertile. They concluded that wheat germ must contain a new fifth vitamin, which they called Vitamin E. Evans and his associates then went to work to isolate their new vitamin in a pure state from wheat germ oil. In 1936 they succeeded in obtaining three different crystalline derivatives. One of them, identified as *alpha-tocopherol*, a higher alcohol, possessed the power of stimulating reproduction characteristic of crude wheat germ oil. In 1938 the Swiss chemist, Karrer, succeeded in synthesizing alpha-tocopherol. Thus this latest addition to the vitamin family became available commercially in synthetic form some 17 years after its existence was first suspected.

Vitamin E occurs naturally in wheat germ oil, and in several other vegetable oils such as corn oil, olive oil, cottonseed oil, and palm oil. It is also found in green vegetables, particularly lettuce, and in meat, milk and butter. This vitamin does not dissolve in water and it resists high temperatures so that cooks need not worry about its destruction in the cooking process, but it is rapidly destroyed when food becomes rancid.

VITAMIN K

Vitamin K, the blood clotting vitamin, was discovered by the Danish biological chemist, Henrik Dam. While attempting to find out if chickens could synthesize cholesterol, he noted that they developed cutaneous and intramuscular hemorrhages. He was at the time feeding them on a synthetic diet of casein, starch, salt, marmite and cod liver oil. The blood of the chickens with the hemorrhagic tendency clotted much more slowly than normal blood. This was due to a lowering of the prothrombin content, the other constituents of the blood being normal.

Dam and his associates found during several years' work that the cause of this hemorrhage diathesis was a deficiency in a dietary factor occurring in hog liver, hemp seed, and certain seeds and vegetables. In 1935 Dam proposed the name Vitamin K, or the coagulative vitamin, for the new substance.

The next step in isolating the vitamin was made by Herman J. Almquist and E. L. R. Stokstad at the University of California College of Agriculture. In 1936 they prepared a highly concentrated extract of the vitamin from alfalfa, and the following year from fish meal and rice bran. In 1939 the structural formula of Vitamin K was worked out and its synthesis achieved independently in two different American laboratories by R. W. McKee and his associates at St. Louis University School of Medicine, and L. F. Fieser and his associates at Harvard University.

Vitamin K is present in a wide variety of food stuffs and it is not at all clear as yet what significance if any the vitamin has in the normal diet. It has acquired prominence from the fact that it is of crucial value in certain diseases in which there is a hemorrhagic tendency, particularly biliary disease. Ever since surgeons began to operate upon the biliary tract, the bleeding tendency which results from obstructive jaundice and certain other disorders of the liver has thwarted them. Countless patients have bled to death or have been denied a necessary gallbladder operation on this account. In 1935, a New York chemist, A. J. Quick,

and his associates presented data to show that patients with obstructive jaundice and the bleeding tendency had an abnormally
low level of prothrombin in their blood, just like Dam's chickens.
Quick therefore suggested that this deficiency in prothrombin in
human beings might be due to a lack of Vitamin K. Dr. E. D.
Warner and his associates at the State University of Iowa shortly
afterward treated jaundiced patients with the new vitamin and
showed that it corrected their hemorrhagic tendency. In the two
years that have since elapsed Vitamin K has taken its place as an
indispensable part of the surgeon's armamentarium. It has also
been found that this vitamin will cure a hemorrhagic diathesis
that occasionally affects newborn babies.

DOES OUR DIET CONTAIN ENOUGH VITAMINS?

Everyone asks himself, "Do I get enough vitamins in my diet?"
From what we have written of the history of vitamins it should be
clear that our knowledge regarding them is too recent and too
incomplete to permit any final answer to such a question. The
chemists are attacking the problem with such energy and skill
that it is certain that more vitamin fractions will be discovered.
The clinicians, on their part, have shown that grave deficiencies
of certain of the known vitamins exist in the impoverished regions
of the south, and among the poor of our great cities. Pediatricians
in general agree that it is wise to supplement the diet of infants
and children with Vitamins A and D, particularly during the winter months. A committee of the National Research Council studying the broad question of the prevalence of malnutrition has
recently concluded that "dietary inadequacies and malnutrition of
varying degrees are of frequent occurrence in the United States
and that the nutritional status of an appreciable part of the population can be distinctly improved." A recent study of the diets of
industrial workers carried out under the direction of the Council
has shown that even when good food was provided for the workers, the majority chose poorly balanced meals.

In Europe and Asia, in the countries ravished and stripped of foodstuffs by the German and Japanese armies, severe forms of malnutrition and vitamin deficiency have no doubt developed, and the next generation will bear the irreparable mark of these crimes.

Before the present war began, however, it is fair to say that the average man in the United States, and in certain of the more fortunate European countries, was better fed, both as to variety and quantity of foodstuffs, than ever before in history. Descriptions of the diet of the laborer in Great Britain a hundred years ago leave no doubt of the great improvement in diet that has occurred. Andrew Combe, the Scottish authority on diet, wrote in 1842 that many of the poor townspeople were living largely on potatoes and porridge. Their main standby was bread, with which they consumed large quantities of tea because it gave them a deceptive feeling of warmth. Very little meat was eaten, for it was much too expensive. Milk was also too expensive to buy, and what there was of it was unbelievably bad. The diet of the average man has improved not only because his economic condition is better, but because modern methods of preserving foodstuffs and the ease of transportation have made them available to all. It is interesting to speculate whether this improved diet has been responsible for the marked increase in man's physical stature that has occurred during the last half century. In 1927 Horace Gray found that American boys born of American-born parents had increased two inches in height during the preceding fifty years. The Harvard anthropologist, Gorton T. Bowles, has compared the measurements, made since 1880, of some sixteen hundred fathers of Harvard students, with those of their sons. The fathers had a mean height of 68.6 inches, while the sons averaged 70 inches in height. Similar studies at Wellesley, Vassar, Smith, and Mount Holyoke Colleges revealed that present day daughters were 1.1 inches taller than their mothers.

When we compare these figures with what we know about the height of man in earlier centuries it becomes apparent that this recent rapid increase in stature is something new. It is well known that medieval armor is too small for the average man today, and careful studies of the length of the thigh bones from early English graves lead F. G. Parsons to the conclusion that the midland English male of the 13th to the 15th Century averaged 65.75 inches in height. Our earliest American records of stature are those of a New Hampshire regiment of Revolutionary War soldiers. They averaged 67.9 inches. Harvard students from 1836 to 1855 were approximately this same height. Thus it can be said that between the 13th and the 19th Century the height of the average male of the stock from which Americans are chiefly descended increased only about two inches. Yet since 1880 the males of this same stock have increased about an inch and a half in height.

Records from a number of other countries show that this recent increase in stature is a world phenomenon. It has been particularly marked in the Scandinavian countries, and in Holland, but it has also been noted in Japan. It is interesting to speculate upon its cause. The decline in infectious disease, a higher standard of living in every sense, and particularly improvement in the abundance and quality of food are all probably concerned. But it would seem likely that better food has been more influential than other factors, and that some of the vitamins have played an important part.

We should like to know, of course, whether or no this increase in physical stature has been accompanied by an improvement in intellectual ability. This is a difficult question. Numerous observers agree, however, that the average height and weight of students in the higher scholastic ratings are greater than those of students in the lower ratings. Since students today are getting both younger and taller than they were a generation ago it can at least be said that they are changing in the right direction.

PERNICIOUS ANEMIA

PERNICIOUS ANEMIA is one of the most common diseases of the blood. The discovery that it too is a deficiency disease, due to a lack of a necessary blood-building substance elaborated in the stomach, is one of the most interesting of our generation.

In a wide variety of diseases ranging from typhoid fever to chronic nephritis, the number of red blood cells is diminished, causing a so-called *secondary or hypochromic* anemia. The red blood cells contain less hemoglobin than normal, thus the term hypochromic. This kind of anemia disappears when the cause is removed.

But there is a very different form of anemia called *pernicious* or *Addisonian* anemia. It occurs without any accompanying discernible primary cause, and it was in former times invariably fatal. Because the red blood cells in this kind of anemia are larger than normal and are well filled with hemoglobin it is classified as *macrocytic* anemia.

Pernicious anemia was first accurately described in a case report published in 1822 by the Edinburgh physician, James Scarth Combe. It was first clearly distinguished from other forms of anemia in 1849 by the great English clinician, Thomas Addison. For victims of pernicious anemia the road to death was long and hard, being often marked by curious remissions and heartbreaking recurrence of the symptoms.

This disease was conquered in 1926 by an American physician, George Richards Minot. His great achievement was linked with the conquest of diabetes, which was a landmark for the year 1922, for in 1921 Minot himself had discovered that he had diabetes. Despite the most careful dieting his tall thin figure seemed to those who sat in his classes to grow taller and thinner. He was evidently losing ground, and if insulin had not been found, Minot would certainly not have lived to discover the cure for pernicious anemia. He was one of the first to take insulin.

His diabetes controlled, he was able to return to work with renewed vigor at his specialty, diseases of the blood. For Minot's conquest of pernicious anemia was not the brilliant lightning stroke of an amateur; it was the carefully considered reasoning of a highly trained specialist who had spent his life studying diseases of the blood. Minot's inheritance in family and medical tradition, and his training, were the quintessence of all that Boston could give a man of his generation. He was born on December 2, 1885. His great-grandfather, James Jackson, was one of the founders of the Massachusetts General Hospital and a leading figure in early New England medicine. His great-uncle, Francis Minot, was an early physician to the hospital; his cousin, Charles Sedgwick Minot, was a famous anatomist; and his father, James Jackson Minot, was also a distinguished physician at the Massachusetts General.

Graduating in 1912 from the Harvard Medical School, George Richards Minot served his interneship at the "General." There in his father's wards he began at once to focus his attention upon patients with diseases of the blood, and particularly upon those with pernicious anemia. In 1915 he began a careful study of the diets of victims of pernicious anemia in an attempt to determine whether or not a dietary deficiency of some sort could be found. He discovered that many of them did in fact have peculiar habits of eating. Another fact suggesting a dietary deficiency to Minot was the similarity between certain of the symptoms of pernicious anemia and those of the known deficiency diseases, sprue, pellagra, and beri-beri. Soreness of the tongue, for instance, is common to all. Minot also knew that achlorhydria, that is, an absence of hydrochloric acid in the gastric juice, is a constant accompaniment of pernicious anemia, and he wondered whether this disorder of the digestive system had something to do with the disease.

In 1919, as a result of studies of bone marrow from pernicious anemia patients, carried out with the collaboration of Dr. James Homer Wright, the pathologist at the Massachusetts General, Minot arrived at a new concept of the fundamental nature of the blood disturbance in the disease. Dr. Wright was an authority on the structure of the blood cells, having devised the method of staining them for microscopical study that is still used in most American laboratories today. He taught Minot to see that the abnormal red blood cells that crowded the bone marrow in pernicious anemia were young immature cells. Thus Minot came to believe that something was needed to make these immature cells grow to normal cells. This concept fitted with the idea of a *deficiency* of something in the body that Minot's clinical observations had repeatedly suggested. It was radically different from the generally accepted concept of the disease, which taught that abnormal blood *destruction* was the primary factor.

In his search for the missing "something" that pernicious anemia patients lacked, Minot came across a number of references to the value of liver as a food. The great English expert on tropical disease, Patrick Manson, had shown in 1883 that liver feeding helped patients with sprue and pellagra. In 1922 George H. Whipple at the University of Rochester School of Medicine had done a series of feeding experiments on dogs made anemic by bleeding, in which he showed that liver was exceptionally valuable in restoring the blood to normal. Whipple's dogs had, of course, only secondary anemia, for it is impossible to produce pernicious anemia experimentally.

These were some of the facts which led Minot, in the fall of 1923, to begin asking a few of his patients to try eating liver regularly. It had been his custom for years to give his patients the most detailed instructions about diet. Now he suggested that in addition to the usual amounts of green vegetables, fruits, and red meat, they take 125 grams of liver every day. As the year 1924, and the spring of 1925 went by, Minot noted that these patients did better than he would have expected. In all there were ten of them who had taken liver with some regularity and they were all surprisingly well. Minot permitted himself no more than speculation, however.

He determined to put liver therapy to a real test and he asked Dr. William P. Murphy, a young internist on the staff of the Peter Bent Brigham Hospital to join him in this undertaking. Dr. Murphy, like Minot himself, was specially interested in diseases of the blood. He went to work wholeheartedly at the difficult task of getting patients to take large amounts of liver daily. The treatment had to be carried out on patients who were often critically ill, in the face of the frank skepticism of some of their colleagues, and the open criticism of some of the others. By May 1926 Minot and Murphy had treated 45 patients, and had proved beyond all doubt that liver would cure pernicious anemia. In many of the patients symptomatic improvement was obvious within a week. Soon they craved food, and color appeared in their faces. Within 60 days their red blood counts had risen to approximately normal levels. Some of the patients thus restored to health had been desperately ill, unconscious and unable to take any food, when the treatment was begun. It is of interest to add that when Murphy wrote a follow-up report of these original 45 patients ten years later, 31 were still living. Eleven had died, not from pernicious anemia but from some unrelated condition.

Minot and Murphy reported their discovery before the Association of American Physicians on May 4, 1926. It was soon confirmed in clinics in many parts of the world.

The next task Minot and Murphy attacked was the preparation of a concentrated extract of the blood-building substance in liver. In this they were aided by Dr. Edwin J. Cohn of the Department of Physiology of the Harvard Medical School. Although the exact chemical nature of the potent substance remained unknown, Cohn soon made an extract which could be taken by mouth, thus relieving patients of the necessity of eating large amounts of whole liver. Chemists in various parts of the world now attacked the problem and soon extracts were made that could be given intramuscularly. When administered in this way the extracts proved to be from 30 to 50 times as potent as when given by mouth. Today the patient with pernicious anemia can be treated entirely by these intramuscular injections. Once his anemia is controlled he need only have an injection of 1 cubic centimeter of the extract repeated once every few weeks. Under this kind of a regime he lives on in good health as far as his anemia is concerned.

Quite apart from this direct boon to victims of pernicious anemia, Minot's discovery has led to much new knowledge of the physiology of blood formation. Early in his liver feeding he found that within a few days after the administration of an adequate amount of liver substance the blood stream is flooded by young red blood cells (reticulocytes). This response came to be used as a test for effective therapy.

The blood-building material has since been found to exist not only in liver, but to a lesser extent in stomach tissue and in kidney, brain, and placenta. William B. Castle, working in Minot's clinic in 1928, carried out interesting experiments in which he demonstrated the peculiar role of the stomach in the causation of pernicious anemia. Withdrawing his own gastric juice after eating meat (not liver) he showed that this gastric juice contained the same active blood-building substance as liver. In the individual with pernicious anemia, therefore, there must be some sort of specific defect in the gastric secretion which prevents an essential reaction from taking place between the gastric juice and certain constituents of food. In the normal individual this reaction furnishes the supply of "liver extract" necessary to maintain normal blood formation.

Minot is one of the few surviving men who have made great original medical discoveries. As the leading authority on diseases of the blood, he continues an active and productive life in Boston, crowned with honors, including the Nobel Prize, and admired throughout the world.

DIABETES

Diabetes is another common disease which modern medicine has discovered how to control. It is the most frequent of the so-called diseases of metabolism.

The beginning of our modern understanding of this disease dates back to the opening year of the American Revolution, when Matthew Dobson, physician to the Liverpool Infirmary, discovered that the urine, which is passed in too great an abundance in this disease, contains sugar. This discovery led the way to attempts to control the disease by limiting the amount of sugar in the diet, a method which was not very successful.

And so the matter stood for another hundred years, until in 1889 the experimental attack on diabetes was begun by a Russian physician, Oskar Minkowski, then a young assistant to Professor Naunyn at the University of Strassburg. Minkowski removed the entire pancreas in a dog and discovered that severe diabetes at once developed which persisted until the animal succumbed a few weeks later. He also found the sugar content of the blood elevated.

The next step was made in 1900 by Eugene L. Opie, recently professor of pathology at Cornell Medical School, but at that time a young instructor in pathology at Johns Hopkins. Studying the microscopical sections of the pancreas of a little girl who had died of diabetes, Opie saw that the islands of Langerhans were so degenerated that they could not be identified. These islands of cells of a special kind had been first described in 1869 in a doctoral thesis by a young Berliner, Paul Langerhans, who later became a distinguished pathologist. No one suspected their function, however, until Opie noticed that they were damaged in those who had diabetes. His observation led the English physiologist, Sir Edward Schäfer, in 1916, to postulate the theory that these special pancreatic cells produced some form of internal secretion that controlled the metabolism of sugar.

During the first two decades of the century countless experiments were done in laboratories all over the world in an attempt to find a cure for diabetes, but without avail. Some of these experimenters had the most elaborate facilities and worked patiently for years. Many had tried to prepare an extract of the pancreas that would relieve the excessive excretion of sugar, but none had succeeded. In 1921 a young Canadian surgeon, without any special training in research or in diabetes, but with a real idea, discovered how to make an extract that worked, and in so doing achieved one of the greatest medical triumphs of all time. His name was Frederick Grant Banting.

Banting was born in Alliston, Ontario, on November 14, 1891. He entered the medical school of the University of Toronto in 1912, but felt his patriotic duty so strongly that he enlisted as a private in the army in 1915. He was ordered back to finish his medical training. Graduating in 1916 he at once joined the Canadian Army Medical Corps and was sent to France. He was wounded at Cambrai in September, 1918, and was awarded the Military Cross for gallantry on the field.

Returning to Canada in 1919, he served as resident surgeon at the Hospital for Sick Children in Toronto. In July, 1920, he settled down to practice in the city of London, Ontario. There practice was unbearably slow. In Banting's own words: "After observing the conventional office hours of 2 to 4 P.M. and 6 to 8 P.M. for 28 consecutive days, my first patient presented himself. At the end of the month I had four dollars on the books."

In the fall of that year, when the Western Ontario Medical School opened, he succeeded in obtaining an appointment as demonstrator in anatomy and physiology. While preparing a lecture on the relation of the pancreas to diabetes on the evening of the third of October, he came across an article in the November number of *Surgery, Gynecology and Obstetrics* which was to prove of fateful consequence to him. This was a report of a rare case of stone in the pancreatic duct by Moses Baron of the department of pathology of the University of Minnesota. Baron pointed out that the blockage of the pancreatic duct by the stone had caused atrophy of the pancreatic cells *excepting those of the islands of Langerhans.* Diabetes had not developed, death resulting from other causes. Baron had reproduced this syndrome experimentally in the dog, by tying off the pancreatic duct.

Banting was struck by the thought that here was a method of preparing an extract of the cells of Langerhans that might actually relieve the excess secretion of sugar. He relates how, obsessed by this idea, he got up at two in the morning and wrote three sentences in his note book: "Ligate pancreatic ducts of dogs. Wait 6 to 8 weeks for degeneration. Remove the residue and extract." He went forthwith to Toronto and talked about his idea with his friends, and with the professor of physiology in the medical school from which he had graduated, Dr. J. J. R. Macleod, whom he had not known before. Macleod was not encouraging. He asked Banting what he could hope to accomplish when the best trained physiologists had failed to prove that there was an internal secretion from the pancreas. But Banting was determined to try. He persuaded Macleod to give him a place to work, ten dogs, an assistant for two months, and facilities for doing blood and urine sugar estimations.

He was fortunate in securing as an assistant a second year medical student named Charles H. Best, who not only was a trained chemist able to make the tests for sugar in the blood and urine that were necessary for the experiment, but who quickly became an enthusiastic and determined collaborator.

Banting and Best operated on their first dog on May 16, 1921. Their first attempts to obtain atrophy of the pancreas failed because Banting's too tightly tied ligature around the pancreatic duct cut through it and permitted re-establishment of its continuity. Finally, however, on July 27th, they had available a dog with a well atrophied pancreas. Removing it and preparing a watery extract of it, they injected it into the blood stream of a dog whose pancreas had been removed and who was dying of diabetes, his blood loaded with sugar. Within two hours the dog's clinical condition was much improved. His blood sugar had fallen to one half its former level. The miracle had happened! They had prepared an extract of the islands of Langerhans that burned up the sugar accumulating in diabetic blood and relieved the disease at least for a while.

Spurred on by their success, Banting and Best now worked frantically improving their chemical methods of extracting, and searching for a better source of "isletin," as they named the extract. Finally, in November, 1921, Banting in his reading came across the fact that the pancreas in new-born infants is composed largely of Langerhans cells, and it occurred to him that he might be able to secure a potent extract from the pancreas of calf embryos. He tried it and succeeded. The next step, the discovery that a potent extract could be prepared from the pancreas of the adult cow if the extraction was made with alcohol rather than salt solution, followed from continued attempts to improve the method of extraction. The alcohol inactivated the pancreatic juice in the extract, checking its destructive action upon the internal secretion or hormone elaborated by the islands of Langerhans. Banting and Best now had an unlimited source of "isletin" and they were able to keep their diabetic dog patients alive by means of injections of it for a long time. By January, 1922, they had kept their Dog No. 33, a black and white collie whose photograph we show, alive for 70 days.

Banting's first human patient was his close friend, Joe Gilchrist, a Toronto physician, who had been a classmate in medical school. Gilchrist had developed diabetes a few years previously and was now steadily losing weight and strength despite the

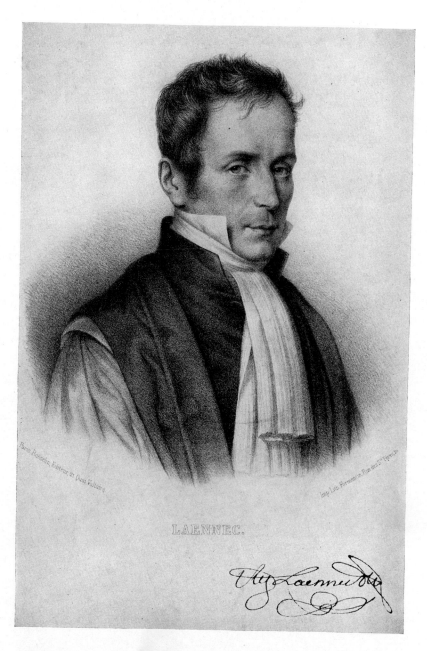

LAENNEC.

He began the study of medicine at Nantes at the age of fourteen years and seven months. From then on, until his death at the age of 45, he worked at it with an intensity and brilliance which we can scarcely comprehend. At the age of 25 he had made his mark in Paris as a teacher, written a treatise on pathology, and become the editor of a medical journal. His knowledge of disease was already enormous.

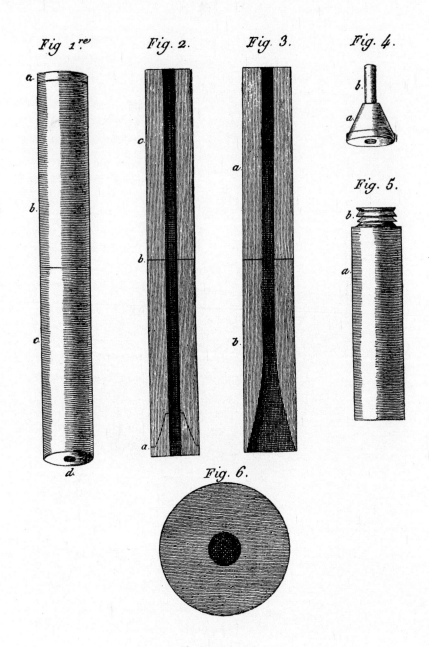

The Plate Showing the Stethoscope in Laennec's
De l'auscultation médiate

most careful dieting. He became the human rabbit at whose expense Drs. Banting and Best first learned the dangers of over- and under-dosage of their new hormone. Banting recounted that he believed no man ever had blood withdrawn from his veins as many times as Gilchrist. His courage was undaunted. What a joy to Banting when he saw that the hormone was really helping his friend!

But this was a particularly trying time for Banting. Now that he was on the brink of success, the whole project was threatened by a lack of funds. He had spent all the money he had saved and all that he had borrowed. He needed a much larger supply of the hormone for his therapeutic experiments but there seemed no way of getting it. Professor Macleod, who had been abroad while Banting and Best made their great discovery, was now taking a hand in the laboratory study of the new hormone, but he did not offer to help Banting with his difficulties. It was Macleod, by the way, who insisted that the new hormone be named "insulin" rather than "isletin" as Banting wished.

Fortunately, at this juncture another department of the University of Toronto, the Connaught Laboratories, came forward and provided Banting with the facilities and the help he needed. Best took up the problem of producing an adequate supply of insulin in the Connaught Laboratories. By the summer of 1922 he had succeeded in producing a sufficiently large and sufficiently purified supply so that the value of the hormone in the treatment of patients could be proved. Banting and Gilchrist worked out this proof at a clinic for diabetics which they established in connection with the Soldiers Civil Re-establishment at the Christie Street Hospital in Toronto. Despite many difficulties they succeeded in controlling the disease in all of their soldier patients, thus laying the foundation for the modern diabetic regime.

Although the ultimate cause of diabetes still escapes us, Banting's discovery has changed the prospect for the diabetic patient from that of starvation and eventual death to that of a comparatively normal life. It is a special boon to child diabetics. Before insulin they rarely survived to adult life. Today they have every prospect of living to old age.

The discovery, unlike some other medical discoveries of recent times, was quickly recognized and utilized in medical practice. It was January, 1922, when Banting controlled the diabetes of his famous Dog No. 33. By January, 1923, insulin was being successfully used in the treatment of human diabetes in a number of clinics in Canada and the United States.

With the true humanitarian spirit of modern medicine, neither Banting nor Best took any financial profit from their great discovery. They assigned their patent rights to a Committee of the University of Toronto. This committee acted merely to protect the public from exploitation by assigning the manufacturing rights only to dependable commercial firms. In the United States Eli Lilly & Company of Indianapolis was commissioned to prepare and standardize insulin. They provided large amounts to the medical profession without charge while the clinical methods of using the drug were being tested. Soon insulin was available at a small cost everywhere.

Banting was showered with honors from all over the world. In 1923 the Nobel Prize for Medicine was awarded jointly to him and Macleod. Banting resented the fact that his devoted collaborator Best was not included in the award, and he divided his prize with him. He was knighted in 1934. At the University of Toronto a Banting-Best Department of Medical Research was created in 1923 and Banting was installed as Director. He gathered about him a group of young men devoted to research, for he was always interested in and helped every young man who appealed to him for an opportunity to investigate medical problems.

In his new post Banting continued the laboratory research that he loved until the present war interrupted him. In 1939 he donned the King's uniform again and concentrated his attention on military medicine. On February 21, 1941, while he was flying to England on a mission for the Canadian government, his plane crashed in the wilds of Newfoundland and he was killed. Thus perished the man who, more than any other physician of his generation, brought relief to the sick. His life was a model that all medical students might well look to. He carried out in deeds the philosophy he once expressed in words: "The greatest joy in life is to accomplish. It is the getting, not the having. It is the giving, not the keeping."

DISEASES OF THE HEART
AND BLOOD VESSELS

As our control over infectious diseases has increased, and as our understanding of some of the diseases of metabolism has advanced, some of the other organic diseases, particularly those of the heart and kidneys, have come into greater prominence. Heart disease is today by far the most frequent cause of death in this part of the world, being responsible for one out of every six or seven deaths. At the turn of the century, tuberculosis outnumbered it in importance, but today the latter has fallen far behind. The relative importance of heart disease as compared with several of the other chief causes of death is well shown in the accompanying chart (from *Heart Disease*, by Paul D. White).

This increase in the mortality of heart disease has occurred to a large extent in old people, because today there are so many more old people to get heart disease, now that infant mortality and the mortality of the infectious diseases of childhood and youth have been so wonderfully reduced. After the age of 45 the incidence of heart disease rises sharply to reach a peak at 70.

We are apt to think offhand today that no important advances have been made in recent times regarding heart disease. To appreciate how false this attitude is let us look back at the predicament of a patient with heart failure a hundred years ago. His physician would have felt his pulse and listened to his heart with the newly popularized stethoscope, and might indeed have diagnosed accurately the presence of incompetency of the mitral valve. But he would have had no conception of the grave import of the irregularity in force and rhythm of his patient's pulse. *Auricular fibrillation* was not then recognized. For dropsy he would have prescribed diuretics and purgatives. He might or might not have prescribed small amounts of digitalis. If the drug was given at all it was because of its diuretic action, and not because of any special effect on the heart itself.

During the last half century three new and important technical aids in the study of cardiac function have been devised which give the modern physician a considerable advantage over his predecessors who had only the stethoscope. We may appropriately begin our historical review of heart disease by describing these new instruments.

The first to be developed was the blood pressure apparatus or *sphygmomanometer*. In older times physicians had of course appreciated the fact that the blood pressure varied in different individuals, and had attempted to measure these differences by feeling the pulse. They found this method not sufficiently accurate.

In 1876 the Parisian physiologist, Étienne Jules Marey, was the first to devise an instrument for measuring and recording blood pressure. He sealed the forearm in a glass vessel containing water and measured the pressure required to obliterate the pulse, the oscillations of which were recorded on the revolving drum of a kymograph. This method proved unsatisfactory.

The first instrument that really worked was devised by Samuel von Basch, a native of Prague, who accompanied the unfortunate Emperor Maximilian to Mexico and served as his personal physician until his execution in 1867. On his return to Vienna, von Basch published an interesting account of his experiences, and went to work at experimental pathology and physiology, in which he made many valuable contributions. In 1881 he devised a small instrument consisting of an outer glass bulb with an elastic membrane stretched across its mouth and an inner mercury manom-

eter, which, when placed over the radial artery at the wrist recorded the pressure required to obliterate the pulse. He gave it
the name, *sphygmomanometer*. Although awkward to manage, it
gave the first approximately accurate readings of arterial systolic
pressure.

Ten years later Scipione Riva-Rocci, a young assistant in
medicine at Turin, devised the modern blood pressure apparatus, in which a rubber cuff is placed around the arm above the
elbow and inflated with air, measuring the blood pressure within
the brachial artery in millimeters of mercury. This simple measurement has become an essential part of every physical examination. Patients probably pay too much attention to it, not realizing
that anxiety, like excitement, exercise, eating, smoking, and
fatigue, all tend to elevate the blood pressure somewhat.

The second of the important new methods of studying the
heart was roentgen ray examination. Francis H. Williams of Boston led the way in this development. Williams was both a physicist and a physician, having graduated from the Massachusetts
Institute of Technology in 1873 and from Harvard Medical
School in 1877. He was an attending physician at the Boston City
Hospital in 1895 when Röntgen's discovery startled the world,
and he plunged at once into the study of the application of the
new rays to medicine. He was aided in the physical aspects of this
work by his brother-in-law, William H. Rollins, in the Rogers
Laboratory at M.I.T. In 1896, with a Crookes tube placed beneath the patient's cot, he traced the outlines of the heart by
means of the fluoroscope in a series of patients at the Boston City
Hospital. Soon thereafter he used this method to diagnose thoracic aneurysms, pericardial effusion, cardiac hypertrophy, and
transposition of the heart. He made the sage prediction that
fluoroscopic examination would be "especially useful in diseases of
the heart and lungs." Time has indeed confirmed this early opinion, for fluoroscopic examination of the heart has today won a
place as perhaps the most useful of the various methods of
visualizing cardiac function.

Williams' work gained for him the post as the first roentgenologist to the Boston City Hospital. In 1901 he published *The Roentgen Rays in Medicine and Surgery*, a classic early treatise on the subject. It is of interest to add that unlike many pioneers in roentgenology, who sustained burns which eventually led to death from metastatic epithelioma, Williams suspected the potency of roentgen rays from the first and protected himself carefully. He lived to the ripe age of 84.

Soon after roentgen ray films of the chest began to be taken, clinicians found that various measurements of the contour of the heart and great vessels gave them considerable assistance. In this way a permanent record is obtained of the size of the various chambers of the heart involved in hypertrophy or dilatation, and of the changes in the heart valves and the great vessels.

In order to obtain an image of the heart corresponding more exactly to its true size, Alban Köhler of Wiesbaden in 1908 suggested taking films at a distance of two meters from the x-ray tube. At this distance the rays are almost parallel and the distortion of the image due to their divergent course is insignificant. Köhler called such films *teleroentgenograms*. The method has been widely adopted.

Another refinement of roentgen ray study of the heart is so-called *kymograph,* a method of recording on films the amplitude and character of the cardiac pulsation, which was popularized a decade ago by the Munich roentgenologist, Plicart Stumpf. This ingenious method uses a lead screen with narrow slits which moves across the film during the exposure, lasting through several cardiac cycles.

The *electrocardiograph* is the third and the most important instrument that has been devised to record cardiac function. As long ago as 1678 the great Dutch anatomist and physiologist, Jan Swammerdam, demonstrated to the Grand Duke of Tuscany that the muscle in a frog's leg contracted when stimulated with an electrical current. But it was not until 1856 that the Würzburg anatomists, Albert von Kolliker and his associate, Heinrich M.

Müller, showed that when the frog's heart contracted it produced a small electric current. This heart current of laboratory animals was extensively studied during succeeding years, always with the thorax opened and the heart exposed.

Augustus Désiré Waller in 1887 discovered that this heart current could be demonstrated *outside the body* in the human being by simply placing an electrode on the front of the chest and another in the back and connecting them to a capillary electrometer. Waller was the son of an eminent English physiologist. The son was trained in medicine at Aberdeen, Scotland, and in London, where he in turn chose physiology as a career.

The capillary electrometer was not a satisfactory instrument for recording this delicate heart current because the inertia of the mercury produced a lag in its response. Willem Einthoven, professor of physiology at Leyden, in 1903 solved this difficulty by adapting the galvanometer for this purpose. His instrument consisted of a very delicate silver-coated quartz fiber stretched across a narrow gap between the poles of a stationary electric magnet. The feeblest heart currents caused deflections which could be recorded graphically. This instrument was accurate and practical and was shortly introduced in hospitals. Einthoven himself made pioneer studies of cardiac physiology with it, and in 1924 was awarded the Nobel Prize for his work.

Today electrocardiography is an essential step in the examination of every patient suspected of having heart disease. Although the electrocardiogram may still remain normal when serious heart disease is present, it is often abnormal, and is then of considerable help to the examiner. Portable electrocardiographs have recently been devised which can be carried to the patient's home, making the method of examination available to all.

RHEUMATIC HEART DISEASE

In the damp cool climates of the north temperate zone, in the British Isles and in New England, rheumatic heart disease is by far the most frequent type of heart disease. Paul White estimates that 40 per cent of all heart disease in Boston is of this type. In tropical climates the disease is so rare that children who acquire it in northern climates have sometimes been sent there to avoid further hazard from it.

The syndrome of rheumatic heart disease as we today conceive of it is a complex one. It includes chronic as well as acute involvement of the heart by the rheumatic infection, usually beginning in childhood or youth. The infection manifests itself in a variety of forms, which include not only typical rheumatic fever, but tonsillitis, chorea, and scarlet fever.

The elementary fact that heart disease is related to rheumatic fever was first recognized by English clinicians towards the end of the 19th Century. Matthew Baillie, Scottish nephew and pupil of the great William Hunter, in 1812, in the second edition of his classic treatise, *The Morbid Anatomy of Some of the Most Important Parts of the Human Body*, wrote that "on some occasions the heart will become enlarged from rheumatism attacking it," and added in a footnote that, "Dr. Pitcairn has observed this in several cases, and is to be considered as the first person who made this important observation." David Pitcairn was a well known London practitioner and friend of Baillie's. *The Morbid Anatomy* was dedicated to him. The book became justly famous, for it was the first textbook devoted strictly to pathology, and the atlas which supplemented it contained beautiful copper engravings.

The relationship of tonsillitis to rheumatic fever was first emphasized by the keen French clinician, Armand Trousseau, in 1861 in his *Clinique Médicale de l'Hôtel Dieu*. Trousseau pointed out how this type of sore throat was apt to be associated with the stiff neck, joint pains, and lumbago of rheumatic origin.

Chorea, popularly called St. Vitus' or St. Guy's Dance, because the irregular, imperfectly coordinated, involuntary movements characterizing the disease recalled the ecstasies of pilgrims at the Shrine of St. Guy, is also related to rheumatic fever. This relationship was recognized and carefully studied by several French pediatricians about the middle of the 19th Century. In 1866, Henri L. Roger, chief at the Hôpital Sainte-Eugénie in Paris, asserted in an important paper on the subject that "the coincidence of chorea and rheumatism is so common a fact that it ought to be regarded as a pathological law, just as much as the coincidence of heart disease and rheumatism."

Subcutaneous nodules, developing most often over the elbows, the knees or the ankles, are another phenomenon of the rheumatic syndrome. These nodules were described in 1868 by Thomas Hillier in his book, *Diseases of Children*. He saw them in his patients at The Hospital for Sick Children, in Great Ormond Street, London. It was not until 1881, however, that Sir Thomas Barlow, a distinguished pediatrician at this same hospital in the succeeding generation, emphasized the great importance as a sign of rheumatic fever of these tiny nodules which so easily escaped detection.

It remained for another pediatrician at the Great Ormond Street Hospital, Walter B. Cheadle, to fit all these different clinical phenomena together into the syndrome of rheumatic fever as we know it today. Before Cheadle settled down in London to devote his life to the diseases of children, he had already won fame as an explorer. In 1862, after completing his undergraduate studies at Cambridge and obtaining his M.B. at St. George's in London, he accompanied Viscount Milton on his journey on foot across North America through the northern passes of the Rocky Mountains. On their return in 1864, they wrote an account of their journey that became one of the most popular travel books of the time, going through many editions. Back in London Cheadle devoted himself to pediatrics, becoming an attending physician at The Hospital for Sick Children in 1869. There he saw much rheumatic fever, and studied all its manifestations intently.

His interest in the disease was intensified by the fact that it struck one of his own sons. Years later he included the boy's case in a series of case reports as follows: "Series VII—F.M.C.—a boy of seven had acute articular rheumatism, with tonsillitis, in 1878. There was no endocarditis or pericarditis or other manifestation —arthritis and tonsillitis only; and for several years there was complete quiescence of rheumatic activity. Then in 1883, or five years after the arthritis, purpura rheumatica appeared; this was unaccompanied by any other phase. Then, about one year later, chorea and emotional attacks occurred. Finally, he had tonsillitis, recurring frequently and severely for four or five years."

In 1888 Cheadle was asked to give the Harveian Lectures and he used the opportunity to present his conception of the rheumatic syndrome. The lectures were published in book form the following year, with the title, *The Various Manifestations of the Rheumatic State as Exemplified in Childhood and Early Life.* This work marked a great step forward in the understanding of rheumatic fever. Cheadle was the first to grasp the fact that the arthritis, the subcutaneous nodules, the tonsillitis, the erythema, the chorea, the anemia, the pleurisy, and the pericarditis and endocarditis, occurring in varying sequence and severity in children, were all part of the same "rheumatic state." He recognized that in the great majority of cases permanent damage to the heart results. This occurs in the form of inflammatory changes in the heart valves which most commonly result in scarring of the mitral valve, preventing it from closing properly, or in the form of injury to the heart muscle with consequent hypertrophy and dilatation of the weakened organ. Cheadle also recognized that some cases of scarlet fever are associated with rheumatic fever.

Cheadle included in his book drawings of the microscopical appearance of the lesions in the heart valves and of the subcutaneous nodules. He pointed out that the proliferation of fibrous tissue and the infiltration of inflammatory cells produced a similar picture in both tissues, and he concluded that *"the materies morbi* of rheumatism, whatever its nature,*"* sets up changes of this kind in the fibrous tissues of the joints, the tendons, the pericardium, and the endocardium.

This broad concept of rheumatic fever has been confirmed by many careful students of the disease since Cheadle's time. The concept has a practical value in that it enables the alert pediatrician to diagnose rheumatic fever at a relatively early stage and to put the child to bed until signs of activity of the disease have disappeared. Cheadle urged the great importance of enforcing absolute bed rest for these children. He believed that this was the best means of minimizing the damage to the heart. Today this is still the most important part of the treatment.

Considerable progress has since been made, however, in the laboratory study of rheumatic fever. In Cheadle's time, and up until the turn of the century, pericarditis and endocarditis were the only well recognized forms of heart involvement. The former condition, in which effusion and fibrosis develop in the pericardium, is not very common in cases of rheumatic fever, but it is such a striking change that pathologists have long been familiar with it. The latter condition, in which tiny vegetations of thrombotic origin form along the edges of the heart valves, has been generally recognized since the Parisian internist, Jean-Baptiste Bouillard, published the first adequate description of it and named it "endocarditis" in his *Traité Clinique des Maladies du Coeur*, which appeared in 1835. Bouillard, as a young man, was a great admirer of Napoleon, and enlisted in a Hussar regiment when the Emperor returned from Elba. After Waterloo he took up his medical studies again. He was trained by the distinguished pathologist Jean-Nicolas Corvisart, who inspired in him a special interest in diseases of the heart. Bouillard became professor of medicine at Paris at the early age of 35 and published his great book on the heart only four years later.

It is only during the last generation that the damage done by rheumatic fever to the heart muscle itself has been brought to light. In 1904 the Marburg pathologist, Ludwig Aschoff, described in the heart muscle a special kind of inflammatory nodule which is characteristic of the rheumatic process. These nodules have come to be known as Aschoff bodies. Alvin F. Coburn of New

York, one of the keenest present day students of the rheumatic state, has recently shown (1932) that these nodules are not the earliest tissue change, but rather the late reaction following initial hemorrhage and necrosis. The heart, following this kind of injury, often dilates and eventually fails. Extensive bacteriological studies of the lesions of rheumatic fever have led such authorities as Coburn to the conviction that a hemolytic streptococcus is probably the bacterium chiefly responsible. But many of the bacteriological aspects of the problem remain unsolved.

HYPERTENSIVE HEART DISEASE

High blood pressure, and the changes in the heart consequent to it, form another frequent and important type of heart disease. Paul D. White estimates that hypertension is a primary or secondary factor in one third of all cases of heart disease in New England, and that in the United States about 100,000 people die annually as a result of it.

The clinical recognition of hypertensive heart disease was of course made possible by the introduction of the blood pressure machine into clinical medicine, and is therefore recent. While von Basch was taking the first approximately accurate readings of blood pressure in Vienna with the little machine that he devised in the early 1880's, Clifford Allbutt in England, and Henri Huchard in France were independently attacking the same problem. They adopted von Basch's and Riva-Rocci's new sphygmomanometers when they became available, and undertook to record and classify the new clinical observations they were able to make. They found at the beginning that there were individuals who had markedly elevated blood pressure, but showed no apparent arteriosclerosis or kidney damage, which generally accompany such a condition. The signs of kidney disease that were expected to develop in these patients sometimes failed to appear, and after keeping track of them for years it became apparent to all three of the investigators that they were dealing with a hitherto unknown disease, the primary feature of which was a markedly elevated blood pressure. Von Basch called it "latent arteriosclerosis," Huchard, "pre-sclerosis," and Allbutt, "hyperpiesia." Allbutt finally became convinced of the genuineness of the disease after watching a woman with high blood pressure for eighteen years, until she finally died of an apoplectic seizure with a large and dilated heart but no clinical evidence of kidney disease. He published his conclusions in 1895, two years after Huchard had presented rather similar opinions in his book on diseases of the heart and blood vessels. Allbutt's great work *Diseases of the Arteries,* which appeared in 1915, included much additional information. These writings drew the attention of medical men everywhere to the significance of high blood pressure. The primary form of the disease, without clinical or anatomical evidence of antecedent nephritis or urinary obstruction, has come to be known in the United States as *essential hypertension,* or *hypertensive heart disease.*

It is believed by some cardiologists that our modern high speed mode of life is responsible for the prevalence of this disease. They infer that the excessive nervous tension under which many of us live leads to a chronic state of constriction of the arterioles throughout the body. This results in increased resistance to the circulation of the blood, to which the heart responds by raising the blood pressure. We have of course no historical test of this indictment of modern living, for the blood pressure apparatus came into general use about the same time that the automobile did. We simply do not know what blood pressures were in the horse and buggy age when it was permissible to take two hours for lunch and when there were no radios and motion pictures to keep us up late at night.

Both Allbutt and Huchard attributed high blood pressure to excessive eating of meat and drinking of alcoholic liquor. Mention of gluttony recalls the tremendous quantities of food and drink consumed by the well-to-do in England and France during the 18th and 19th Centuries. J. C. Drummond and Anne Wilbraham in their recent interesting book, *The Englishman's Food,* recount some of this dietary history. An ordinary dinner given by Rev. James Woodforde on April 19, 1768, might be taken as an example of the daily fare of those days. It consisted of "A roasted Shoulder of Mutton and a plum Pudding—Veal Cutlets, Frill'd Potatoes, cold Tongue, Ham and cold roast Beef, and eggs in their shells. Punch, Wine, Beer and Cyder for drinking." Special dinners of those days were much more elaborate, and included fish and fowl in addition to the usual variety of meats. Dinner was often served in mid-afternoon, and the eating and drinking went on for hours. The gentleman of those days aspired to be known as a "four bottle man." He drank prodigious quantities of claret or burgundy with his dinner, and port or madeira with his dessert, often staying at table until he fell under it.

Today the well-to-do certainly consume a great deal less meat than they did in those days, yet high blood pressure is common among them. It is also frequent among the poor. Modern students of the problem have not indeed been able to find any convincing scientific proof that gluttony or a high meat diet causes essential hypertension. It may be that proverbs of folk-lore that have warned us against these things are quite wrong. Some of them are expressive, however, for example, "Much meat, many maladies," and "The glutton digs his own grave with his teeth."

A most interesting experiment regarding a meat diet was carried out by the Arctic explorer Vilhjalmur Stefansson. Stefansson lived for seven years in the Arctic with the Esquimos, following their mode of life and eating nothing but meat. During these years he was at the peak of health. Some years later in New York he volunteered to undergo a carefully controlled experiment at the Russell Sage Institute of Pathology at Bellevue Hospital. He lived exclusively on meat from February, 1928, to March, 1929. Intensive metabolic and laboratory studies before and at the end of the experiment showed no change in Mr. Stefansson's blood pressure, and no evidence of damage to his kidneys. It should be added that studies that have been made of blood pressure among the Esquimos show them to be remarkably free from hypertension, despite the fact that they live on meat alone and often gorge on it.

Although our clinical knowledge of hypertensive heart disease is recent, and certainly relatively incomplete, the pathological changes in the heart and blood vessels that accompany high blood pressure have been recognized for a long time. The massive enlargement of the heart and the thickening of its walls that develops is the natural response of muscle to increased work. In 1784, Matthew Baillie in his *Morbid Anatomy* wrote: "Sometimes the heart is enlarged to twice or thrice its natural size." Laennec, who gained fame by the discovery of the stethoscope, had a profound knowledge of the pathology of the heart as well as the lungs, and in his *De l'auscultation médiate* (1819) he included a clear description of the physical signs in "hypertropia" of the heart and of the gross appearance of the enlarged thickened heart itself.

As hypertension continues, complex changes occur in the blood vessels. The aorta dilates, and the arteries and arterioles throughout the whole body thicken. Arteriosclerosis often develops. In the aorta, in the coronary arteries to the heart, and in the arteries of the brain and other viscera, scarring and the deposition of lime salts occur, narrowing the lumen of the vessels. These changes in the great vessels were clearly described as long ago as 1761 by Giovanni Battista Morgagni, in the autopsy reports from Padua which he included in his famous work *De sedibus et causis morborum.*

Although these blood vessel changes were obvious enough after death there was no way of visualizing them in life until the London neurologist, William Richard Gowers, in 1876, discovered that the arteries in the retina of the eye, viewed with the ophthalmoscope, showed definite changes in patients with high blood pressure. The retinal arteries are seen to be much narrowed and there may be tiny hemorrhages into the retina. Today the internist has another method of detecting arteriosclerosis, especially

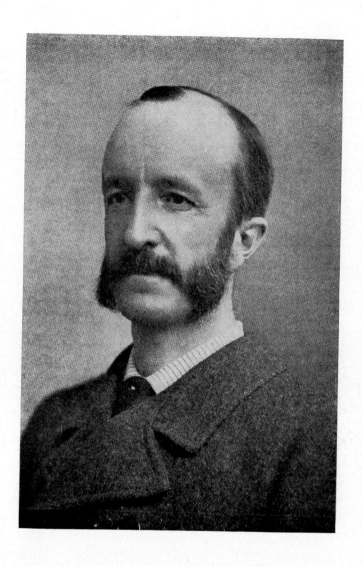

Edward Livingston Trudeau

He went to the Adirondacks to die but lived a long and useful life during which he founded the sanitarium that bears his name and developed our modern method of treating tuberculosis.

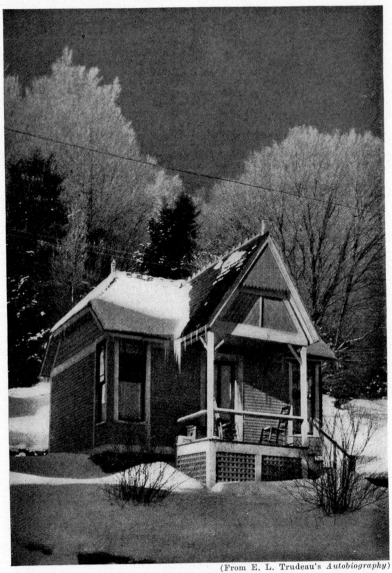

(From E. L. Trudeau's *Autobiography*)

"The Little Red"

The first cottage built at the Trudeau Sanitarium.

when it is advanced. The lime salts in the sclerotic vessels show in roentgen ray films.

Hypertension may lead to death either as a direct result of failure of the overburdened heart musculature, or indirectly from apoplexy when a sclerotic artery in the brain bursts, or when the coronary arteries which supply the heart itself become thrombosed, or when kidney function fails.

No specific cure has been found for these complications, but encouraging progress has recently been made in the experimental attack on the basic problem of hypertension. In 1910 it was proved by Ernst Rautenberg, in experiments done in the department of medicine at Königsberg, that blocking one of the ureters in rabbits produced hypertension. In the years that followed a great variety of experiments of this kind were done, mostly on dogs. It was not until 1937, however, that Tinsley R. Harrison and his associates at Vanderbilt University showed that hypertension produced by ligation of the ureter is due to a decreased blood flow through the kidney, and that the mechanism of this effect is a humoral rather than a nervous one, for it is not prevented by preliminary denervation of the kidney.

In the meantime, Harry Goldblatt, at Western Reserve University in Cleveland, had carried out a series of ingenious experiments on dogs and monkeys. By means of a special silver clamp which he applied to the renal arteries, occluding them and reducing the blood flow through them to any desired degree, he produced hypertension of maximum severity and prolonged duration. Moreover, the animals developed enlarged hearts and arteriosclerosis similar to the lesions occurring in human beings with hypertension. Here then was a perfect experimental means of reproducing the disease as it occurs in man.

Many investigators attacked the problem, using Goldblatt's technique, after its publication in 1934. Several of them found that removal of the normal kidney, in animals in which the vessels to the other kidney had been clamped, hastened and intensified the rise in blood pressure. This led them to infer that normal kidney tissue is concerned in some way in preventing the rise in blood pressure. Working on this hypothesis efforts have been made to lower elevated blood pressure by injection of an extract prepared from normal kidney tissue. Reports of some success with this kind of treatment have not as yet been confirmed, but the experiments are being watched with interest.

CORONARY DISEASE AND CORONARY THROMBOSIS

Everyone today is impressed with the prevalence of disease of the coronary arteries—most of all physicians, for they themselves seem to develop it with an extraordinary frequency. It is possible that the disease is actually increasing, but it is more likely that we have merely learned how to diagnose it more accurately. White found it in 37 per cent of a large series of patients with heart disease. Coronary disease is an old man's disease, 90 per cent of the cases occurring in individuals over 50 years old, most of whom are males. Areas of fatty softening develop in the lining of the coronaries; fibrosis and calcification follow, with narrowing of the lumen. Its blood supply being thus limited, the heart reacts, at times when it is under special stress, with so-called *angina pectoris.*

The first good medical description of angina pectoris, and one which has scarcely been improved upon since, was written in 1768 by William Heberden, a distinguished London physician whose scholarship was admired by no less a critic than Samuel Johnson, whom he attended as a physician. Heberden wrote of *Pectoris Dolor,* as he called it, as follows: "Those who are afflicted with it, are seized while they are walking (more especially if it be uphill, and soon after eating) with a painful and most disagreeable sensation in the breast, which seems as if it would extinguish life, if it were to increase or continue; but the moment they stand still, all this uneasiness vanishes. In all other respects the patients are, at the beginning of this disorder, perfectly well . . . the pain is sometimes situated in the upper part, sometimes in the middle, sometimes at the bottom of the os sterni, and often more inclined to the left than to the right side. It likewise very frequently extends from the breast to the middle of the arm. . . . The termination of angina pectoris is remarkable. For, if no accidents intervene, but the disease goes on to its height, the patients all suddenly fall down and perish almost immediately."

Heberden gave no suggestion, in this masterly description of the disease, that he knew its cause. But at least one of his contemporaries understood it. He was Edward Jenner, of vaccination fame. In 1777 John Hunter, the founder of experimental and surgical pathology and the most prominent surgeon of his day, began to have attacks of angina pectoris. Jenner had been a favorite pupil of Hunter's in London and when he settled down in Gloucestershire he continued to carry out experiments for Hunter, supplying him with a great variety of wild life, from eels to hedgehogs. When Jenner discovered that Hunter had angina pectoris, he wrote off to Dr. Heberden as follows: "When I had the pleasure of seeing him (Mr. Hunter) at Bath last autumn, I thought he was affected with many symptoms of the Angina Pectoris. . . . Though in the course of my practice I have seen many fall victims of this dreadful disease yet I have had only two opportunities of an examination after death. In the first case I found no material disease of the heart, except that the coronary artery appeared thickened. As no notice had been taken of such a circumstance by anybody who had written on the subject, I concluded that we must still seek for other causes as productive of the disease: but about three weeks ago, Mr. Paytherus, a surgeon at Ross, Herefordshire, desired me to examine with him the heart of a person who had died of Angina Pectoris a few day before. Here we found the same appearance of the coronary arteries as in the former case. But what I had taken to be an ossification of the vessel itself, Mr. P. discovered to be a kind of firm, fleshy tube, formed within the vessel itself, with a considerable quantity of ossific matter dispersed irregularly through it. . . . The importance of the coronary arteries, and how much the heart must suffer from their not being able to perform their functions, (we cannot be surprised at the painful spasms), is a subject I need not enlarge upon . . ."

It is a strange fact, however, that a hundred and thirty-four years elapsed from the date of Jenner's fundamental observation until further progress was made in the understanding of the natural history of coronary disease. It was not until 1912 that James B. Herrick, professor of medicine at Rush Medical College in Chicago, published a paper which threw new light on the disease. Herrick showed that the obstruction of a coronary artery or one of its large branches is not always immediately fatal, as had previously been thought to be the case. He described the symptoms of such a non-fatal occlusion as resembling those of acute serious abdominal disease—with nausea and vomiting, ashy countenance, cold sweat, and a feeble pulse. Herrick recognized that the clinical picture of coronary occlusion is often complex and variable. He stressed the importance of absolute rest in bed for these patients.

In the thirty years since Herrick drew attention to this new aspect of coronary disease, much has been learned concerning it. It is now known that the occlusion of a coronary by a fresh blood clot or thrombosis is a relatively common phenomenon. The area of heart muscle supplied by the occluded vessel becomes infarcted, that is, the muscle fibers die because their blood supply is cut off. When the infarct is not too large, and the immediate shock is not overwhelming, the patient survives and the area of damaged muscle is replaced by scar tissue. This leaves a weakened area in the heart wall, and the heart often enlarges in an effort to compensate for the injury.

Internists have become so familiar with coronary thrombosis today that many mild cases are diagnosed. Most of the patients survive; one authority on the disease reports that the immediate mortality is only from 15 to 25 per cent. With prolonged rest in bed—at least one or two months—and careful and gradual convalescence, it has been found that these patients have a good prospect of surviving for years. Some are able to take up their work again, if it is not too strenuous, and lead useful lives.

As a matter of fact John Hunter, whose coronary disease we have mentioned above, lived with the disease from 1773 until 1793. During these 20 years he worked as hard as any surgeon ever worked, and made many contributions of lasting importance. Sir James Mackenzie, who has been regarded as the founder of modern cardiology, himself had coronary disease. He had a coronary thrombosis in 1908 when he was 55 years old, but recovered and worked very hard for 17 years more, during which he had numerous small thromboses. It was not until 1925 that he succumbed to a final thrombosis which produced an infarct at the apex of his heart.

No therapy of much value in relieving the acute pain of an attack of angina pectoris was found until Thomas L. Brunton in 1867 discovered that amyl nitrite was remarkably effective. He knew from pharmacological experiments that the drug would lower blood pressure by dilating blood vessels, and knowing that blood pressure rose during attacks of angina, it occurred to him to combat the pain by having the patient inhale a few drops of the drug. When he made this merciful discovery Brunton was house physician at the Royal Infirmary at Edinburgh, and was only 23 years of age, having received his Bachelor of Medicine degree only one year before. Brunton subsequently established a laboratory for pharmacology and physiology at St. Bartholomew's in London, where important research was done. He never gave up his interest in the heart and took an important share in the experimental study of digitalis in the 1870's and 1880's.

A variety of surgical measures to stop the pain of severe angina pectoris have been tried, but the only one which has stood the test of time is alcohol injection of the dorsal nerve roots. Blocking of the first five thoracic roots was introduced by Felix Mandl of Vienna in 1925, and it has been taken up in a number of American clinics. The alcohol, which is injected into the vicinity of the nerve root, blocks cardiac pain by destroying the sympathetic nerve connections between the dorsal root and the dorsal ganglion. The technique of the injection is difficult, and the injection fails in a good many cases. But most patients are benefited to some degree, and many are completely relieved of their pain.

HEART FAILURE—SIGNS AND TREATMENT

We have discussed the development of our knowledge of the three main types of heart disease as regards their causation and pathology. In all three—rheumatic heart disease, hypertensive heart disease, and coronary disease—the heart may eventually fail to perform its vital function. In most instances, when it begins to fail, it gives evidence of its weakening by irregularities in its rate, by the development of edema, shortness of breath and other physical signs. Naturally the early detection and proper evaluation of these signs is of great importance in terms of proper treatment.

The discovery of methods of treatment long antedated the discovery of the prognostic significance of the various signs of disturbance of heart function. The most valuable of all drugs for heart failure, digitalis, was introduced into medical practice by William Withering, a country doctor practicing in Shropshire. An old woman in the community used a secret concoction of herbs with such success in the treatment of dropsy that her method of treatment attracted Withering's attention. He was a skilled botanist and quickly perceived that the active ingredient was the purple foxglove, *digitalis purpurea,* a plant with purple flowers and small pointed green leaves common in the British Isles. It was in 1775, a year in which Withering's feelings were stirred with sympathy for the American rebels, that he first made a decoction of the leaves of digitalis and began to use it in patients with edema and ascites, common symptoms of heart failure. The treatment was so successful that it was taken up by his friends in Birmingham and Edinburgh, and Withering found it necessary to write a monograph describing his experience with the drug. This work, entitled *An Account of the Foxglove,* was published in 1785, and remains one of the great medical classics.

Withering did not understand how the drug acted. Indeed, he failed to realize its special value in edema due to heart failure as compared with edema due to other causes. Yet his was one of the most important therapeutic discoveries of all time. Withering himself had a strenuous and trying life. In 1791 his house was attacked by a mob because of his sympathy with the French revolutionists and he had to flee with his possessions hidden in wagons covered with straw. At this time he was suffering from advanced pulmonary tuberculosis, from which he died in 1794. He was a cultivated gentleman and a distinguished scholar, and highly successful in the practice of medicine. When he was dying, his chief medical rival said sarcastically, "Alas, the flower of English medicine is Withering."

Although digitalis was at first used in the treatment of a wide variety of diseases, particularly in tuberculosis, by the middle of the next century it came to be generally realized that the drug had no value for disease other than cardiac. But as regards its use in heart failure, there was still no unanimity of opinion. Most of the physicians who did use it gave it in such small doses that it had little or no effect. Others did not use it at all. The experimental study of the action of digitalis, which began to make headway about this time, seemingly had little effect upon this state of affairs. In 1855 Edmé-F.-A. Vulpian of the University of Paris, a leader in experimental pathology in his day, demonstrated the specific action of digitalis on the frog's heart. He showed that the drug, given in a minimal lethal dose, first slows and then completely arrests the heart beat. This phenomenon was studied a good deal in France and Germany during the following years. In 1883, Oswald Schmiedeberg, professor of pharmacology at Strassburg, confirmed and elaborated this digitalis effect, showing that several other plants of the digitalis group, including oleander and Canadian hemp, also possessed it. It was in Schmiedeberg's laboratory a few years later that Arthur R. Cushny, a young Scotsman, began a series of experiments with digitalis which added considerably to the knowledge of the mode of action of the drug. Cushny continued his study of digitalis when he was appointed professor of materia medica and therapeutics at the University of Michigan in 1893, and in 1905, when he went to University College, London, as professor of pharmacology. Cushny and his contemporaries studied the effects of the drug on the dog's heart, recording the contractions directly, and also measuring intracardiac pressure. They showed that although digitalis slowed the heart rate, the force of its contractions was so increased that the net result was a greater output of blood.

These researches during the last half of the 19th Century did not have much influence on the therapeutic use of digitalis. Cushny indeed stated in his monograph on digitalis, written some years later, that "during the 19th Century very little progress was made in the use of digitalis in disease, and what was written by its advocates in 1810 might be quoted as representing the general view in 1900." Medicine was passing through a period when emphasis on pathology dominated thought. Physiology was not popular.

With the beginning of the new century, however, the physiological approach to the problems of disease came to the fore, and the man who, more than any other single individual, was responsible for this was a general practitioner who passed most of his life in the Lancashire factory town of Burnley. He was James Mackenzie, called "the beloved physician" by his biographer, R. McNair Wilson, in the moving book of that name.

Mackenzie was born on a Scottish farm in 1853. Stern necessity dominated his youth. Graduated from Edinburgh University in medicine in 1878, he served one year as resident physician at the Edinburgh Royal Infirmary. He then went to work as a general practitioner in Burnley.

He did a good deal of obstetrics, and he soon was involved in a tragedy that led him to turn his attention specially to heart disease. One of his young women patients died suddenly of heart failure during delivery. Mackenzie had thought her heart normal. He was profoundly distressed, and began to study with special care the signs and symptoms relating to the heart in his patients. He found many changes in the size and position of the heart, murmurs of several types, and variations in rate that he did not understand. He reviewed what had been written on these questions and got but little help. At this date (1883) the diagnosis of the different types of valvular disease of the heart had long since been fairly well worked out on the basis of the murmurs that the lesions of the valves produce. These murmurs in themselves, however, are not a sufficient guide to the functional state of the heart, for it was well known even in Mackenzie's time that many patients who had them suffered no apparent ill effects. The different types of abnormal heart rhythm are more important signs, and concerning these very little was known when Mackenzie began his work. He concluded that the only way to find out what any particular symptom really meant was to make as careful and complete a record of it as possible and then "wait and see." This philosophy was the basis of his thirty years work in general practice at Burnley, and with it he made some of the most important advances of modern medicine.

In order to distinguish the different types of abnormal heart rhythm more clearly, Mackenzie utilized a little instrument, invented some years previously, called the sphygmograph. This was strapped onto the wrist and traced the beats of the pulse on a strip of smoked paper. But Mackenzie soon found that these tracings of the pulsation in the radial artery were not enough: he still could not tell which abnormal rhythms were dangerous and which were harmless. He therefore worked out a method of simultaneously recording tracings of the pulsation in the jugular vein in the neck and the radial pulse. The former gave him a record of the beating of the right auricle and the latter traced the beats of the left ventricle. His watchmaker at Burnley devised a little machine for making these tracings which Mackenzie called a polygraph. It was equipped with pens which made the tracings in ink and was so small that he could carry it in his pocket and make tracings in the patient's home.

His polygraph soon helped him understand the meaning of some of the irregularities of the heart that had perplexed him. In 1890 he identified a common type of irregularity in which the radial pulse misses occasional beats. Mackenzie discovered that when a beat is thus dropped, the ventricle makes a weak premature contraction (now called an extra-systole) which is not perceived in the radial pulse, while the auricle maintains its normal rhythm. "Waiting and seeing," he found that this kind of irregularity was entirely harmless, for the patients who had it continued hale and hearty.

In 1897 Mackenzie identified a serious and common form of irregularity in which the pulse is rapid and entirely irregular both in force and rate. With his polygraph he found no evidence of auricular contraction at all and concluded that the auricles were paralyzed, the ventricles going on beating irregularly. Although Mackenzie's pupil, Thomas Lewis, and the Germans, Rotherberger and Winterberg, working quite independently, in 1909 proved by means of electrocardiographic studies that this type of irregularity is due to fibrillation rather than paralysis of the auricle, Mackenzie deserves the credit for identifying it and for recognizing its grave import. For it usually developed when the heart began to fail seriously, and few of his patients survived for long with it.

Mackenzie found that auricular fibrillation usually responded remarkably well to digitalis. If the drug slowed the pulse the patient was soon benefited, and if enough digitalis was given to keep the rate below 80, the patients were often able to carry on a limited amount of activity for years. This discovery established the use of digitalis on a sound basis for the first time. The correctness of Mackenzie's clinical deductions was quickly confirmed experimentally, the strength of digitalis preparations was standardized, and the drug came into its own as one of the few indispensable medicines.

But these interesting discoveries were not Mackenzie's most important contribution to medicine. His insistence upon reliance on common sense rather than on elaborate laboratory data in the interpretation of disease is more fundamental. He was distressed when his polygraph became popular, because he did not wish overemphasis placed on any single method of examination. He taught that the best test of the condition of the heart was its capacity to respond to effort, and that this was best ascertained from the patient's own statement as to how far he could walk without distress, etc.

In 1902, when he was 49, Mackenzie published his first book, *The Study of the Pulse*. It quickly brought him recognition among those foremost in the study of the heart throughout the world, many of whom came to Burnley to see him. His views did not make much headway, however, among the rank and file of English physicians. Spurred by the crusading spirit, Mackenzie at the age of 54 decided to go to London and present his ideas personally. He was welcomed on the staff of several hospitals, and was soon recognized as the leading consultant for heart disease. In 1909 he published his next important book, *Diseases of the Heart*. The group of eager students of heart disease who gathered around him came to be known as the Mackenzie school. They not only made many important discoveries, but they established cardiology as one of the modern medical specialties. Thomas Lewis was the most gifted of Mackenzie's pupils. After Mackenzie left London, Lewis became the leader of the group, and added fame to it.

For Mackenzie eventually tired of London, even though recognition of every sort came to him. He was knighted in 1915, and had more patients than he could care for, yet he longed to get back to general practice where he could study the early symptoms of disease. In 1919 he retired to St. Andrews in Scotland, where he established an Institute for Clinical Research. There with a group of able associates he began a thorough and comprehensive study of the significance of obscure symptoms of common diseases. At St. Andrews he wrote his important monograph on angina pectoris, the disease which caused his death in 1925, seventeen years after he had his first attack of anginal pain.

With characteristic objectivity Mackenzie requested that his heart be studied after his death. Both coronary arteries showed advanced sclerosis, and there were numerous small scars in the muscle of the heart left by the repeated thromboses that occurred during the seventeen year period between his first coronary thrombosis and his death. Mackenzie's last contribution to medical knowledge, that is, his own case history, was therefore a valuable one.

An advance in the therapy of heart disease since Mackenzie's time has been in the use of quinidine, one of the alkaloids similar to quinine derived from Peruvian bark. The discovery that quinidine has a signal power of restoring normal rhythm to the heart in auricular fibrillation came about in an interesting way. Karl Friedrich Wenckebach, noted Viennese cardiologist, in 1914 reported that he learned of it from a patient who had for years been able to stop his attacks of auricular fibrillation by taking a small dose of quinine. In 1918, Walter Frey, cardiologist at Kiel University, discovered that quinidine is more effective in restoring normal rhythm than quinine.

NEPHRITIS

When we recall that the kidneys are the chief organs through which the blood stream excretes the waste products of cell metabolism, it is not strange that kidney lesions are among the most serious, forming one of the most important causes of death.

The first sign of disturbed kidney function to be discovered was albumin in the urine. This observation was made by an American loyalist physician, William Charles Wells, who had been born in Charleston, South Carolina, but settled in London after the Revolution. There he became physician to St. Thomas' Hospital. He was an original thinker and made a number of important contributions to medicine, biology, and physics. It was Wells who, in 1814, first put forward the correct explanation of the manner in which dew is formed. Two years previously he had written a paper entitled, *On the Presence of the Red Matter and Serum of Blood in the Urine of Dropsy, which has not Originated from Scarlet Fever.* Here for the first time, in a series of case reports, Wells showed that dropsy, i.e., edema, was sometimes accompanied by albumin in the urine, and that these symptoms were associated with alterations in the kidneys. He was not certain that these kidney lesions were the cause of the dropsy and albuminuria, but he suspected that they were. Fortunately, the test for albumin which Wells used, and which is still the one generally used today, namely boiling the urine, is not sensitive enough to detect the small amount of albumin normally present in the urine. This normal amount is eliminated from the blood plasma as the blood circulates through the glomeruli of the kidney, the minute tufts of bloodvessels through the walls of which the filtration of waste products takes place. When the glomeruli have been damaged by disease, their efficiency as a filter is impaired and they allow relatively large amounts of albumin to pass into the urine.

It remained for a great English physician, Richard Bright, to establish beyond all doubt the relationship of albuminuria and edema to diseased kidneys. Bright had been trained in Edinburgh, and began practice in London where he became physician to Guy's Hospital. He was one of the first to see the necessity of correlating the clinical picture of disease with the pathological findings, and he became skilled in both disciplines. In a series of masterly case reports written in 1827 he not only described with exactness the clinical symptoms of nephritis and the gross pathology of the kidneys, but he made the fundamental distinction between degenerative disease of the kidney, and acute and chronic inflammatory disease.

Edema was the symptom which first drew Bright's attention to nephritis, and his work made it possible for the first time to distinguish its several forms. After Bright, edema due to kidney disease and to cirrhosis of the liver were distinguished from edema due to cardiac disease, whereas previously they had all been grouped together. This is one of the most fundamental differential diagnoses in all medicine. Nephritis has been known as Bright's disease ever since, and no eponym was more justly given.

In 1842 Bright had two clinical wards at Guy's Hospital set apart for the special study of renal disease. A consulting room and a laboratory were included, thus forming a separate unit for the study of a special disease, quite in the manner in which certain diseases are being attacked in our modern hospitals today. Bright served 23 years at Guy's during which time he made many new observations concerning a variety of diseases. When he died of arteriosclerosis at the age of 69, he was the most celebrated of all English physicians of his day.

It was an interesting historical coincidence that only one year after Bright had described nephritis, urea, which is the chief product of protein catabolism in the human body and the main waste product which the kidney eliminates, was synthesized. The pioneer German physiological chemist, Friedrich Wöhler, made it by heating ammonium cyanate. This was the first time that a substance occurring naturally in the body had been artificially made in the laboratory—a step so epoch-making that its effect has been compared to that of Darwin's theory of the origin of the species, and to Pasteur's demonstration of the parasitic origin of pestilences. It was the beginning of the synthetic chemistry which is today carrying us far into the secrets of some disease processes.

Among the physicians of Bright's era who were attempting to apply new chemical knowledge to the problems of clinical medicine, Robert Christison, professor of materia medica at Edinburgh, was outstanding. Christison had been stimulated to study nephritis at the Edinburgh Infirmary by Bright's work. An able chemist, he soon saw the need of studying the concentration of urea in both the blood and urine in nephritis. The chemical methods for the estimation of urea in the blood available in his day were only of the crudest sort. Yet in 1829 Christison was able to make the fundamentally important observation that urea was increased in the blood and decreased in the urine in chronic nephritis because the damaged kidneys could no longer eliminate it satisfactorily. Ten years later Christison wrote a monograph *On Granular Degeneration of the Kidneys* which added much to the knowledge of the clinical, pathological, and chemical aspects of nephritis. Among other things he pointed out the severe anemia that develops in nephritis, the accumulation of urea in all the body fluids, its diminution in the urine, and the grave prognostic significance of the progressive lowering of the specific gravity of the urine.

The next phase of the development of the knowledge of kidney disease was the microscopical one. When Bright first described nephritis the microscopical structure of the normal as well as the diseased kidney were still largely unknown. But when the new compound microscope came into use a few years later, great advances in the understanding of kidney disease were made with it. This work was done both in England and in Germany, and independently. The English contribution was made by William Bowman, who came to King's College in London in October, 1837, at the age of 21 to begin his three years' study for membership in the Royal College of Surgeons. He brought with him a compound microscope which his former master at the Birmingham General Hospital, where he had served for five years as an apprentice surgeon, had presented to him. Bowman was also a skilled dissector and an expert draughtsman. He was at once enlisted by Professor Todd at King's College in the task of describing the microscopical structure of the skin, all the sensory organs, the nerves, muscle, bone and cartilage, all of the glands, the lungs, liver and kidneys, for a new textbook. As he did this work, Bowman made many new and original observations. He got to the kidneys in or before 1841. The tubular structure of the kidney was in part already known, and the glomeruli had been identified, but the latter were supposed to have no connection with the renal tubules. The great Johannes Müller, the father of histology, had asserted this in a very positive manner. Bowman, in a beautiful study of injected specimens, proved that the intracapsular space of each glomerulus is continuous with the lumen of a tubule— that the glomerulus must be regarded as the beginning of the renal tubule. He concluded that urine is formed by secretion of waste products from the blood by the tubule cells into the lumens of the tubules, then washed out of the tubules by a saline stream flowing down from the glomeruli. Bowman communicated his observations on the kidneys to the Royal Society in February, 1842, and was awarded a Royal Medal. He hoped to become professor of surgery at Kings' College but was disappointed and turned to ophthalmology.

Meanwhile in Germany another equally brilliant young mi-

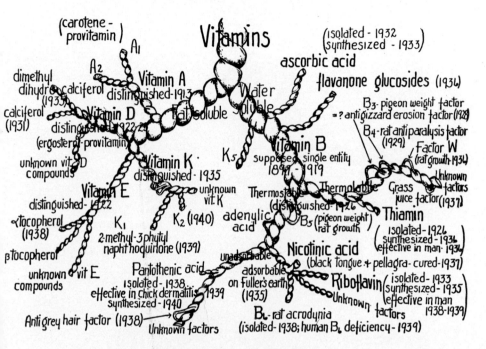

(From Speis, T. D., Hightower, D. P., and Hubbard, L. H.: "Some Recent Advances in Vitamin Therapy," *J.A.M.A.*, 115:292–297, 1940)

Diagrammatic representation of the interrelationship of the vitamins. They are schematically differentiated into the water-soluble and the fat-soluble fractions; the latter group is further separated into its thermolabile and its thermostable components. Certain of these substances have been shown to be essential to human nutrition and effective in the treatment of specific deficiency diseases. The physiologic properties of many are as yet undetermined.

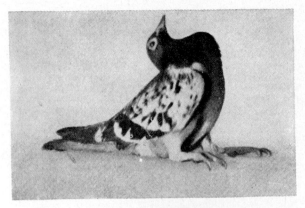

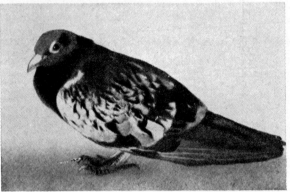

Experimental Beri-Beri Cured with Crystalline Vitamin

After Eijkman's discovery that beri-beri could be produced experimentally in fowls, pigeons were used for many of the studies of the disease. Funk, in 1912, was the first to prepare a crystalline vitamin extract from yeast which relieved the symptoms of beri-beri miraculously. The pigeon in the upper figure shows the spastic paralysis of acute beri-beri resulting from a diet of polished rice. In the lower figure the same pigeon is seen to be completely recovered three hours after the intramuscular injection of 8 milligrams of crystalline extract of yeast.

croscopist was also studying the kidney. He was Jacob Henle, who had been a favorite pupil of Johannes Müller. Henle became professor of anatomy at Zurich in 1840, at the age of 31, and the following year reported a microscopic study of the urine. He saw in it certain short cylindrical objects, some transparent, others granular, others containing epithelial cells or fat droplets. These so-called *casts* had been seen in the urine before but their origin had not been traced. Henle showed that they came from nephritic kidneys, for he found them in the urine and then in the kidneys of the same nephritic patient at autopsy. It soon became apparent that granular epithelial or fatty casts signified degenerative changes in the tubular epithelium of the kidney.

Henle made a number of other important microscopical observations regarding the kidney. In his *Handbuch der rationellen Pathologie* (1847) he presented the first extensive description of the microscopical changes in the kidneys in Bright's disease. He described what he regarded as an exudation of fibrin between and into the tubules, which later organized, contracted and produced cirrhosis of the kidney. He unfortunately failed to describe important changes in the glomeruli and concluded that they were not involved by nephritis. In 1862, many years later, Henle made still another important contribution regarding the kidney. He identified and described a portion of the urinary tubule which had hitherto escaped notice—since known as the loop of Henle.

The physiologists, too, were stimulated to study the kidney by Bright's work. One of these was a young prosector at Marburg named Karl Friedrich Wilhelm Ludwig. Destined to be one of the great pioneers in modern physiology, he was only 25 years old and just beginning to work in physiology when in 1842 he conceived the theory that urine is formed by filtration of a cell-free, protein-free fluid containing all the constituents of urine, through the walls of the glomerular capillaries, and that this filtrate in its passage down the renal tubule is concentrated by reabsorption from the tubule. This was, of course, an entirely different theory of urine formation than Bowman had advanced, but we shall see that time eventually proved Ludwig to be right.

In England Bright's work had stimulated comprehensive and prolonged study of nephritis, and the fruits of these efforts now began to be presented. In 1852 George Johnson, also of King's College, London, published an important book, *On Diseases of the Kidney*. It contained many original observations regarding both the clinical and pathological features of nephritis, and included the first comprehensive microscopical description of the glomerular changes. The swelling and thickening of the capillary loops of the glomeruli in the acute stage, and the fibrosis of the glomeruli in the later stages of nephritis, were all described. Johnson realized that a number of different disease entities had been included by the term, Bright's disease, and he identified amyloid and fatty degeneration of the kidney as separate types.

With the enormous development of microscopical pathology during the last half of the 19th Century, a voluminous literature grew up regarding the classification of the various forms of nephritis. The final classification of all disease was by now generally recognized to be dependent primarily upon microscopical morphology, and the refinements of histological technique produced such a profusion of descriptive interpretations that in a complex disease like nephritis a multitude of classifications were developed. It was not until 1914 that the classification generally accepted today was worked out by Franz Volhard, a clinician, and T. Fahr, a pathologist, of Mannheim. These men integrated their experience with nephritis to produce a classification that has been of great practical value. It was presented in a monograph, *Die Brightsche Nierenkrankheit*, remarkable for its clarity and for its beautiful colored illustrations. Their classification grouped the varied conditions originally included under Bright's disease into three broad classes: (1) the nephroses—degenerative conditions like amyloid disease; (2) the nephritides—inflammatory conditions; (3) arteriosclerotic disease of the kidney. Classification of disease, even when imperfect, has the advantage of permitting students to group their cases into categories which have similar features. It is by studying such groups of cases that progress in diagnosis and therapy is largely achieved.

Since the turn of the century there has been a revival of interest in physiological research and a corresponding decline of interest in pathological research in most branches of medicine. In the study of kidney disease this physiological approach has been particularly fruitful. One of the first advances in this direction came through the study of blood pressure in nephritics. Clifford Allbutt was a pioneer in this work. He was stimulated to begin his studies of blood pressure by Burton Sanderson, the distinguished professor of physiology at University College, and his subsequent extensive studies of circulatory disease emphasized the physiological point of view. Allbutt and his contemporaries found early in their studies that elevation of blood pressure is a cardinal symptom of chronic nephritis. As the disease continues the blood pressure tends to become higher and higher, until it not infrequently exceeds 200 mm. systolic and 120 mm. diastolic. The heart hypertrophies. Headache and nosebleeds consequent to the high pressure are common. As the accumulating knowledge of kidney disease has made it possible to distinguish chronic nephrosis from chronic nephritis, it has been found that nephrosis is not ordinarily accompanied by elevation of blood pressure, and the point has become useful in differential diagnosis.

Another important advance in the understanding of the physiology of the kidney came through the modern methods of chemical study of the blood. It took a long time to get to this point: three quarters of a century elapsed between Christison's observation that the blood urea was increased in nephritis and the introduction of blood urea and non-protein nitrogen determinations in clinical medicine.

Hermann Strauss of the 3rd University Clinic at Berlin deserves the credit for this important step. In a monograph on nephritis written in 1902, Strauss emphasized that the study of the blood chemistry was the most important and the most reliable index of kidney function. The reason of course why chemical tests of the nitrogenous constituents of the blood had not been utilized before, and why they were not generally adopted even after Strauss emphasized their value, was that the available chemical methods were not good enough. The first reasonably reliable figures for the urea content of blood had been published between 1850 and 1860, being obtained by a laborious technique borrowed from methods used for urine analysis. The accurate determination of the non-protein nitrogen in the blood was first made possible by Johann Kjeldahl's method of nitrogen determination, which was published in 1883. These methods were not only laborious but they required such a large amount of blood that they were not practical. For instance, the method for determining non-protein nitrogen used by Strauss required from 50 to 70 cc. of blood.

It was therefore a great step forward when Otto Folin at Harvard Medical School in 1912 devised his new colorimetric method for the determination of the nitrogenous constituents of the blood. Non-protein nitrogen, urea, and ammonia could all be determined from a single sample of 2 cc. of blood. Clinicians now began to do these determinations on all nephritics, and from these new data important advances were made in the understanding of nephritis and in its treatment. It now became possible to detect failing kidney function and the accumulation of nitrogenous waste products in the blood before the actual onset of uremia, that terminal stage of nephritis in which the accumulated waste products poison the system and produce a variety of symptoms including drowsiness, headache, stupor, muscular twitchings and coma. Countless patients have been rescued, at least temporarily, from uremia by the finding of an elevated blood non-protein nitrogen.

Although urea is the chief waste product accumulating in the blood when kidney function fails, the non-protein nitrogen, which includes several other waste products, such as uric acid, creatinin, amino-acids, and ammonia, is usually determined instead of the urea. The two determinations give parallel values for practical purposes, but the method for non-protein nitrogen determination is considerably simpler and easier to carry out than that required for urea determination. Folin so simplified and improved his methods of blood analysis as time went on that it is today possible, by using his method, to determine the non-protein nitrogen from only 0.1 cc. of blood. In routine work 1 cc. is ordinarily used.

Another fundamentally important advance in understanding kidney function was being made about this same time by the physiologists. Almost a century had elapsed since Ludwig had put forward his theory of the functional relationship between glomerulus and tubule in the formation of urine. A great mass of experimental data had accumulated, much of which was contradictory. The simple question of how urine was formed remained unanswered. This was the situation when Alfred N. Richards, professor of pharmacology at the University of Pennsylvania, in 1921 devised a new method of studying the formation of urine in the frog's kidney, and with it carried out experiments which answered most of the questions that had troubled physiologists for a hundred years. With infinite delicacy he inserted tiny sharply pointed glass tubes into the intracapsular space of the glomerulus of the frog's kidney and withdrew the fluid filtering out through the walls of the capillary loops. The fluid thus obtained amounted to only one one-thousandth of a cubic centimeter, but this sufficed for both qualitative and quantitative chemical tests. These revealed that the glomerular fluid contains urea, chloride and glucose, indeed all the constituents of blood plasma which might be expected to pass through the capillary walls by simple filtration.

Richards and his collaborators eventually succeeded in the more difficult task of inserting their delicate cannulas into the frog kidney tubules at several different levels, and withdrawing fluid for analysis. These tests showed that as the glomerular filtrate flows through the tubules, the tubule cells re-absorb much of the water as well as other substances like chloride and glucose which the body cannot afford to lose, but allow waste products like urea to pass through. Thus Richards' work has confirmed the theory of kidney function put forward by Ludwig long ago.

This new physiological knowledge has been of very real value to clinicians because it has helped them to understand the mechanism in failure of renal function, and to devise various new tests for measuring it. The non-protein nitrogen content of the blood, which we have described above, is the most widely used and perhaps the most valuable of these tests.

The clinician has today at his disposal another comparatively simple test of renal function which does not require a chemical laboratory. This is the so-called specific gravity concentration test. It is based upon the fact that in chronic nephritis the specific gravity of the urine is lowered, due to the fact that the renal tubules, where concentration of the urine takes place, have been damaged and cannot re-absorb fluid as well as they should. It was the distinguished Parisian urological surgeon, Joachim Albarran who, in 1905, first carried out an extensive study of this concentration phenomenon. He noted while studying the urine from separate kidneys which he had catheterized, that the specific gravity of the urine which he obtained from diseased kidneys varied less than it normally does. He gave his patients large amounts of water to drink and showed that the specific gravity of the urine from diseased kidneys did not change.

The introduction of the specific gravity concentration test into clinical work was due to Franz Volhard. In an article on nephritis which he wrote in the *Handbuch der inneren Medizin* in 1918 he outlined a standard method for carrying out the test and emphasized its advantages as an indicator of the severity of renal damage. Time has substantiated his claim.

It is unfortunately true that no cure for nephritis has been found. Yet if we compare the treatment given today with what was done for these patients in Bright's time, we at once realize that we have come a long way in making the lot of the nephritic an easier one. Bright and his contemporaries cupped, leeched, and bled their patients with great freedom, particularly those with acute nephritis. This certainly did no good and must have often done harm, for these patients were already anemic.

Mercury was also a favorite remedy in those days. It was usually given in the form of calomel, together with some other diuretic like squill or digitalis, and in doses large enough to cause the excessive salivation and sore mouth characteristic of mercurial poisoning. We know today that inorganic mercury is a kidney poison: it causes necrosis of the tubule cells, and the diuresis that follows its use is due to interference with their function of reabsorption. For patients whose renal function is already impaired, this is the worst possible treatment. Bright himself in one of his later papers began to suspect this, for he detailed the case of a woman with advanced and long-standing nephritis,[1] who entreated him to give her something else than mercury, the use of which, she said, had been "attended with the greatest discomfort, and followed by increased debility." Yet Bright continued to give the drug in small doses, and generations of physicians following him continued to give it freely.

Purgatives were another standby of Bright's contemporaries. Such treatment must have been a hard punishment for patients already weakened by bleeding, annoyed by blisters over the loins, and tormented by turpentine enemas given as counter-irritants!

Today all this has fortunately been changed. Guided by the new knowledge of renal physiology our efforts are directed at lightening the task which the kidneys have to perform. Since the waste products of protein have to be excreted via the kidneys to a greater extent than fat and carbohydrates, which can be oxidixed and eliminated by the lungs and skin, the protein intake of victims of nephritis is limited. But it is not excluded entirely from the diet, for the body must have a certain amount of protein to maintain a balance between nitrogen intake and excretion.

The limitation of inorganic salt in the diet is another method

[1] Case XI—Cases and Observations, Illustrative of Renal Disease accompanied with the Secretion of Albuminous Urine, Guy's Hospital Reports, Volume I, 1836.

of relieving the work of the kidneys. In 1902 Fernand Widal, the distinguished Parisian clinician, who earlier in his career had discovered the diagnostic test for typhoid fever which bears his name, carried out studies which showed that sodium chloride excretion is interfered with in nephritis. Accumulating in the blood and tissue fluids, it is an important factor in the causation of edema. Widal showed that restriction of sodium chloride in the diet results in a decrease in edema, and its restriction in the nephritic diet is often advised today. The intake and output of fluid is carefully measured in hospital patients today and in nephritic patients these data have yielded information of great value.

PART THREE

Surgery During the Last Hundred Years

22

THE BEGINNING OF MODERN SURGERY:

EPHRAIM McDOWELL'S OVARIOTOMY

IF WE CONSIDER the modern era of surgery as beginning at the point at which surgeons dared to open the great cavities of the body, the abdomen and the chest, and to operate upon the viscera, rather than being content merely to deal with wounds and disease on the surface of the body and in the extremities, then Ephraim McDowell clearly deserves recognition as the first modern surgeon. For he was the first deliberately to open the abdomen and remove a tumor which he knew would otherwise have killed his patient.

Ephraim McDowell was of Scotch Irish ancestry, and his family represented the best pioneering tradition in colonial times. His grandfather, Captain John McDowell, was killed in an Indian ambuscade in 1742. His father, Samuel, fought in the French and Indian Wars, and served as a colonel during the Revolution. He was a prominent citizen in his home state, Virginia, and it was there that Ephraim McDowell was born on Nov. 11, 1771, the ninth of eleven children and the sixth son. In 1782 his father was appointed by the Virginia Assembly to settle land claims in Kentucky, and took his family across the mountains to the vicinity of Danville. Thus Ephraim, at the age of twelve, came to live in a frontier town on the Wilderness Road to the great unexplored west. It was an environment favoring the development of courage, self-reliance, and common sense, virtues that guided Ephraim to his surgical triumph in manhood.

In 1790, when he was nineteen, Ephraim rode back east over the mountains and began the study of medicine as an apprentice with Dr. Alexander Humphreys of Staunton, Virginia. Three years later he went abroad and entered the medical school of the University of Edinburgh at which his preceptor, Dr. Humphreys, had studied. Ephraim attended two sessions there, but during his second year he came to realize that the anatomy and surgery taught privately by John Bell, the famous Edinburgh surgeon, were superior to any courses given in the University, and he became one of Bell's pupils. We do not know that he inspired McDowell with any special interest in the problem of ovarian tumors, but he must have taught him the importance of a direct and practical approach to surgery, based upon a sound knowledge of normal and pathological anatomy, for Bell was one of the great practical surgeons of his day.

When his money ran out after two years in Edinburgh McDowell had no choice but to return to Kentucky without his degree. He began the practice of medicine in Danville in 1895, and within a short time had all that he could do. He was the best trained surgeon in his community and he undertook all of the standard operations that were done in his day, including such difficult ones as lithotomy, the removal of bladder stone. Before every operation, usually performed on Sunday in his own house, he studied the anatomy and the steps of the procedure with care, and drilled his assistants in what he expected of them.

His great opportunity came in 1809, when he was 38 years old. Called to see a Mrs. Thomas Crawford, sixty miles out in the wilderness from Danville, he found that she had a huge ovarian tumor. Seeing that she was a stalwart soul, he told her that nothing but an operation could help her, and that although no such operative removal of an ovarian tumor had ever before been attempted as far as he knew, he would try the experiment if she would come to Danville. She agreed, and made the journey back to Danville on horseback, with her enlarged abdomen supported by the pommel of her saddle. The journey took her several days, and when she arrived in Danville a decubitus ulcer had formed in the skin over her abdomen from the constant rubbing of the pommel against it.

In his own home, on Christmas Day, 1809, with only his nephew, Dr. James McDowell, to help him, Ephraim made his fateful experiment. Without any anaesthesia, but supported by the fortitude of his patient, who sang hymns while he worked, Ephraim made a long vertical incision on the left side of the abdomen. The tumor was then seen as a huge cystic movable structure, attached by a narrow pedicle. McDowell first passed a ligature around the pedicle and tied it off before he opened the sac. Some fifteen pounds of gelatinous material escaped, giving him room to cut through the pedicle and remove the remaining portion of the tumor. He closed the abdominal wall with interrupted sutures. The whole thing took twenty-five minutes. The tumor which he had removed, including both its fluid and solid parts, weighed a total of twenty-two and one-half pounds.

It is told that while McDowell operated, a crowd of his fellow-citizens gathered outside of his house with the intention of hanging him if his patient should die. The proposed operation had been the chief topic of conversation in the town for several days and opposition to it had reached a high pitch. As the operation proceeded the crowd began to get out of hand, and had actually to be restrained by the sheriff and some of the more level-headed citizens. It dispersed only when word came that the patient had survived.

But McDowell himself well knew that the most dangerous phase of his experiment lay ahead—the possibility of fatal peritonitis, that is, inflammation developing within the abdominal cavity. All that he could do was to put his patient to bed and hope for the best. But Mrs. Crawford withstood this hazard as staunchly as she had gone through the operation. McDowell found her up making her bed on the fifth post-operative day, and he could not keep her from going home on the twenty-fifth day. She went back to her hard life of a frontier housewife completely cured of her trouble, and lived to the ripe age of 79.

The courage that Ephraim McDowell showed in removing for

the first time a tumor from the abdominal cavity can only be appreciated by reviewing the surgical knowledge of his day. Recall first of all that the surgeons of the late 18th Century who taught in the great European centers of medical training understood rather well the natural history of ovarian tumors. They knew that they were often slow growing, cystic, freely movable within the abdominal cavity, and attached only by a relatively narrow pedicle. Even though these features made them the most favorable of all abdominal tumors for surgical attack, and even though they knew that all of the methods of treatment previously used were futile, they dared not attempt to remove them because of their fear of peritonitis. John Bell, in his two volume work *The Principles of Surgery*, completed in 1806, wrote at length about tumors and the operative methods used in removing them, but he did not mention even the possibility of attacking ovarian tumors, or indeed any tumor within the abdominal cavity. Bell was all his life beset by the jealousy and intolerance of his colleagues in Edinburgh, who attacked him on every possible pretext. He could scarcely be expected to make such a hazardous experiment as attempting to remove an ovarian tumor. But his pupil McDowell, schooled in self-reliance by the frontier life, and unhampered by the surgical traditions that prevailed in older communities, dared to try it. The old world had been outstripped by the new!

McDowell did not rush into print. He waited seven years, until he had operated successfully upon two more women for ovarian tumor, before he reported his great achievement. His brief and concise description of his three cases was published in *The Eclectic Repertory*, a Pennsylvania medical journal, in 1817. It was generally ignored, except for doubting comment regarding its veracity expressed by a certain Dr. Henderson in a subsequent number of the *Repertory*. McDowell wrote a sprightly reply defending his report, and added descriptions of two further ovariotomies, which appeared in the *Repertory* in 1819. He still failed to make any appreciable impression on his surgical contemporaries.

In America there were only a half dozen surgeons who dared attempt to remove ovarian tumors in isolated instances during the thirty-two years that elapsed between McDowell's first ovariotomy and the revival and further development of the operation by the Atlee brothers in Lancaster, Pennsylvania.

In Great Britain also McDowell got no recognition. When he sent his report of his first three cases to his American publisher he forwarded a copy of it to his old chief, John Bell, in Edinburgh. But it so happened that Bell was in Italy at the time, seriously ill, and the copy fell into the hands of his successor in Edinburgh, John Lizars. Lizars did nothing with it at the time, but seven years later, in 1823, he attempted ovariotomy for the first time himself. His venture was an unfortunate one, for on opening the abdomen he failed to find any tumor. In the description of his case which he published in 1824 he included McDowell's long ignored report. Lizars did the operation three times during the following year but had so little success that he gave it up, and it was not done again in Scotland for twenty years. The operation was taken up again and developed successfully in 1842 by Charles Clay of Manchester, and he received the credit from his British colleagues for its innovation. Even when the facts were all thrashed over by the successful British ovariotomists of the next generation, they never would acknowledge the importance of Ephraim McDowell's accomplishment.

McDowell continued the life of a busy practitioner as Danville grew and the tide of immigration moved westward. In his fifties he retired to a plantation, where he lived a more leisurely life in the style of a southern gentlemen of his day. A year before he died he wrote that he had done a total of eleven ovariotomies, with only one death. He died in June, 1830, apparently of acute appendicitis. Fate would have it that he, the founder of abdominal surgery, should succumb to a disease which the abdominal surgeons a half century later would learn to control.

23

THE COMING OF ANAESTHESIA

MORE THAN the courage of an Ephraim McDowell was required to give surgeons safe access to the interior of the body. A whole series of technical problems had to be solved. The first of these was the problem of pain.

This was solved by two Americans who, quite independently of each other, in the early 1840's discovered the anaesthetic power of ether. Dr. Crawford W. Long, a Georgia physician, deserves priority for the discovery, for he first operated with ether anaesthesia in 1842. But he did not publicize his discovery, and the credit for making the use of ether known to the world clearly belongs to the Boston dentist, William T. G. Morton, and to the staff of the Massachusetts General Hospital where ether began to be regularly used in 1846. It is an ironic fact that neither Long nor Morton got much reward for their discovery—certainly one of the most merciful in the whole history of medicine.

Now what both Long and Morton discovered was the *use* of ether to relieve pain during surgical operations. They did not discover the power of ether to put people to sleep and to suppress the sensation of pain; these properties had been known for a long time not only for ether but also for nitrous oxide or laughing gas. As early as 1799 Sir Humphry Davy, the English chemist, showed that nitrous oxide produced unconsciousness. He wrote, "As nitrous oxide . . . seems capable of destroying physical pain, it may probably be used with advantage in surgical operations in which no great effusion of blood takes place."

228

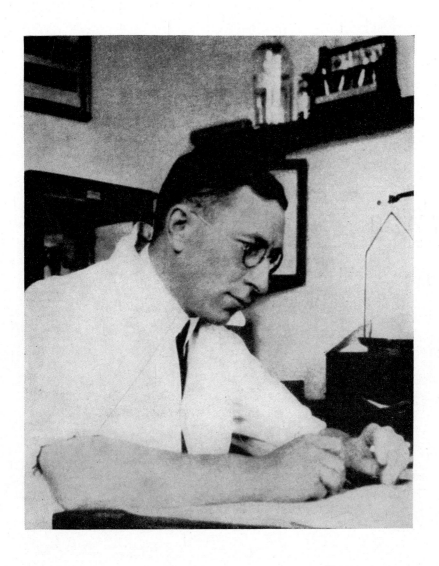

Sir Frederick Banting at Work in His Laboratory

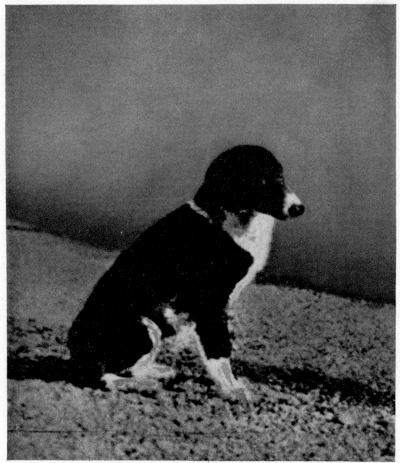

(From Paul de Kruif's *Men against Death*)

Dog. No. 33

The female black and white collie that Banting and Best kept alive with insulin for seventy days after pancreatectomy.

Thirty years after Davy wrote these words, Michael Faraday showed that ether could produce much the same effect as nitrous oxide. These facts became more or less well known, not only to chemists and physicians but also to the public. Medical students inhaled these gases as a routine diversion, and traveling showmen gave demonstrations of their effects. Ether jags were a popular form of dissipation for young bloods.

It seems incomprehensible that no one tried to use these agents to suppress pain in surgical operations during all these years. Surgeons had tried a great variety of other drugs, including opium, hashish, and mandragora, and, of course, alcohol in its many forms. None of these was adequate, and the ordeal of operation was dreaded by surgeon and patient alike. In the trustee's room of a London hospital hangs a bell, which before the days of anaesthesia hung outside the operating theater, where it was rung to summon orderlies and nurses to hold down patients undergoing operations. Imagine the ominous sound of that bell!

When Crawford W. Long finally, for the first time, used ether as a surgical anaesthetic, he was a general practitioner in the little village of Jefferson, Georgia. He was a sociable young man, who amused his friends by giving parties at which he allowed them to inhale ether. He had learned the practice while a medical student in Philadelphia. He noticed that when his friends were intoxicated by the ether they sustained bruises without apparently feeling pain, and he thought of using it to suppress pain in surgery. It so happened that one of these friends, James Venables by name, developed a small tumor on the back of his neck. Long saw this as a chance to test his idea and persuaded him to allow it to be excised under ether. On the evening of March 30, 1842, in his office, before a group of friends, Long etherized Venables with a towel soaked with the drug, and excised the tumor. The experiment was entirely successful. Long fully realized what he had found, and although he hesitated as yet to report his discovery to the medical world in writing, he told his medical friends and his neighbors enthusiastically about it. They ridiculed him. He faced this criticism by trying to test his discovery more thoroughly. He needed a chance to carry out a major operation under ether, but such opportunities came rarely to a general practitioner, and during the next four years he was able to perform a total of only eight minor operations with it. In all, pain was abolished. In a Negro boy who had to have two fingers amputated, he removed one finger under ether and the other without it, with the obvious results.

Then one evening late in 1846, while reading the December number of the *Medical Examiner,* he came across an announcement of Morton's discovery of anaesthesia in Boston. Long still waited three years more before publishing his own account of his use of ether in the *Southern Medical and Surgical Journal.* Although the Georgia Medical and Surgical Association in 1852 passed a resolution naming him the discoverer of anaesthesia, Long received little or no credit during his lifetime. He was a southern gentleman not given to publicity, and the life of a busy practitioner occupied him fully. He did not enter into the bitter controversy waged before Congress in the fifties between Morton and his rival New England claimants for priority, except to write a single letter to his own congressman stating the simple facts of his discovery.

The Civil War and the period of hatred of the South that followed it, blotted out Long's claim to fame. He survived the war, and continued the useful life of a country doctor. But he always felt he had been cheated of credit for his priority in the use of ether. He died suddenly in 1878 while attending an obstetrical case.

William Thomas Morton was a Boston dentist puzzling over the problem of how to pull teeth painlessly when he became interested in ether. There is no clear record as to how he came to think of ether after having tried a variety of other drugs to deaden pain. When he married in 1843, he promised his bride's parents to give up dentistry for medicine, and to this end became an apprentice to Dr. Charles T. Jackson, a well known Boston physician and chemist, who later claimed to have suggested the use of ether to his pupil. Be that as it may, Morton, once having got the idea into his head, kept at it through every discouragement. He tried ether upon goldfish, bugs, and dogs, and finally forced *himself* to inhale it to the point of partly losing consciousness. Finally, in the summer of 1846, he began to give it to patients for tooth extractions. He had difficulties because some of his patients reached only the excitement stage of anaesthesia and became unmanageable, but on the whole he was successful. The *Boston Daily Journal* reported his discovery, and finally Dr. Henry J. Bigelow, surgical chief at the Massachusetts General Hospital, came to Morton to inquire. It should be noted at this point in the story that Morton had carefully concealed the fact that the drug he was using was ether. He had no humanitarian aims in his search: he intended to patent his discovery and make a fortune out of it. He did not allow even Dr. Bigelow to examine the drug, for fear he might discover it was merely ether and steal the idea.

This aspect of the discovery was, of course, distasteful to Dr. Bigelow, but it is a tribute to his common sense and that of his associates at the Massachusetts General Hospital that they nevertheless invited Morton to give a demonstration of his pain-killing drug. This took place on Friday morning, October 16, 1846, in the surgical amphitheater of the hospital. An attentive surgical gallery watched Professor John Collins Warren excise a tumor of the neck, while the patient slept. The operation completed, Dr. Warren turned to the audience and made his famous statement, "Gentlemen, this is no humbug."

In the next few days Morton was asked to administer his drug for a series of operations, including an amputation of the thigh. There was no doubt that the discovery was genuine. Morton now faced a dilemma. The surgeons demanded to know the nature of the drug, which they strongly suspected to be ordinary ether, and Morton dared not reveal it if he intended to patent it. He filed his patent papers and told them that it was ether. Thereupon Oliver Wendell Holmes coined the word *anaesthesia*, and Bigelow reported the discovery in the *Boston Medical and Surgical Journal.*

With the weight of the surgical opinion of the Massachusetts General Hospital behind it, ether quickly came into use throughout the United States, and indeed throughout the rest of the civilized world. October 16th has since been celebrated at the Massachusetts General Hospital as Ether Day, a day on which the alumni of the hospital gather to honor its fame. And well they may, for it is doubtful if any other hospital has presented a more important discovery than that of ether to the world.

Morton, unfortunately, got little satisfaction from the discovery. His patent was at once broken, and he became involved in a tangle of litigation over the patent rights. Both Dr. Charles T. Jackson, his former teacher, and Dr. Horace Wells, a former dental partner, claimed a share in the discovery and a congressional investigation failed to get at the truth of the matter. Morton lost his dental practice and his mental balance as a result of all this.

He refused to give up the hope of making a fortune out of his discovery. But for gifts from friends and scientific groups, he would have starved. Finally, in July, 1868, while in New York making a frantic effort to prove his right to his discovery, he died of a cerebral hemorrhage, penniless and unhonored.

In retrospect it is clear that the unfortunate man deserved full credit for bringing the value of ether before the world, even though he was anticipated in his discovery by Crawford Long.

In England ether anaesthesia was taken up by the Professor of Midwifery at Edinburgh, James Y. Simpson. He, however, was not satisfied that ether was the best drug for the purpose, and set out to look for something better. He shortly discovered the anaesthetic power of chloroform and began to use it with success in his obstetrical practice. He became a violent protagonist for chloroform anaesthesia, not only in obstetrics but in all forms of surgery where anaesthesia was required. Almost single handed he forced its adoption in the British Isles.

The unfortunate aspect of Simpson's work was his choice of chloroform rather than ether. Deaths occurred of course from the injudicious use of both anaesthetics, but it did not take long to accumulate evidence which clearly indicated that while chloroform induced anaesthesia more quickly and easily than ether, it was more dangerous to the patient. In the United States, where both ether and chloroform were used, the greater safety of ether soon became apparent. John Collins Warren in a paper written in 1850 collected reports of eighteen deaths from chloroform and warned against it. Its use was soon generally abandoned in America.

In these early days of anaesthesia there was one man, however, who realized the need of attacking the problems of anaesthesia experimentally. He was John Snow, of whom we have already written in discussing cholera. In 1846 when ether anaesthesia was introduced, he was beginning practice in London, and being impressed by the serious difficulties encountered in anaesthesia, he turned his full time to it, becoming the first specialist anaesthetist. He did much experimental work, laying the foundations of our modern scientific knowledge of anaesthesia. He wrote the first textbook on the subject. Snow fully realized the dangerousness of chloroform, but gave it instead of ether because the surgeons preferred it.

In England, and indeed throughout most of Europe, however, chloroform has continued to be used, even up to the present time, despite the fact that physiologists have long since proved that it must be regarded as a dangerously toxic substance, unsuited for use as an anaesthetic. It not only depresses the heart, but it causes damage to the liver and kidneys which may later cause death.

Local anaesthesia was the next step in the evolution of anaesthesia. Various methods of dulling pain locally, such as applying pressure or freezing with ethyl chloride, had been used without much success. Cocaine was the first substance found to have an inherent and powerful pain-inhibiting action. It is the active principle of the leaves of the coca plant, *Erythroxylon coca*. These leaves, mixed with leaves or ashes, are chewed extensively by the natives of Peru and other South American countries. The drug was isolated chemically as early as 1855, and its power of producing numbness when applied locally to the tongue noted in 1862 by the Viennese pharmacologist Karl Ritter von Schroff. It was not until twenty years later, however, that cocaine was suggested as a local anaesthetic. The man who was responsible was none other than Sigmund Freud, who has achieved notoriety by discovering sex for our generation. His claim to fame for calling the attention of his colleagues at the General Hospital in Vienna to cocaine is sound, however. He did it in a rather general paper on the drug read in 1884. One of his colleagues, a young ophthalmologist, Karl Koller, was the first actually to use cocaine as a local anaesthetic. Taking up Freud's suggestion, he carried out a series of experiments on dogs in 1884, and discovered that he could anaesthetize the eye by simply dropping a one or two per cent solution of cocaine into it. He then used the method for operations on the eye in human beings. The drug quickly came into use among ophthalmologists all over the world. It soon began to be used locally on the mucous membrane of the nose, throat, and larynx, where it was found to give equally satisfactory superficial anaesthesia. Applied on the skin, however, the drug was not absorbed to a sufficient extent to deaden pain. It was therefore injected in dilute solution directly into the tissues where it gave complete anaesthesia in the region injected. Unfortunately, the anaesthesia was of comparatively short duration, although it sufficed for simple operations.

This discovery aroused great interest and experiments were begun everywhere to find new ways of using cocaine. William Stewart Halsted, the great leader of modern American surgery, was then a busy young attending surgeon to the Roosevelt Hospital in New York, having just returned from two years of contact with German surgery. He took up the study of the use of cocaine in the autumn of 1884, shortly after Koller had published his method of using the drug in the eye. Working with his associate, R. J. Hall, Halsted soon showed that injection into the trunk of a nerve produced anaesthesia of the whole region supplied by the nerve. In this way large areas of the body could be anaesthetized. One of the first applications of this method was to block the nerves to the teeth. There was a tragic side to Halsted's discovery. At this early date no one knew that cocaine was a habit-forming drug, and before they realized it Halsted and his associates had become addicts. Several of them were utterly ruined and died in pathetic circumstances. Halsted, with superhuman will power, overcame the addiction, although it cost him more than a year's time to do it.

Another New Yorker, J. Leonard Corning, soon afterwards discovered another important method of obtaining anaesthesia with cocaine. He was a neurologist, and undertook the study of the effect of the drug on the spinal nerves. In 1885, while injecting it into the spine of a dog, hoping that it would travel along the spinal nerves and influence the spinal cord itself, he pierced the dura (the lining of the spinal cord). The cocaine thus mixed with the spinal fluid, producing transient anaesthesia and paralysis of the dog's legs. Later in the same year Corning successfully produced a similar anaesthesia in a man whom he was treating for a neurological condition. He was not a surgeon and made no attempt to use his method for surgical operations. But he realized that he had discovered a new form of anaesthesia and named it *spinal anaesthesia*. The utilization of the method had to await the development of a practical technique for withdrawing fluid from, and injecting substances into, the spinal canal. This was done by Heinrich Quincke of Kiel, who was working with hydrocephalus. The final step in the development of spinal anaesthesia was then taken by the surgeon, August Bier of Berlin. On August 16, 1889, he injected 3 cc. of a 0.5 per cent solution of cocaine into the spinal canal of a man whose foot he had to amputate, and obtained good anaesthesia. Before publishing the method, Bier and his assistant Hildebrandt both took spinal anaesthesia themselves. The method was taken up widely in France and in the United States, but its wave of popularity was soon checked by the occurrence of occasional fatalities.

It was not until the chemists unraveled the chemical structure of cocaine, and were able to synthesize less toxic derivatives of it, that spinal anaesthesia came into its own. A satisfactory compound was finally made by A. Einhorn and his associates at Munich in 1905, and was called novocaine or procaine. It soon replaced all other cocaine derivatives. Spinal anaesthesia has now come to assume an important place in the anaesthetic armamentarium, and in some clinics is used for the majority of operations on the legs and lower abdomen. A serious handicap of this form of anaesthesia, namely its short duration, has recently been overcome by the practice of giving repeated small doses. Thus a continuous spinal anaesthesia which can be kept up for a number of hours has been achieved.

There have been equally important improvements in general or inhalation anaesthesia during recent years. The most fundamental improvement has been the development of the so-called closed system of administration. Ether used to be given by dropping it in an open cone held over the patient's face, but nitrous oxide and oxygen, gases sometimes given alone or supplemented with ether, had to be conducted through a closed system of tubes to a mask fitting tightly over the face. It therefore became desirable to give all inhalation anaesthetics through a closed system, which had the further advantage of enabling the anaesthetist to measure accurately by means of meters the proportions of the various gases used. The use of such a closed system necessitated the development of an apparatus that would satisfactorily absorb the carbon dioxide in the air exhaled by the patient, and add oxygen as required, to the air inhaled. Professor D. E. Jackson of Cincinnati devised such an apparatus for anaesthetizing laboratory animals in 1915. Dr. Ralph M. Waters of the University of Wisconsin was a pioneer in applying this principle in clinical anaesthesia.

He began in 1921 to use a complicated closed apparatus which he has simplified and improved until it, or modifications of it, have come into general use in American hospitals. This closed method enables the anaesthetist to control the vitally important carbon dioxide-oxygen ratio in the patient's respiratory passages with a degree of exactitude hitherto impossible, and to add anaesthetic gases in any desired concentration. Anaesthesia can in this manner be carried on for a much longer time and much more safely than formerly. It is not unusual nowadays for surgeons to operate for as long as four or five hours with this kind of anaesthesia.

Recently several new anaesthetic gases have become popular. The best known of these is ethylene. Its anaesthetic effect has been known since 1864, but its clinical use was first made practical as the result of intensive laboratory and clinical experiments done by Professor Arno B. Luckardt of the University of Chicago during 1922 and 1923. Cyclopropane is another anaesthetic gas recently developed. Both of these gases are in general superior to ether, but they have one disadvantage which has not yet been overcome. They are so highly explosive that despite elaborate precautions a few fatal accidents have occurred with them.

Still another form of anaesthesia which has recently been perfected is intravenous anaesthesia. As long ago as 1872 a French surgeon, Louis-L.-G. Oré of Lyon, produced general anaesthesia by the intravenous injection of an anaesthetic drug. He used chloral hydrate. This was not, however, a satisfactory agent for the purpose. Many of the new synthetic sedative drugs that chemists developed in such large numbers during the first part of our century were tried intravenously, but for one reason or another they were all found to be unsuitable.

The first drug that was found to be comparatively satisfactory for producing general anaesthesia by the intravenous route was N-methylcyclohexenylmethyl barbituric acid, or *evipal* as it was known by its trade name. It was developed in 1932 by the German chemist Hellmut Weese, in the pharmacology laboratory of the *I. G. Farbenindustrie* at Elberfeld. It belongs to the general class of barbiturates, the largest as well as the most valuable class of synthetic sedative drugs. The original sedative of this class, called barbital or *veronal* was developed in 1903 by Emil Fischer, the great Berlin physiological chemist. He called it veronal after Verona, the most restful place he had ever known. Evipal has the special property of producing quickly a deep, quiet sleep which lasts but a short time, just the kind of anaesthesia that the surgeon often desires. Another drug, *pentothal sodium*, closely related chemically to evipal, has a similar action, except that it is more potent. These two barbiturates have recently been used intravenously on a large scale in several American and German clinics to supplement other methods of anaesthesia, and, for certain types of cases where anaesthesia of short duration only is required, they have been used alone. It is as yet too soon to know what place in the anaesthetist's armamentarium these drugs will eventually take.

THE

CONQUEST OF SURGICAL INFECTION:

LISTER AND HIS FOLLOWERS

ALTHOUGH PAIN had been banished from the operating room, the specter of infection still remained in pre-Listerian days. Erysipelas, pyemia, septicemia and hospital gangrene were endemic in most surgical wards. No patient was safe from these dread complications. As late as 1872, W. S. Wylie, describing conditions at Bellevue Hospital in New York, wrote: "I saw, while on duty in the wards, patients die from septic diseases contracted in the wards after the slightest surgical operations or injuries. From forty to sixty per cent of all amputations of limbs proved fatal."

The man who changed all this was Joseph Lister. Lister was born near London in 1827 of a Quaker family. His father, Joseph Jackson Lister, as an amateur student of science, made important discoveries in optics which led to the production of the achromatic microscope lens and the evolution of the modern microscope. Joseph thus grew up in a fortunate home atmosphere, and was given the best medical education available, at University College in London. He next went to Edinburgh as assistant to James Syme, the professor of surgery, whose daughter he later married. Syme was one of the great surgeons of his day. Under his tutelage Lister matured as a surgeon, and also carried out important research concerning inflammation and blood coagulation.

At the age of 33, Lister went to the University of Glasgow as Professor of Surgery. There, as surgeon to the Glasgow Royal Infirmary, with 80 surgical beds, he faced the responsibility for the frightful consequences of wound infections. Almost all operative wounds became infected. Of the amputations, which constituted almost 20 per cent of all operations, about 40 per cent were followed by fatal infections.

Seeking for a solution of this paramount problem, Lister became interested in 1865 in Pasteur's work. He was particularly impressed by Pasteur's demonstration that organisms that produce fermentation and putrefaction are carried on particles of dust in the air. Assuming such air-borne germs to be the cause of wound infections, Lister decided to try to prevent infection by excluding the air from wounds with a dressing containing a material capable of destroying the floating particles. His colleague, Dr. Thomas Anderson, the professor of chemistry, provided him with crude carbolic acid for this purpose. With it Lister made his first antiseptic dressing in March, 1865. The case was a compound fracture of the leg, the sort of wound which previously had almost invariably become infected, often with fatal results. He washed the wound out with the carbolic solution, and applied a piece of lint soaked with the solution over it. Healing was astonishingly good and Lister was encouraged to try this method in other cases. By March of 1867, he was able to report a total of eleven cases of compound fracture treated by the antiseptic method, with nine recoveries, one amputation, and one death. This was an unprecedented result.

In the meantime Lister had begun to apply his new method to operative wounds such as amputations. They healed so well that he dared to cut his ligatures short in the depths of his wounds, rather than leaving them hanging from the wound as had been the custom, so that they could be pulled out during the period of suppuration that almost inevitably ensued.

In April, 1867, he was able to write: "Since the antiseptic treatment has been brought into full operation . . . my wards, though in other respects under precisely the same circumstances as before, have completely changed their character, so that during the last nine months not a single instance of pyemia, hospital gangrene, or erysipelas has occurred in them." Lister was only 40 when he wrote these words.

The antiseptic doctrine did not have a sympathetic reception in England. It was attacked particularly by Sir James Y. Simpson of chloroform fame, who saw in the doctrine only a method of using carbolic acid, quite overlooking the fundamental underlying discovery that infection in wounds was due to germs which could be excluded and destroyed by proper handling of the wound. Lister nevertheless went ahead with his experiments to improve his method. After a while he stopped using undiluted carbolic acid to purify recent wounds because he found that it caused superficial sloughing. A five per cent watery solution proved to be strong enough for his purposes.

He next discovered a method of preparing antiseptic catgut by soaking it in liquefied carbolic acid and oil, that made it absorbable and relatively sterile. He tied the carotid artery of a living calf with catgut prepared in this manner, and when the calf was killed a month later he found the catgut gone, and the site of the ligature occupied by a ring of tough fibrous material. From his Christmas holiday in 1868 to the end of his active life, Lister was constantly experimenting and improving his ligatures at a cost in sheer labor that cannot be adequately appreciated.

The Anti-Vivisectionists, who exerted a powerful influence in England during this period, repeatedly attempted to prevent Lister from continuing his important animal experiments. But even in the face of a personal appeal from Queen Victoria herself that he condemn vivisection, he did all that he could to foster it, and testified before a Royal Commission that his discovery of absorbable catgut could not have been made without it.

Lister's continued efforts to avoid air-borne infection led him in 1870 to begin spraying the air of the room in which an operation or dressing was being done, with a 1:40 solution of carbolic acid. This was a trying ordeal for the surgeons because the carbolic vapor numbed their hands and sometimes poisoned them badly.

English surgeons in general remained hostile to Lister's doctrine. Some of them gave the antiseptic method a perfunctory trial and then dismissed it. The rigors of the carbolic spray did not help Lister's cause. As late as 1880 in all the British Isles there were only one or two clinics where his methods were used. Never was a prophet less honored in his own land.

But abroad, particularly in the German university clinics, Lister's methods were promptly and thoroughly tested, his results duplicated, and his discovery confirmed. Carl Thiersch, professor of surgery at Leipzig, began to use Lister's methods in 1867, with the result that hospital gangrene was abolished in his large clinic. In 1870 the brilliant Richard Volkmann returned from the Franco-Prussian War to his professorship at Halle, to find his hospital full of wounded soldiers, with pyemia and erysipelas rampant. All his efforts to improve conditions failed, and he thought of closing the hospital. Then in November, 1872, he tried Lister's method. Infections disappeared like magic and he became one of Lister's most vigorous proponents. Professor J. N. Nussbaum at Munich was the next important convert. In his hospital at Munich gangrene had developed in no less than 80 per cent of all wounds. In 1875 he began to use Lister's methods and within a short time gangrene, pyemia and erysipelas disappeared. In 1875 Nussbaum wrote a little book describing his experience, which was widely read and translated and helped to spread Listerism on the Continent. This was the first presentation of Lister's doctrine in book form. Lister himself never wrote a book.

These German surgeons not only adopted Lister's methods of controlling surgical infections, but they greatly improved upon them. Between 1880 and 1890 they developed the essentials of our modern aseptic technique, which are quite different from Lister's antiseptic methods. They were able to do this because bacteriological research was making great advances in Germany in these years, and provided exact methods for solving the wound infection problem. Lister, in Britain, lacked such expert bacteriological assistance.

This new bacteriology had been begun by Robert Koch, as we have said before. While practising in the little town of Wollstein, Germany, Koch carried out fundamentally important experiments in which he studied and classified the bacteria in artificially produced infections in mice and rabbits. By staining the bacteria with aniline dyes, he was able to distinguish them clearly. His findings were presented in a small but epoch-making book, *Untersuchungen über die Aetiologie der Wundinfectionskrankheiten* (Studies of the Etiology of Wound Infections) which appeared in 1878. This work won him fame and a place in the government service as a bacteriologist. Koch realized that the greatest handicap to progress in classifying bacterial disease was the lack of a method of isolating the different strains of bacteria and growing them in pure culture. In 1880 he solved this problem with the invention of the poured plate method for culturing bacteria, in which solid gelatin provided a transparent and solid surface on which bacteria could be grown in single colonies.

With this method bacteriologists were able, in the course of a few years, to identify the chief bacteria responsible for infections in operative and traumatic wounds, and to work out methods that would prevent their entry into wounds. Much of the work was done in Ernst von Bergmann's surgical clinic at the University of Berlin. There, in 1883, Friedrich Fehleisen proved by inoculation experiments on both animals and human beings that streptococci were responsible for erysipelas. Others worked out the role of staphylococci in wound infections. It was found that the bacteria present in the air were, for the most part, harmless. The dangerous, or so-called pathogenic bacteria, were conveyed to wounds by the hands of surgeons and nurses, or by instruments or dressings. Studies of the comparative efficacy of different methods of destroying bacteria showed that most of the chemical antiseptics were unreliable. The carbolic acid that Lister relied on to sterilize his hands, instruments, and dressings, failed to destroy ordinary bacteria if they were clumped together and enclosed in fatty or albuminous matter. Even 1 to 1,000 corrosive sublimate was ineffective under these conditions. The spores of certain bacteria were found to be even more resistant. Twenty-four hours' exposure to 5 per cent carbolic was required to destroy anthrax spores, for example. Koch himself took an important part in these studies, and he deserves the credit for showing that heat is much the best method of destroying bacteria.

Hugo Davidsohn, working in Koch's laboratory, proved in 1888 that boiling for five minutes was sufficient to destroy all bacteria and spores. In von Bergmann's clinic, therefore, chemical antiseptics were for the most part abandoned, and sutures and instruments were sterilized by boiling them in water to which a little soda to prevent rusting had been added.

The problem of disinfecting the patient's skin and the operator's hands had of course to be solved some other way. Lister simply dipped his hands in strong carbolic, and began operating. When Carl Eberth, the professor of bacteriology at Zurich, showed in 1875 that the skin fairly teems with bacteria, which hide in the glands in its depths and come to the surface in perspiration, it was obvious that a better method of sterilizing the skin had to be found. Hermann Kümmell, in the surgical clinic at Hamburg, proved that thorough scrubbing with soap and water, using a good brush, was more effective than any chemical antiseptic. Furbinger, in von Bergmann's clinic, demonstrated the importance of mechanically cleaning beneath the fingernails.

All of these practices were soon adopted in most German clinics. In 1892, Carl Schimmelbusch, one of von Bergmann's assistants at Berlin, wrote a book, *Anleitung zur aseptischen Wundbehandlung* (The Aseptic Treatment of Wounds) in which the new aseptic technique was fully described. The chief emphasis was on meticulous mechanical cleanliness of everything that came into contact with the patient, rather than upon disinfection with chemicals. Instruments and all material brought into the operating

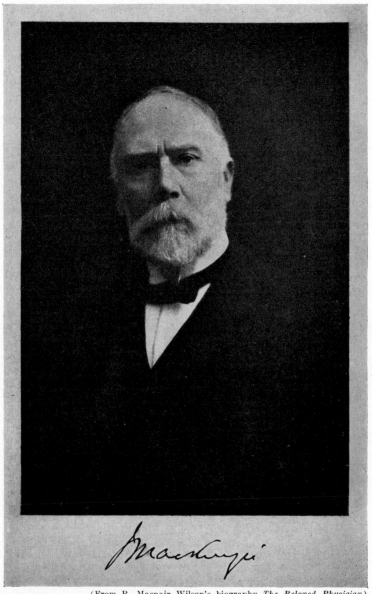

(From R. Macnair Wilson's biography *The Beloved Physician*)

Sir James Mackenzie

While doing general practice he carried out clinical research of great and lasting value.

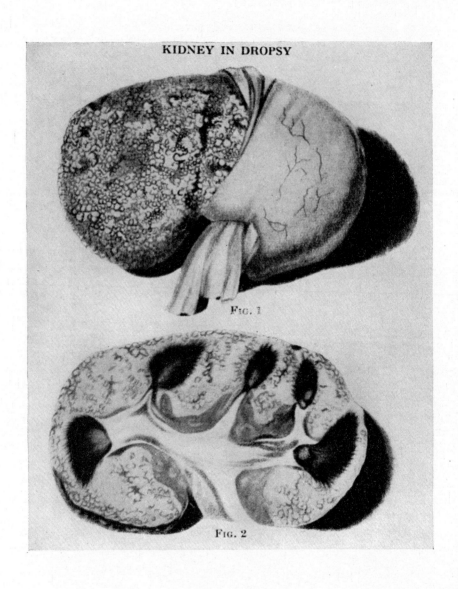

KIDNEY IN DROPSY

Fig. 1

Fig. 2

Bright's Disease

Bright's great work on the kidney was illustrated by excellent lithographs, "executed under his own immediate superintendence." Figures 1 and 2 from Plate III, reproduced here, show the gross appearance of the kidney in chronic nephritis.

room were sterilized by boiling or by steam. The operators and nurses scrubbed their hands and arms with soap and water a specified length of time. They then donned sterile gowns. The patient's skin was similarly prepared and draped with sterile coverings. Wounds were dressed with simple absorbent gauze, which had been sterilized by steam. This is essentially our present day technique, with the exception of a few details which we will refer to later.

Despite the triumph of Lister's doctrine in Germany, his methods spread but slowly throughout the world. His house surgeons who saw for themselves what he achieved were his most influential disciples, and of course there were not many of these. Dr. Archibald E. Malloch of Hamilton, Ontario, who served as Lister's house surgeon in 1868, brought Lister's teaching back to Canada and used it with success. Dr. David W. Gandell of Louisville, Kentucky, treated a series of 30 cases with Lister's methods in 1869. Dr. Henry O. Marcy of Boston spent the summer of 1870 with Lister in Edinburgh and on his return attempted to introduce Lister's technique in Boston. Henry I. Bigelow, the distinguished surgical chief at the Massachusetts General, tried it in a perfunctory way, and failing to obtain results, dropped the method.

In 1876, when Lister toured the United States, and described his method at the International Congress of Medicine in Philadelphia, he found almost no one using it, and encountered strong opposition from many surgeons. At the Congress he spoke for two and one-half hours explaining his doctrine. As a result of this exposition, Drs. W. H. Van Buren and Stephen Smith, in New York, and W. W. Keen in Philadelphia, began to use his methods, but they were not able to make much impression on their colleagues. As late as 1883, in a discussion of a paper on Lister's doctrine before the American Surgical Association, leading surgeons from many parts of the United States almost without exception condemned his methods, saying that they had tried them and had no success with them. The truth was, of course, that they had not tried them out with the requisite attention to detail and so they failed. The late J. M. T. Finney, one of America's most distinguished surgeons, wrote a revealing description of the "antiseptic" technique carried out in the operating rooms at the Massachusetts General when he was a house officer there in 1888. The surgeons, when they operated, donned black Prince Albert coats which were covered with spots of dried blood and pus. The instruments, all having wooden handles, were either soaked or wiped off in carbolic solution, or else no attempt at all was made to sterilize them. The wounds were sponged with sea sponges, used over and over again.

It remained for younger American surgeons who had learned something of the new science of bacteriology and had seen Lister's methods succeed in Germany, to make them work in America. Prominent among these was William S. Halsted, who returned to New York in 1880 after two years in German clinics. In his work at Bellevue and Roosevelt Hospitals, he followed Lister's technique and did much to establish its principles in New York. Halsted gave publicity to Schimmelbusch's book when it appeared in 1892, and adopted sterilization by heat at Johns Hopkins, where he was then Professor of Surgery. Hunter Robb, an associate of Howard A. Kelly, the distinguished chief of the gynecology clinic at Hopkins, where this aseptic surgical technique was rigorously followed, wrote a little book describing it in 1895. This excellent presentation of the subject was the first in English, and it had an important influence.

Rubber gloves were also introduced by Halsted. At Johns Hopkins, in 1889, the nurse in charge of his operating room, Miss Caroline Hampton, complained that the solution of mercuric chloride, in which the hands were rinsed following scrubbing, caused dermatitis. Since, as Dr. Halsted stated in an explanation of his concern for Miss Hampton's hands some years later, she was an unusually efficient woman, he went to New York and got the Goodyear Rubber Company to design a pair of rubber gloves for her. These proved very satisfactory, and soon their advantage from the viewpoint of protecting the patient from infection became obvious and everyone wore them. Since Dr. Halsted and Miss Hampton were married shortly after this glove episode, it would appear that this discovery, certainly one of the most important means of avoiding wound infections, was not entirely the result of scientific zeal.

Another important item of the surgeon's paraphernalia, the face mask, was introduced in 1896 by Johann von Mikulicz. His colleague at Breslau, the bacteriologist Flügge, had proved that even during quiet speech droplets containing pathogenic bacteria are sprayed from the mouth into the surrounding air. Flügge suggested that these droplets might be a cause of wound infection, and von Mikulicz devised a face mask to overcome this danger. It was a simple gauze band that covered the mouth and nose. It was some years before surgical masks were generally adopted, but their employment is now known to be an important part of the aseptic ritual, for numerous instances have come to light where unmasked surgeons with sore throats or colds have infected their patients' wounds. In von Mikulicz's time the mask had one important additional advantage: it restrained the flowing beard which surgeons of that day usually wore.

The last country to grant recognition to Lister was his own. Although he was given honorary degrees by both Oxford and Cambridge in 1880, and was made a baronet in 1883, British surgeons continued to doubt the obvious facts of his conquest of wound infection. It was not until 1890 that he was praised in *The Lancet,* that bulwark of British medical opinion. By that time the majority of his colleagues had been converted. Halsted summed up the matter when he said that America learned antiseptic surgery from Germany, and England learned it from America.

Viewed from the perspective of a generation that takes aseptic surgery for granted, and sees the surgeon with modern aseptic technique invade every part of the body, Lister becomes one of the giants of medical history, worthy of rank with such men as Virchow and Pasteur. Although his antiseptic methods have all been superseded by better ones, he slew the dragon of wound infection. His followers have merely picked the dragon's bones.

The problem of wound infection is not yet wholly solved, but progress is being made. Infections continue to occur despite the elaborate technique used to prevent them. In hospitals where the problem is being seriously attacked, however, encouraging improvement is seen. At the Presbyterian Hospital in New York, for instance, the total percentage of all infections in clean operative wounds (including both trivial and serious infections) has fallen from 14 per cent in 1925 to 2.6 per cent in 1939. This improvement has been achieved by increasingly careful attention to details of aseptic technique that have been well known for at least twenty-five years. The recent discovery of new and incredibly efficient bactericidal agents—the sulfonamides—may soon make it possible to banish wound infection almost entirely.

THE CONTROL OF HEMORRHAGE

WITH PAIN and the danger of infection overcome, the surgeon of fifty years ago was almost ready to begin his modern conquest of disease. One serious operative hazard remained—that of hemorrhage.

The surgeons of earlier days, as we have already shown, were to a large extent limited to opening abscesses and amputating limbs. In amputations bleeding had to be controlled, for in most cases several vessels of large caliber are cut across. The tourniquet was invented in 1674 by Marel at the siege of Besançon, and solved the problem of temporary control of bleeding. During the following century ligatures for the larger vessels began to come into general use, the vessels being caught with a hook or a crude kind of artery forceps and tied with strong waxed thread of silk or linen. The surgeon of pre-anaesthetic days operated very rapidly, for every moment prolonged the patient's agony. Many were so skillful as to be able to complete a major amputation in as little as four or five minutes. Under these circumstances there was time to tie only the largest blood vessels. Bleeding from the smaller ones was absorbed by the compression dressing.

When anaesthesia freed the surgeon in terms of time, these slapdash habits of operating persisted. But as soon as aseptic technique made it possible for surgeons to operate within the abdomen, they had to begin to work more carefully and deliberately, for a single mistake in dealing with the vitally important viscera might be fatal. The first requisite in this new kind of surgery was gentleness in the handling of these delicate internal tissues. The second requisite was complete control over bleeding. The surgeon had to be able to make his field of operation entirely dry of blood, so that he could see what he was about, and so that there would be no subsequent internal hemorrhage. For this purpose more delicate artery clamps, and ones that would lock tight, were necessary. Jules Péan of Paris and Spencer Wells of London, both pioneers in ovariotomy in their respective countries, devised improved hemostats for use in clamping vessels and popularized their use. Péan invented his clamp in 1862 and Wells invented his in 1872. Both instruments closely resembled the large-sized 6-inch curved hemostat in use today, having ring handles and a ratchet lock.

When in the 1870's and '80's the pioneers in abdominal surgery began to venture to do extensive procedures upon the stomach, bowel, and other viscera, they made increasing use of these new hemostats. William S. Halsted, a leader in the new hemostasis, summed up his experience in his *Operative Story of Goitre*, as follows: "On my return from Germany in 1881 I was impressed with the fact that our surgeons were greatly handicapped in most of their operations by lack of proper instruments, particularly of artery clamps. These were insufficient in number and design. . . . Rarely had I seen in our country, prior to my first visit to Europe (1879) more than one artery clamp at a time left hanging in a wound. Clamps were too few for this—four to three or even two being considered ample for an operation. Few hospitals, in New York at least, possessed as many as six artery clamps in 1880. I recall vividly an operation in Vienna performed by Mikulicz in 1879 in Billroth's clinic. Americans, newly arrived in Austria, were greatly amused at seeing perhaps a dozen clamps left hanging in a wound of the neck while the operator proceeded with his dissection, and were inclined to ridicule the method as untidy or uncouth. Slowly it dawned upon us that we in America were novices in the art as well as the science of surgery."

Halsted, in 1878, designed a new hemostat to meet his own

high standard of hemostasis. It was smaller than previous hemostats, and with the fine point that Halsted finally designed for it, had the important advantage of grasping a small vessel more exactly, without including a large bite of the surrounding tissues. This hemostat, now generally called the "Halsted" clamp, is today the standard instrument in clinics where the best surgery prevails. It is not unusual to use several hundred of these clamps in an extensive operation. These clamped vessels, later tied with the finest silk or catgut, are no hindrance to wound healing.

But the control of bleeding itself has not been the only advantage of this kind of surgical technique. Halsted wrote in this regard: "The artery forceps, adequate in number and design, undoubtedly played a very important role in the strikingly rapid progress in the art of operating made by surgeons, the world over, in the final quarter of the past century. The value of the artery clamps is not likely to be overestimated. They determine methods and effect results impossible without them. They tranquillize the operator. In a wound that is perfectly dry, and in tissues never permitted to become even stained by blood, the operator, unperturbed, may work for hours without fatigue. The confidence gradually acquired from masterfulness in controlling hemorrhage, gives to the surgeon the calm which is so essential for clear thinking and orderly procedure at the operating table."

We have already told how a type of hemorrhage occurring in jaundiced patients, and hitherto presenting one of the most serious hazards of operation in these cases, has been recently shown to be due to a lack of Vitamin K. There is every prospect that further advances in our knowledge of the chemistry of blood coagulation will be made, bringing the surgeon ever nearer to his goal of bloodless surgery.

SURGERY GROWS UP

THE MOST IMPORTANT CONQUESTS

OF MODERN SURGERY

To ILLUSTRATE the enormous development of surgery during the last fifty years, it is interesting to compare the figures for the numbers and types of operations performed today with those of fifty years ago. In the Presbyterian Hospital in New York in the year 1889 there were a total of 130 beds. Ninety-seven of these were for patients with surgical diseases. During that year a total of 402 operations were done. These included:

          86 for incision of abscess
          20 amputations
           1 for appendicitis
          11 for hernia
           6 for cancer of the breast

No operations were performed on the thyroid or the gallbladder. The abdomen was opened 32 times. Thirteen of these laparotomies were for the removal of uterine or ovarian tumors. There was not a single instance of removal of a cancer of the gastrointestinal tract. There were 60 deaths, a mortality of 16.5 per cent.

In 1939, fifty years later, when the total number of beds in the Presbyterian Hospital and its private wing, Harkness Pavilion, was 587, the number of ward beds for general surgery was 128. Urology, ear, nose and throat, and gynecology and obstetrics were now separate services. The total number of operations performed on the general surgical service during 1939 was 3,259. These included:

60 incisions of abscess
23 amputations
245 for appendicitis
249 for disease of the gallbladder
245 for hernia
294 for thyroid disease
60 for cancer of the breast
144 for cancer of the stomach and bowel

The total number of deaths was 68, a mortality of 2.1 per cent.

These figures show that the most frequent operations of the old era, incisions of abscess and amputations, now form an inconsequential part of the surgeon's work. The enormous growth of surgery has been chiefly concerned with new kinds of operations, most of them for internal diseases. The surgeon has learned to attack disease in almost every part of the body, sometimes under the most trying conditions. We have no space here to describe in detail what he has accomplished. But since almost one half of the modern surgeon's work is made up of the six most frequent types of operations which we have listed above, we will give some space to each of them.

APPENDICITIS

Even though our grandfathers never heard of appendicitis, it would be incorrect to regard appendicitis as a new disease. All that has happened is that the modern surgeon has learned how to recognize it and what to do for it.

When, in the 18th Century, physicians began to make careful autopsy studies of internal disease, reports of what we now know to have been inflammation of the appendix began to appear. In most of these cases the inflammation had gone on to the point where the appendix had burst and an abscess formed around it, or there was severe infection of the whole peritoneal cavity. It was no longer apparent that the disease had begun in the appendix, and the condition was called perityphlitis, meaning inflammation of the region of the cecum. The early stages of appendicitis continued to remain a mystery for a long time to come, for surgeons in those days could not open the abdomen in the living to learn what was wrong. The various abdominal conditions causing vomiting and pain were thus all hopelessly confused.

But as is so often the case in the history of the development of knowledge, there were a few great minds who saw the light ahead of their time. In 1812, James Parkinson, the London physician whose name we associate with the first description of paralysis agitans, wrote a good account of a fatal case of appendicitis in a boy of five. At autopsy a piece of hardened feces was found impacted in the inflamed appendix. It had caused obstruction, perforation, and generalized peritonitis. In 1827, a young Parisian physician, François Mélier, wrote an article on appendicitis that showed remarkable understanding. He described five cases of acute appendicitis, and also a case of late appendicitis in which a large abscess had formed around the cecum and appendix. Mélier grasped the fundamental fact that this kind of abscess resulted from acute inflammation and perforation of the appendix. He even suggested that if the diagnosis of appendicitis could be definitely established it might be possible to operate! For his time this was indeed a bold and prophetic suggestion.

It was many years before operation was practised, and then at first it was attempted only in the late cases in which an abscess had formed. The credit for this innovation belongs to Willard Parker, professor of surgery at the College of Physicians and Surgeons in New York. In 1843 he successfully diagnosed and incised and drained an appendiceal abscess in a colleague of his, Dr. T., of Brooklyn. By 1867 he had operated upon three more similar cases, with success in all. He therefore concluded that surgical drainage was indicated in such cases, and that it should be done after the fifth and before the twelfth day of illness. He had learned to recognize appendicitis in its early acute stage, but either it did not occur to him to operate at this stage and remove the appendix or he did not dare to attempt it in those early days of abdominal surgery.

Parker's recommendation attracted some attention, particularly in New York, and during the next twenty years "Parker's operation," as it was called, was done in sporadic cases without any real advance in the understanding of appendicitis being made. Then, in 1886, Reginald Fitz, of Boston, presented his masterly study of the disease, which cleared up the confusion regarding its nature and placed its diagnosis on a firm foundation of fact. Fitz, after graduation from the Harvard Medical School in 1868, and an interneship at the Boston City Hospital, went to Germany to study, like so many other young men of his time. There he came under the influence of the two great founders of modern pathology, Carl Rokitansky of Vienna and Rudolph Virchow of Berlin. When he returned to America after two years, he had a good knowledge of the gross and microscopical appearance of disease, and an appreciation of the fact that progress in the understanding of disease must come through correlation of clinical and pathological findings.

Fitz began teaching pathology in Harvard Medical School and was given charge of the pathological laboratory at the Massachusetts General Hospital. It was there that he made his keen studies of appendicitis, following the manifestations of the disease both in the wards and in the autopsy room. The fundamentally important point that Fitz grasped was that several conditions developing in the right lower abdomen and known as typhlitis, peri-typhlitis, and perityphlitic abscess, were merely different manifestations of the same underlying pathological condition, namely, inflammation of the appendix. He therefore called the disease appendicitis, the name by which it has been known ever since. Fitz clearly outlined the symptoms as well as the pathology of the disease, and concluded from the 466 cases he studied that operation was the proper treatment and that it should be done much earlier than Parker had recommended.

Stimulated by Fitz's teaching, surgeons now began to diagnose cases of appendicitis correctly, and to operate upon them and remove the inflamed appendix. This was first done successfully in 1887 by Thomas G. Morton of Philadelphia and by Henry B. Sands of New York. In both of their cases, however, the disease had advanced to the stage where the appendix was found at operation to be perforated. Sands became much interested in the problem of diagnosing appendicitis in an earlier stage, and during the year 1888, he succeeded in making the diagnosis and removing the inflamed organ before perforation had occurred in several cases.

Although Sands' untimely death occurred during the same year, his assistant, Charles McBurney, carried on his important studies of appendicitis at Roosevelt Hospital. It was McBurney who, in 1889, defined anatomically the special area in the right lower part of the abdomen which is specially tender in many cases of appendicitis, and which has since been known as McBurney's point. It lies "between an inch and a half and two inches from the anterior spinous process of the ilium on a straight line drawn from that process to the umbilicus." McBurney described the symptoms and signs of early appendicitis with great accuracy, and emphasized the necessity of immediate operation.

This teaching was quickly accepted and successfully applied by a number of prominent American surgeons, including Maurice Richardson, John Homans and E. R. Cutler of Boston, Nicholas Senn and J. B. Murphy of Chicago, and J. M. Baldy of Philadelphia. After 1890 appendectomy became a common operation.

The basic principles of the diagnosis and treatment of the disease have not undergone much change since then. As the public has become familiar with the fact that abdominal pain and vomiting may mean appendicitis, and has learned to call a doctor and abstain from taking cathartics which aggravate the disease, and as surgeons have learned that immediate operation is essential, the mortality from appendicitis has steadily fallen. Under proper circumstances, the death rate following operations for appendicitis today should be less than one per cent.

It is a sad fact, however, that such ideal circumstances do not always exist. There were in the United States during the last registration year for which mortality figures are available (1936) a total of 16,480 deaths from appendicitis. This is a mortality rate of 12.8 per hundred thousand. The conclusion is inescapable that the great majority of these deaths were preventable, and that they were due to ignorance on the part of both the public and the medical profession.

GALLBLADDER DISEASE

Stones in the gallbladder, and some of their sequelae, were well known to the early anatomists and pathologists, who found them in great variety in the bodies that they dissected. Since modern studies have shown that between 20 and 25 per cent of all adults have gallstones, and that probably an equally large proportion of adults have inflammatory changes in the gallbladder without stones, it is not surprising that medical men have long been aware of gallbladder disease.

As long ago as 1863, a London physician named J. L. W. Thudichum wrote a book on the subject containing many of the essentials of our modern knowledge of the form and variety of gallstones, the pathological changes resulting from them, and the clinical signs of their presence. He knew that many people with gallstones have no symptoms at all from them, that some are troubled by rather vague indigestion, while a few experience the attacks of terrible colicky pain in the right upper part of the abdomen which result when stones formed in the gallbladder become lodged in the duct leading from it to the intestine, or when the gallbladder becomes acutely inflamed. Thudichum knew the fatal consequences of rupture of the distended gallbladder, and of gallstones blocking the main (or common) bile duct, thus preventing the flow of bile from the liver to the intestine and causing jaundice. But all that he could do for these evils was to administer opium or choloroform for the pain of the acute attack, and send his convalescent patients to Vichy or Karlsbad to be purged in the hope that their gallstones would finally pass through the bile duct into the intestine. Surgeons of his day had begun to attempt such simple lower abdominal operations as the removal of ovarian cysts, but they dared not attack lesions in the more vital upper portions of the abdomen.

The first instance of incision and drainage of a distended gallbladder, indeed, was done under the mistaken impression that the tumor was an ovarian cyst. The operator was John S. Bobbs of Indianapolis: the date June 15, 1867. The tumor filled the right side of the abdomen. Bobbs opened the peritoneal cavity and incised the cyst-like tumor. Clear fluid (retained bile) and many gallstones escaped. The opening in the gallbladder was then closed and the patient recovered.

Eleven years later, in 1878, Marion Sims, the great American gynecologist, correctly diagnosed a distended gallbladder and deliberately drained it. This operation, to which Sims gave the name cholecystostomy, now began to be done with increasing frequency. The English ovariotomist, Lawson Tait, by 1885 had done it fifteen times. One of the earliest of these operations in America was done by William S. Halsted under particularly trying circumstances. In 1881, when he was but 29 years old, and had just begun his surgical career in New York, he was called to see his aged mother in Albany. He found her very ill, jaundiced, and with a tumor and great tenderness in the region of the gallbladder. Halsted recognized that cholecystostomy was the only thing that would save her life, and since none of the distinguished consultants who saw her dared attempt it, he decided to carry it out himself, even though he had never before done the operation. In the middle of the night in his mother's home he operated upon her, incised the gallbladder, which was found distended with pus, and extracted seven stones. Mrs. Halsted was much improved, but her symptoms recurred and she finally succumbed to the disease after two years. Years later Halsted described the details of this first operation of his on the gallbladder before the Johns Hopkins Hospital Medical Society, without indicating that the patient was his mother.

This recurrence of symptoms has proved to be the great disadvantage of mere drainage operations on the gallbladder. Follow-up studies have shown that symptoms persist or recur in about half of the cases. When patients are very ill it is often impossible to attempt anything more than cholecystostomy, but surgeons gradually came to realize that a better method of treatment must be found.

Carl Langenbuch, surgical chief at the Lazarus Hospital in Berlin, was the first to dissect out the gallbladder and its duct, thus removing the focus of infection and stone formation. This was in 1882. He realized that this operation (cholecystectomy) was preferable because it was much more likely to achieve permanent cure, and he urged others to attempt it. Langenbuch's German colleagues took up the operation, and by 1890 the distinguished Swiss student of gallbladder disease, L. G. Courvoisier, professor of surgery at Basel, was able to collect reports of 47 cholecystectomies in his important book on gallbladder disease. Cholecystectomy began to be done by the leading abdominal surgeons in England and America a few years later, and has steadily gained favor since. Today it is the operation of choice for gallbladder disease, and its technique has been so much improved that its mortality has been reduced to around two per cent.

The problem of stones obstructing the common bile duct was a more serious one, for surgical manipulations of this vital and delicate structure are more difficult and dangerous. Courvoisier, in 1890, was the first to incise the duct and extract stones from it successfully. The Americans, Halsted and McBurney, soon added important technical improvements to the operation, and urged exploring the common duct whenever there were signs of its being obstructed. This procedure gradually won recognition, and today has become one of the most important resources of the surgeon operating on the biliary tract.

HERNIA

Hernia, the protrusion of an intra-abdominal structure through a point of weakness in the abdominal wall, was an unsolved problem until fifty years ago. The most frequent type of hernia, the groin or inguinal hernia, incapacitated many a stalwart man, and all that surgeons could do was to fit the patient with a truss which pressed upon the hernia opening and kept the hernia from protruding. Nevertheless the hernias at times came out, or, to put it more correctly, down through the inguinal canal, and could not be put back. Such incarcerated hernias, if they contained intestine, were often accompanied by intestinal obstruction which led to death.

In the 16th Century, daring surgeons such as Pierre Franco and Ambroise Paré began to operate upon such extreme cases, opening the hernial sac, enlarging the ring of the opening in the abdominal wall, and replacing the intestines within the abdomen. Between 1803 and 1807 the great English surgeon, Sir Astley Cooper, published his beautifully illustrated works on hernia, in which all the essentials of our modern clinical and anatomical knowledge of the disease is embodied. They contained nothing, of course, regarding the operative repair of hernia, because before Lister's antiseptic methods made abdominal surgery safe, surgeons dared not attempt such elective operations.

When, in the 1870's, the era of abdominal surgery began, many surgeons attempted to cure hernias. Several types of operations were used. The simplest consisted of merely cutting down on the hernial sac (i.e. the layer of peritoneum which constitutes the innermost covering of a hernia), ligating it, and excising it, without any attempt to repair the defect in the abdominal wall. Auguste Socin, professor of surgery at Basel, reported a series of 75 such operations in 1888, claiming favorable results. A more

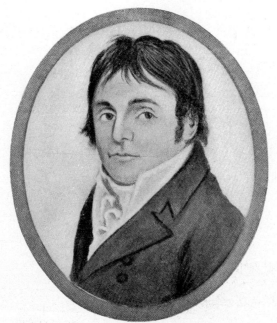

(From M. T. Valentine's
Biography of Ephraim McDowell)

A Medallion Portrait of McDowell Painted
When He Was a Student in Edinburgh

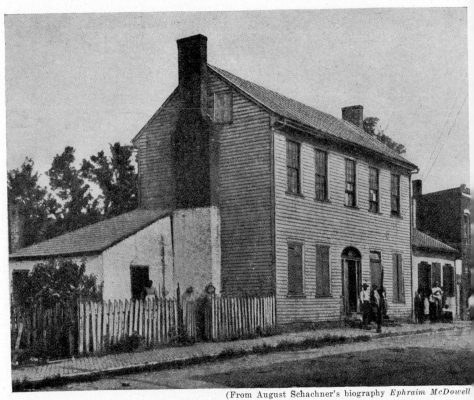

(From August Schachner's biography *Ephraim McDowell*

The House in Lexington, Kentucky, Where McDowell
Performed the First Ovariotomy

ambitious method of hernia repair was devised in 1878 by Vincenz Czerny, then professor of surgery at Freiburg. This consisted of ligating and excising the sac at its neck, and attempting to repair the defect in the abdominal wall by suturing its outer edges (the pillars of the external ring of the inguinal canal) together in a very simple manner.

Credit should go to William T. Bull, professor of surgery at the College of Physicians and Surgeons in New York, for showing that neither of these methods was much good. In 1890 he reported the follow-up results in a series of 134 hernia operations he had performed. After from one to four years, 40 per cent of the patients operated upon by Socin's and by Czerny's methods had recurrence. Bull concluded that these results did not justify operative attempts to cure hernia, and he advised the use of a truss. The majority of his contemporaries agreed with him.

This was the state of affairs in 1889, when Eduardo Bassini, professor of surgery at Padua, and William S. Halsted at Johns Hopkins, independently of each other, devised an operation that does cure inguinal hernia. Although their operations differed in some details, they both included the same fundamental feature, namely, wide incision and exposure of the whole length of the hernial rent, dissection and excision of the hernial sac, and careful sewing up in layers of the muscles and fasciae of the abdominal wall. Halsted and others subsequently devised certain improvements in the operation, such as special ways of overlapping the flaps of muscle and fascia in order to add to the strength of the repair. This operation today can be done with a mortality of less than one per cent, and the recurrence rate probably varies between 5 and 10 per cent. It has restored countless men to an active working life who in earlier generations would have remained truss-bound invalids.

GOITER

It was just a little over one hundred years ago (1836) that T. W. King at Guys' Hospital in London saw and described for the first time the elementary units of which the thyroid gland is composed—the follicles, filled with a translucent material called colloid. As the result of a long series of clinical and experimental studies, we now know that this gland secretes and supplies the body with a hormone which is of vital importance to body economy. This hormone was isolated and identified as an iodine-containing compound in 1915 by the American chemist, E. C. Kendall, who called it thyroxine. It was subsequently (1927) synthesized by the London chemists, C. R. Harington and G. Barger. Our knowledge of the physiology and chemistry of the thyroid is intimately bound up with the story of the surgeons' efforts to remove safely enlargements of the thyroid—so-called goiters.

There are certain regions of the world where a large proportion of the inhabitants, both human and animal, have goiters. The incidence is highest in mountainous regions, but it is also considerable in certain non-mountainous regions, such as the Great Lakes district of the United States, the plains of Lombardy, and the southwestern counties of England. It has become clear that the one feature that these goiterous regions have in common is a low concentration of iodine in the soil and drinking water.

When the body lacks iodine in youth, the thyroid gland hypertrophies and forms the so-called simple goiter. This was proved in 1920 by David Marine of the Montefiore Hospital in New York, who has made many important contributions to our knowledge of the thyroid gland, and his associate, O. P. Kimball of Cleveland. For experimental purposes they divided the school children of Akron, Ohio, where about half of the young people develop simple goiters, into two groups. To one group they gave a small amount of iodine. With this treatment only a very few of the children developed goiters, and in many of those who had them they decreased in size. The children of the control group who did not receive iodine went on to develop goiters with the usual frequency. When those who have developed the so-called simple goiters in youth reach adult life, their goiters may become nodular, and form tumors which have to be removed surgically because they are unsightly or because they grow so large that they interfere with breathing. Iodine is of no help with goiters of this kind.

The history of surgical attempts to deal with these tumors, which was carefully traced by Halsted, goes back to the 16th Century. Even after the advent of anaesthesia, fear of hemorrhage deterred surgeons from operating on goiter, for the thyroid is one of the most vascular organs of the body. The bolder ones, nevertheless, persisted. Between 1850 and 1877 some 190 operations were done, with a mortality of almost 20 per cent. Most of these patients died of sepsis.

The surgical conquest of goiter is due in large degree to Theodore Kocher, who, in 1872, at the age of 31, became director of the surgical clinic at Bern, Switzerland. The high incidence of goiter at Bern gave him an unusual opportunity to study the disease. Lister's methods had just been adopted by Kocher's Swiss, German, and Austrian colleagues, and the specter of infection in operative wounds banished. Kocher, who was a master technician as well as a keen thinker, devised new methods for obtaining satisfactory surgical exposure of the thyroid, for controlling hemorrhage, and for avoiding damage to the nerves of the larynx. In 1883 he reported his first ten years' work, a total of 101 goiter extirpations, with a mortality of 12.8 per cent. In this famous paper he not only described the essential features of the modern technique for removing thyroid adenomas, but he identified a new clinical condition which he called *cachexia strumipriva*. All but two of a series of 18 patients in whom he had removed the entire thyroid, developed a syndrome characterized by lethargy, puffiness of the face, dryness of the skin, etc. Kocher rightly concluded that this was due to a lack of thyroid secretion.

This condition, which today goes by the name of myxedema, had first been described in 1874, as it occurred spontaneously in adults, by the London clinician, Sir William Gull. He correctly regarded it as analagous to cretinism in childhood. It was not until

1891, however, that George R. Murray of Manchester, England, proved that myxedema could be relieved by the administration of an extract of sheep's thyroid. Since then dried extract of the thyroid gland has proved to be helpful in a variety of conditions in which there is a deficiency of thyroid secretion.

Kocher, in the meantime, had made further progress in thyroid surgery. By 1895 he was able to report that he had operated upon more than 1,000 cases of goiter. In the 900 cases done since his 1883 report, the mortality was only a little over one per cent. His success was so striking that German and Austrian surgeons quickly adopted his methods, and added further improvements to the operation. Halsted and C. H. Mayo brought Kocher's methods to America in the late 80's. The former not only did important experimental research regarding both the parathyroid and thyroid glands, but perfected the technique of the operation that is done today throughout the world.

There is another type of thyroid disease in which surgery has proved to be of great value. This is hyperthyroidism, often called exophthalmic goiter because protrusion of the eyes is a prominent symptom. This disease was first described by Caleb H. Parry, a clinician in Bath, England, in 1828. It is often referred to as Graves' or Basedow's disease, because of the descriptions that these men wrote of it some years later. In this disease the thyroid becomes enlarged and produces an excess of secretion, which causes a toxic state characterized by irritability, palpitation of the heart, loss of weight, weakness, sweating, and exophthalmia.

Patients with hyperthyroidism take an abnormally large amount of food and still lose weight. The Marburg clinician, Friedrich Müller, in 1893 first offered a satisfactory explanation for this paradox. He concluded that the thyroid hormone speeds the burning up or oxidation of food in the body, increasing the rate of metabolism. More oxygen is consumed, more carbon dioxide produced. In 1895, Adolf Magnus-Levy of Frankfurt proved by measuring the rate of gas exchange in the air breathed that this increase in oxidation rate actually occurs. The American chemist, F. G. Benedict, in 1918, developed a practical portable apparatus that measures these gas exchanges with a high degree of accuracy. This determination, called the basal metabolism test, has come to be the most reliable laboratory method of estimating the degree of thyroid activity, and is of great help to clinicians.

In hyperthyroidism iodine has a temporarily favorable effect. This fact was discovered accidentally by the great Parisian clinician, Armand Trousseau, in 1863, when by mistake he prescribed iodine rather than digitalis for a young woman with acute hyperthyroidism. Nevertheless, iodine was little used for the disease until after 1923 when H. S. Plummer of the Mayo Clinic clearly showed the great advantage of supplementing surgical treatment with a preliminary course of iodine therapy.

Surgical excision of a part of the hyperactive thyroid, the best treatment yet found for hyperthyroidism, was developed for the most part by the same German and Swiss surgeons who developed the successful methods of treating nodular goiter. Since the surgery of hyperthyroidism is more hazardous, it developed more slowly. Von Mikulicz, in 1885, was the first to perform a partial removal of both lobes of the thyroid for hyperthyroidism—the prototype of our modern operation. By 1900 he was able to report a series of 18 operations with a mortality of 5.5 per cent. In America, William S. Halsted and C. H. Mayo took up the operation about the turn of the century and soon proved its value. By 1908 the latter had operated upon 234 cases of hyperthyroidism with a mortality of 6 per cent.

As time has gone on, a better understanding of the altered physiology in this disease, and refinement of operative technique, have reduced the mortality to only a fraction of what it was. Indeed, if operations for all forms of goiter are taken together, a mortality of less than half of one per cent is well within the limits of reasonable attainment today. When it is recalled that the thyroid is one of the most vascular organs in the body, this is a noteworthy accomplishment, and one of which surgeons may well be proud.

CANCER OF THE BREAST

Cancer of the breast is the second most frequent form of malignant tumor in women, and since the breast lends itself well to surgical removal, surgeons from time immemorial have attempted to cure this disease by excision. It is improbable that these crude attempts of ancient times ever achieved cures.

Before Listerism the danger of sepsis in a large wound was so great that surgeons did as limited an operation as possible. The practice was to remove only the part of the breast containing the tumor. The axilla, where the lymph nodes are situated to which cancer of the breast often spreads, was not entered except when it contained obviously enlarged nodes. We know today that this kind of an operation could have had little or no chance of success. This was fully recognized by the surgeons of pre-antiseptic times, and most of them therefore advised against operation. The two leading surgical text-books of the day, that by Adolf Bardeleben of Greifswald (1865) and that by Sir James Paget of London (1870), both contained the statement that cancer of the breast could not be cured by operation.

Another deterrent to surgical attempts to cure cancer was the belief that the disease was a generalized and multi-centric one from the beginning. On this basis, it was argued that it was of no use to remove one focus because other primary and wholly independent foci would inevitably appear. The German surgeon, Carl Thiersch, and the German anatomist, Wilhelm Waldeyer, proved by careful microscopical studies that this conception of the origin of cancer was wrong, that it begins as a single primary focus, and that if this is removed completely, as is often possible, complete and permanent cure can be obtained. They showed that when cancer appears in distant parts of the body, these are so-called *metastases* from the single original primary focus, i.e., small groups of cancer cells which have broken away from the primary focus and spread through the lymphatic and blood vessels. Thiersch proved this for skin cancer in 1865, and Waldeyer in

Thiersch proved this for skin cancer in 1865, and Waldeyer in 1872 showed that it was also true for all types of internal cancer, including cancer of the breast.

Armed with the knowledge that cancer of the breast was a local disease, surgeons could now attack it more radically with some hope of cure. Charles H. Moore of the Middlesex Hospital in London was one of the first to recognize this opportunity. In 1867 he advocated removal of the whole breast, together with axillary tissues if they seemed involved, in one piece and without cutting into the tumor. Moore's operation was a considerable improvement over previous methods, but it received little or no attention in England.

In Germany, Richard von Volkmann, the brilliant professor of surgery at Halle, who had introduced Listerism into his country, introduced a similar operation in 1873. He removed the entire breast, together with a wide area of the overlying skin, the fascia covering the underlying pectoralis major muscle, and the axillary lymph nodes. This operation soon became the standard one in German and Austrian clinics. For the first time cures began to be obtained, although they were still few. For instance, in Volkmann's clinic between 1874 and 1878 a total of 200 of these operations was done. Only eleven per cent of the patients were well three years later.

In the United States, Samuel W. Gross of Philadelphia adopted Moore's principles of treatment, and extended them in that he practiced dissection of the axilla in every case. In 1880 he published a book on mammary tumors that became well known.

All of these efforts, however, were far short of the limits to which the surgical attack on the disease could be carried. This final step was made by William S. Halsted, of whom we have written so much. He was uniquely equipped for this task. He had mastered the problems of sepsis and hemorrhage, and his art of gentle and meticulous operating permitted him to carry out dissections that were far more extensive than anyone had attempted before. Realizing the need of being as radical as possible in attacking breast cancer, he began in 1889 to perform an operation which was planned to remove all of the tissues of the breast and axillary region that could be removed with safety. Included were a large area of skin, the subcutaneous tissues and fasciae over a wide area, the entire breast, both of the pectoral muscles, and all of the lymph nodes and interstitial tissues of the axilla. The defect on the chest wall which remained was covered with a skin graft. This operation has not, and probably never will be, improved upon. With this so-called radical breast operation Halsted at once obtained results which far surpassed anything his predecessors had obtained. In the first place, the incidence of local recurrence of the cancer in the field of operation fell to 6 per cent in Halsted's first fifty cases, as compared with 50 to 60 per cent in the German case series in which Volkmann's operation was done. In the second place the frequency of permanent cure was greatly increased. Today it is fair to say that counting all cases, early and late, about one-third are cured, while two-thirds of the early cases can be cured by radical operation.

As time has gone on, it has become increasingly apparent that early diagnosis of this subtle disease is more important as regards cure than anything else. This means that every woman who detects a lump in her breast must immediately consult her physician and that he in turn must at once take steps to *prove* the nature of the lump so that appropriate treatment can be given. There are a variety of harmless tumors of the breast which require only local excision, while even the smallest cancer should be treated with radical operation. In advanced cases of breast cancer the clinical signs are proof enough of the nature of the disease, but in the earlier cases the microscopical appearance of the tumor is the only reliable proof. Surgeons of Halsted's day unfortunately had no method for making a microscopical diagnosis at the time of exploratory operation upon breast tumors. They had to rely upon the naked eye appearance of the piece of the tumor that they removed and although they were very skillful, they sometimes made mistakes.

Biopsy, or the removal of a small piece of the tumor for microscopical examination and proof of its nature preliminary to treatment, has come into use in general surgery only recently. The idea of biopsy was developed by the Berlin gynecologist, Carl Ruge, in 1878. He showed that many early cancers of the uterus could not be diagnosed in any other way. The method was taken up by German gynecologists, and in the early 1890's by Howard Kelly in his newly organized gynecological clinic at Johns Hopkins. Both in Berlin and at Johns Hopkins at about this time the frozen section method of preparing the biopsy specimens was introduced, and its advantages quickly appreciated. By this method, in which the specimen is rapidly frozen with carbon dioxide, a thin section can be cut and stained and mounted on a glass slide within three or four minutes. In this way the pathologist can render an immediate diagnosis, rather than having to wait a week while the section is being prepared in the usual way. Freezing tissues to make quick sections had been developed originally in 1865 by the great German pathologist, Julius Cohnheim.

General surgeons were slow to appreciate the advantages of biopsy in the treatment of tumors. In 1905, L. B. Wilson, pathologist to the Mayo Clinic, began to use the frozen section method for surgical biopsies, and its value was quickly recognized by the Mayos. Their influence has had an important effect in fostering the method in American clinics, where its merit is generally recognized today.

The practical importance of biopsy in the control of breast cancer can scarcely be overestimated, for it provides a method of detecting the early, and curable, cases. There is no longer any excuse for delay in diagnosis and treatment. All that the surgeon has to do is to follow the simple rule of biopsying every tumor of the breast, no matter how small and innocuous it may seem.

CANCER OF THE STOMACH AND BOWEL

About one-half of all cancer develops in the stomach and bowel. Arising thus within the interior of the body where it cannot be seen by the patient, causing definite symptoms in most cases only after it is far advanced, and situated in one of the most dangerous regions of the body from the view-point of the surgeon, this form of cancer presents a problem which is far more difficult than that of breast cancer. Yet progress has been made with it even against these odds.

Resection of portions of the stomach or intestine could not be done, of course, until a satisfactory method of suturing together the cut ends of the digestive tube had been worked out. It is a curious fact that such resections were done experimentally in dogs a long time before they were carried out successfully in human beings. As early as 1810 Daniel K. T. Merrem of Giessen, Germany, searching for a method of treating gastric cancer, resected part of the stomach with success in one of three dogs. He employed the crudest sort of technique and it is amazing that he succeeded at all. Antoine L. Lembert, a Parisian surgeon, carried out experiments on dogs in 1826, which were of fundamental importance. He found in suturing the cut ends of the intestine together that his anastomosis succeeded when the outer, or so-called serosal, surfaces of the bowel were united. All of the methods of intestinal anastomosis since devised have been based on this underlying principle. The method was first used in human beings in connection with wounds of the intestine and in resection of strangulated hernia, for in those days surgeons never opened the abdomen except in an emergency.

When the German surgeons of the 1870's who adopted Listerism began to attempt operations within the abdomen, one of the first problems they attacked was that of cancer of the stomach and bowel. In Vienna, Theodor Billroth, one of the most brilliant surgeons of his time, saw that excision of the cancerous stomach was feasible and set two of his young assistants, Gussenbauer and Winiwarter, to work on the problem of removing part of the stomach in dogs. They did this successfully in 1876. In 1881 Billroth performed the first successful gastrectomy on a human being. Through his work with gastric as well as other forms of cancer, Billroth laid the foundations for the modern surgical attack on the disease.

Billroth was a man of wide interests, but his special love throughout his entire life was music. In Vienna he became a close friend of Brahms, and they exchanged a long series of interesting letters, beginning in 1865 and ending with Billroth's death in 1894. Although the letters dealt chiefly with music they give a picture of the cultural life in Vienna in its great period.

During the next few years many continental surgeons, most of them Germans and Austrians, removed cancers of the stomach. Their results, however, were very discouraging. The American pathologist, William Welch, reviewed them in 1885 and found that in a total of 37 gastrectomies there had been 27, or 73 per cent, operative deaths. Of the ten patients who survived the operation, no one had lived longer than eighteen months. Welch drew the pessimistic conclusion that the disease was incurable.

The surgeons have since proved that he was wrong. Today, some sixty years after gastrectomy was first done, it is being performed with steadily increasing frequency and safety. One large American clinic has reported a total of 127 patients alive and well ten years after resection of gastric cancer. It should not be inferred from this, however, that the cure ratio is satisfactory, for the truth is that only about two per cent of all those who develop the disease are cured of it. This is to a large extent due to the fact that the disease is so far advanced when the patient first comes to the surgeon that resection can be done in only about one out of five cases. The early symptoms of the disease are notoriously vague. The two important diagnostic aids, x-ray examination and gastroscopy, are relatively reliable, but they cannot be applied until the patient develops symptoms which drive him to his doctor. The fact that both of these methods of examination are technically difficult and expensive results in their being utilized less frequently than they should be.

The gastroscope, the most recently perfected aid in the diagnosis of lesions of the stomach, has received much attention of late. The first gastroscope, an angulated, rigid tube provided with mirrors through which it was possible to see the inside of the stomach, was devised by Mickulicz in 1881. In 1932, Rudolf Schindler, of Munich, perfected an instrument with a highly developed optical system which was flexible, and therefore more easily introduced into the stomach. The gastroscope is no doubt helpful in the diagnosis of gastric lesions, but owing to the difficulties mentioned above, it does not solve the problem of early diagnosis.

Once the patient, on the operating table, is found to have a stomach cancer which is early enough to be resected, his chances of cure are considerable. It is a great tribute to surgical technique that the mortality for this difficult operation has steadily fallen, until today it is around 5 per cent in clinics where there are special facilities for it. It has been found with this, as with other particularly technical forms of surgery, that better results are achieved by specialization. Of those who survive the operation, about one in four is cured.

These facts about gastric cancer are a challenge to modern medicine. In the United States registration area, somewhere between forty and fifty thousand persons die from the disease each year. In terms of the magnitude of the problem, the funds available for research in the United States regarding the cause and cure of gastric cancer are ridiculously small, certainly less than a hundred thousand dollars a year. One of the great automobile manufacturers probably spends considerably more in perfecting a new type of carburetor.

Cancer occurs in the small intestine so rarely that it has little practical importance, but it develops in the large intestine (colon) with considerable frequency. The disease is more frequent at the lower end of the large bowel, that is, in the rectum, than in its upper part. It often causes symptoms such as bleeding, constipation or diarrhoea, or obstruction, while it is still in an early enough stage for surgical attack. X-ray examination, and, for the cancers of the rectum, local examination and the proctoscope when skillfully used, are indispensable diagnostic aids which can be relied upon to detect these tumors.

As early as 1844, a Lyonnais surgeon, Jean François Reybard, successfully resected a part of the sigmoid colon for cancer, but there were no further successes until the 1870's when German surgeons adopted Lister's antiseptic technique and began to attempt all sorts of formidable operations within the abdomen. Several of them shortly attempted to resect cancers of the colon, but probably the first to succeed was Vincenz Czerny, professor of surgery at Heidelberg. After several failures, he brought a patient through the procedure alive in 1879. By 1884 a total of eighteen such operations had been done, with eight fatalities.

The next generation saw great improvement in the technique of bowel resection. Innumerable new methods of anastomosing the bowel were developed. The really important advance came, however, from experimental studies carried out on dogs by William S. Halsted at Johns Hopkins. In 1887 in a series of careful experiments he proved that the essential point in suturing the bowel is to include a bit of the submucous layer of the intestinal wall in the suture. This is the one strong and tough layer of the intestinal wall. It is, by the way, the layer of the intestine from which sausage casings and catgut have been made from time immemorial. Until Halsted called attention to the importance of this layer in intestinal anastomosis, surgeons did not even know that it existed.

Another important advance in dealing with bowel cancer has been the development of methods for relieving the obstruction of the bowel that the cancer often produces, before proceeding with resection. This may be accomplished by making an artificial outlet for the bowel through the abdominal wall, a so-called cecostomy or colostomy. Recently a new method of relieving obstruction that can be used with much benefit in certain of these cases has been developed by William O. Abbott of the University of Pennsylvania. This consists of passing a long, thin, multi-channelled tube down from the nose through the esophagus and stomach to the point in the bowel where it meets the obstruction.

All of these advances have combined to make the surgical attack on colon cancer relatively successful. Recent data from leading clinics show that radical resection can be carried out in about half of these cases, with an operative mortality of not more than ten per cent. From forty to fifty per cent of those who survive are permanently cured.

The surgical problem of cancer of the rectum is a more difficult one. Jacques Lisfranc, a brilliant Parisian surgeon of the Napoleonic period, was the first, in 1826, to excise the rectum for cancer. His resection, however, was of very limited extent, carried out through the perineum, that is, from the outside only. The scope of this perineal resection was gradually extended after antiseptic surgery made extensive operations safer. In 1885, Paul Kraske, professor of surgery at Freiburg, introduced a method in which a portion of the sacrum was removed to give the operator better access to the diseased rectum. This operation was widely used for more than a generation. Unfortunately, it had the same defect as other exterior or perineal operations for rectal cancer. The resection was of necessity of such limited scope that recurrence of the disease usually followed. In carefully studied series of cases, the recurrence rate approximated 90 per cent.

William Ernest Miles of London was perhaps the first to realize that a much more radical operation was required, including not only the rectum and anus together with a wide zone of the surrounding tissues, but the pelvic colon and its mesentery as well. It is in this mesentery that the lymph nodes lie to which metastases from rectal cancer often extend. This operation, a truly formidable dissection, had to be done in two parts, the first within the abdomen and the second from the outside through the perineum. It was therefore called the abdomino-perineal method. Miles began to perform it in 1907. A few years later the operation was taken up by Daniel F. Jones of Boston, who did much to demonstrate its advantages in the United States. Gradually surgeons have everywhere come to adopt it, or similar abdomino-perineal methods, for rectal cancer. Today the operation is being done on about two-thirds of all those who come for treatment with rectal cancer. The operative mortality varies from ten to fifteen per cent. More than fifty per cent of those who survive the operation are permanently cured. When it is recalled that the limited operation in use 35 years ago cured less than ten per cent, this is seen to be no mean accomplishment.

SURGICAL SHOCK

As MODERN surgeons, freed from the handicaps of pain, infection, and hemorrhage, have become increasingly bold, attempting the formidable operations that we have described in the previous pages, they have met a new enemy—shock. This is the state of general collapse that may follow any severe injury or wound, either accidental or operative. It is often fatal, and even today remains a serious surgical problem.

In former times military surgeons knew this condition well, for not only were the wounds they saw severe, but the victims often lay neglected on the battlefield for a long time—a combination of circumstances particularly favoring shock. Henri François Le Dran, the great early 18th Century French surgeon who served Louis XIV in the Wars of the Spanish Succession in Flanders, described the symptoms of shock or "commotion," as he called it, in his celebrated 1740 treatise on gunshot wounds. He listed them as numbness, a feeling of heaviness, universal coldness, syncope, and vomiting. Following the custom of his day, Le Dran bled these patients—certainly the worst form of treatment that could have been devised.

It was not until a century later (1826) that the knowledge of the subject was advanced by a remarkable book written by Benjamin Travers, senior surgeon to St. Thomas' Hospital in London. The word shock had not yet come into general use and Travers entitled his work, *An Inquiry Concerning that Disturbed State of the Vital Functions Usually Denominated Constitutional*

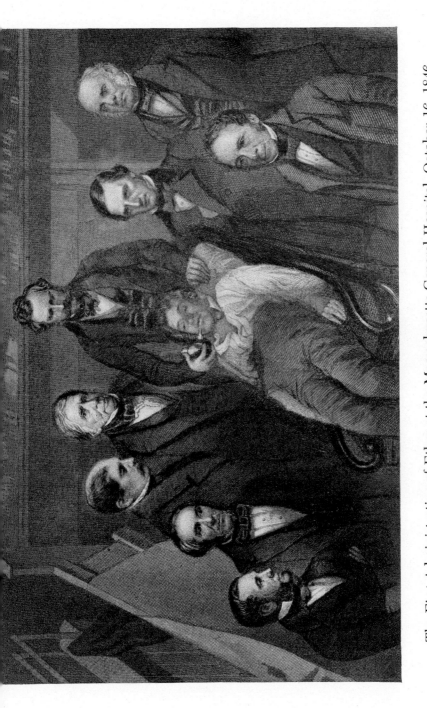

The First Administration of Ether at the Massachusetts General Hospital, October 16, 1846

The artist, who sketched the scene from imagination, included the following (left to right): Henry J. Bigelow, A. A. Gould, J. Mason Warren, John Collins Warren, Morton, Samuel Parkman, S. D. Townsend, and George Hayward.

Irritation. He described with great clarity a long series of cases of shock, most of them fatal, following burns, fractures, severe contusions or lacerations, operations, and hemorrhage. He summed up the symptoms with the following masterly phrases, "universal pallor and contraction of surface, shuddering, very small and rapid pulse, astoundment of the mental faculties, generally a dilated pupil, shortened respiration, dryness of the tongue and fauces; indistinctness, and at length cessation of the pulse at the wrist, stupor, oppressed and noisy respiration, coldness of the feet and hands, involuntary twitchings, relaxation of the sphincters, confirmed insensibility, stertor, and death."

Travers advocated such simple remedies as cordials or brandy in gruel and warned against the blood-letting and purging that were then universally employed. He even suggested blood transfusion, thus anticipating our modern shock therapy by almost a century.

Nevertheless, as late as 1855 we find the great authority on military surgery, G. J. Guthrie, still advocating bleeding for shock in his *Commentaries on the Surgery of the War in Portugal, Spain, France and the Netherlands, from the Battle of Roliça in 1808, to that of Waterloo in 1815; with additions relating to those in the Crimea in 1854–1855.* In this celebrated work (paragraph 344) he tells the story of an officer shot through the chest who developed shock. For this he was bled three times during the first night, and no less than 26 times more during the following fifteen days of his illness! By some miracle he survived both the wound and the bleedings.

With the rapid development of operative surgery in the 1880's and 90's, shock became a problem that surgeons could no longer ignore. It was the predominant factor in the high mortality of surgical procedures of this era. It was soon observed that, in abdominal operations particularly, rough handling of the tissues and prolongation of the procedure were often followed by shock. Important experimental studies of the mechanism of shock were carried out on dogs between 1895 and 1899 by George W. Crile of

Cleveland. He proved that tearing, stretching, and crushing methods of operating, or what he called the *carnivorous* type of surgery, produce shock, and that sharp dissection and meticulous hemostasis, protection of the tissues with warm, moist coverings, and avoidance of too deep anaesthesia, are the important safeguards against it. As time has gone on, the truth of these observations has been amply confirmed.

The First World War, and its terrible toll of injuries, brought the problem of shock acutely to the fore. The physiologists and surgeons of the Allied countries, in particular, attacked it with vigor. As the result of careful clinical studies, it was now proved that a marked fall in blood pressure is the most reliable sign of shock. The peripheral blood vessels become constricted and the rate of blood flow through them is greatly slowed. The volume of blood is reduced by a process not yet fully understood, with the result that the blood is abnormally concentrated. This state of inadequate circulation cannot be tolerated for long by the more vital parts of the body, such as the brain, and death becomes inevitable if the shock is not promptly relieved.

In this period of active study of the shock problem, two predominant schools of thought developed regarding its cause. Walter B. Cannon, the Harvard physiologist, as the result of his extensive clinical and experimental studies, became the chief advocate of the toxic theory. This theory explains shock as due to toxins of some kind derived from the injured tissues. The other school of thought attributed shock to the escape of blood, particularly its fluid part—the plasma—from the blood vessels into the tissues at the site of the injury. This latter theory has gained support during recent years, both as the result of recent experimental work and because it fits so well the clinical observation that the best treatment for shock consists in replacing the lost blood volume by transfusion or by infusion with saline solution. These two forms of supportive treatment have come to be used more and more not only in the treatment of shock, but in other conditions. It is difficult to exaggerate their importance in modern therapy.

The idea of blood transfusion is, however, very old. Soon after Harvey worked out the circulation of the blood, a number of daring physicians began experimenting with the feasibility of injecting various fluids into the blood stream, both in animals and in man. In 1659, Sir Christopher Wren, the celebrated English architect, who was also a member of the recently organized Royal Society, began such experiments. Johann Sigismund Elscholtz of Berlin published an account of similar ones in 1665. The first transfusion done upon a human being was performed in France, in 1667, by Jean Denys of Montpellier, physician to Louis XIV. The patient was a young man suffering with a severe fever. The carotid artery of a lamb was prepared and inserted into one of the patient's veins. Although this patient had no ill effects from the transfusion, others done during the next few years in England and France were so frequently followed by disaster, as might indeed be expected, that the practice was forbidden in France by the highest court.

For more than a century nothing more was heard of blood transfusion. Then it was taken up again in England. In 1818 James Blundell, physiologist and obstetrician of St. Thomas' and Guy's Hospitals in London, devised a special apparatus consisting of a funnel-shaped receptacle into which was built a syringe that forced the blood along a tube to the recipient's vein. He used this both in animal experiments and to transfuse human beings with human blood.

Although Blundell was unable to show that these transfusions were beneficial, his work stimulated continental physicians to take up the problem. In France and Germany, during the remainder of the 19th Century, transfusions still continued to be done occasionally. In 1876 one writer was able to collect reports of a total of 381 transfusions with human blood, and 154 transfusions with animal blood. There were a considerable number of fatalities recorded, and transfusion did not increase in popularity.

The invention of the hypodermic syringe, with its hollow pointed steel needle, encouraged the development of all types of subcutaneous and intravenous medication. Alexander Wood, an Edinburgh physician, was one of the first to inject morphine under the skin for the relief of pain. He and his contemporaries who began this method of using morphine in the 1830's and '40's administered it either with a needle trochar, or punctured the skin with a lancet and forced the solution into the subcutaneous tissues by pressure with a blunt syringe. In 1853 Wood invented the hollow pointed steel needle which could be inserted through the skin and, when attached to a syringe, made subcutaneous injection of fluids an easy task. It was in the same year that Charles Gabriel Pravaz of Lyon began to treat aneurysms by injecting iron sesquichloride into them, causing coagulation of the blood in them. For this purpose he devised a syringe somewhat similar to that invented by Wood. This syringe quickly came into use throughout the world for subcutaneous and intravenous injection, and was generally known as the Pravaz syringe.

Although the mechanical problem of injecting fluids into the blood stream had been solved, a variety of physiological problems concerning blood transfusion remained. The most important of these, namely the incompatability of animal blood with the human organism was brought to light by Leonard Landois, the distinguished professor of physiology at Griefswald. In a series of experiments, culminating in the publication of his book on transfusion in 1875, he proved that the blood of one species cannot safely be transfused into individuals of another species. This stopped the use of animal blood for transfusion.

But even when human blood was used it sometimes produced serious reactions, and even death of the patient. In 1901, Karl Landsteiner, of Vienna, discovered the cause of these reactions to be substances in the blood which cause the red blood corpuscles to form small groups, that is, to agglutinate, when the blood of one individual is added to that of another. The corpuscles thus agglutinated may undergo hemolysis, that is, they may break up and disappear. This reaction takes place between the serum (the fluid part of the blood after clotting) of one blood and the corpuscles of another.

A few years later, in 1907, Jan Janský, of Prague, showed that human bloods can be classified into four main groups, as regards their agglutinating action upon each other. This classification can be made by means of a rather simple microscopical test. To avoid reactions it was now only necessary to use blood from an individual whose blood group was the same as that of the patient's blood. To make certain of this it has been found necessary, as time has gone on, to cross-match the blood of the donor and recipient directly against each other, but the classification in formal groups is still of value. Recently, Landsteiner and Weiner have identified in blood a new factor, and its corresponding antibody, which is sometimes responsible for hemolytic reactions following transfusion. They have called it the *Rh* factor, because it was discovered through experiments with the blood of rhesus monkeys. It is particularly important in matching blood for obstetrical cases because the mother's blood may have been immunized by the fetus to the *Rh* factor.

It was some years after blood grouping was worked out, however, before technical methods were devised by which the actual process of transfusion could be carried out easily and surely. The great difficulty in this regard was the fact that blood clots very quickly when withdrawn. Crile, who was one of the first modern surgeons to realize the advantages of transfusion, worked out an ingenious method of connecting the donor's artery and the recipient's vein with a cannula, but it was far too difficult and too liable to failure because of clotting to be practical. The first practical method of overcoming clotting was devised by A. R. Kimpton and J. H. Brown of Boston in 1913. They collected the blood directly into a large tube coated inside with paraffin, and then injected it from the same tube into the patient's veins. It was a tricky method, but it worked, and it soon had a wide popularity.

A less capricious method of overcoming clotting during transfusion was worked out during the same year (1913) by the young New York pediatrician Edward Lindeman. Its success depended upon speed and teamwork in the withdrawal and injection of the blood. Cannulas were inserted into the veins of the donor and recipient, and the blood quickly drawn and injected with a battery of a dozen 20 cubic centimeter syringes. This method has become the most popular one among surgeons in the United States. Its youthful inventor was drowned in 1919 at Atlantic City, where he went to deliver an address before the American Medical Association.

In 1914 a new method of avoiding clotting was discovered independently by four different workers, Albert Hustin of Brussels, Luis Agote of Buenos Aires, Richard Weil and Richard Lewisohn of New York. This consisted in the addition of sodium citrate to the freshly drawn blood. This relatively harmless compound prevents clotting entirely, but it probably damages the red blood cells to some extent, a fact which may account for the not infrequent minor reactions following this method of transfusion. This method is so simple, however, that it is the one most widely used throughout the world today.

Recently there has been a tendency to use blood plasma or blood serum rather than whole blood for shock. Plasma is the fluid portion of blood which has been prevented from clotting by the addition of citrate, while serum is the fluid which remains when blood clots. It has been found that both plasma and serum can be given without blood grouping if it is "pooled," that is, if the plasma or serum is collected from a number of donors and mixed together. This avoidance of grouping is a considerable convenience where large amounts of blood are handled. Both plasma and serum seem to be almost as efficacious as whole blood in the treatment of shock. Research is now being carried on to settle this point more definitely, and to determine which of the two is preferable.

The latest development, and one which promises to be of great importance in the treatment of shock under the conditions of modern warfare, is the use of dried or "lyophilized" serum. In 1909, L. F. Shackell, of Washington University School of Medicine at St. Louis, worked out a new method of drying fresh foodstuffs such as meats, fruits, and vegetables. The material was thoroughly frozen and then dried in a vacuum. This process had the advantage of causing a minimum of change in the chemical composition of the materials, which, in addition, could be kept in this way indefinitely. The method was also used by Shackell to dry serum. Modified and improved, it has been designated as the "lyophile" process. It now consists of rapid freezing with dry ice, and dehydration in a high vacuum. When blood serum or plasma is treated in this manner the final result is a yellowish powder which has only a fraction of the bulk of the original blood. Sealed under vacuum it will apparently keep at atmospheric temperature for an indefinite length of time. Thus a warship, for instance, on combat duty in the far Pacific, can be supplied with bottles of such dried plasma or serum which need only the addition of sterile water to make them available for immediate use in treating shock. As a matter of fact our armed forces are now being supplied with large quantities of dried plasma made from blood collected from civilian donors by the American Red Cross.

While blood is certainly the most miraculous of restoratives, simple saline solution has also been of great value in combating surgical shock. The story of the discovery of its usefulness is bound up with the story of cholera, because in that disease the depletion of the body fluids is so striking that there has been a continued search for new ways of restoring them. Thomas Latta, a practitioner of Leith, Scotland, was the first to attempt to replace this lost fluid by the injection of large amounts of saline solution into the veins. In 1832, during the great cholera epidemic that raged through Britain, he gave a desperately ill woman a total of 330 ounces of saline solution intravenously during a 12 hour period. She recovered. The method of treatment was taken up by Latta's colleagues and used with some success. During the next fifty years it was used occasionally both on the Continent and in India for cholera, as well as other desperate conditions, without any clear demonstration of its value.

In 1865, Arnaldo Cantani, professor of medicine at Naples, conceived the idea of injecting saline solution into the subcutaneous tissues rather than into the veins, to combat the concentration of the blood occurring in cholera. He found that he could inject from 1,000 to 1,500 cubic centimeters of fluid in this way over a period of a few hours, and that it was taken up into the blood stream quickly. He called the method *hypodermoclysis*, and it was widely used in the Italian cholera epidemic of 1884. This was the beginning of a method of administering fluids which during recent years has become one of the most frequently employed therapeutic procedures in hospital practice.

The intravenous method of giving saline solution, now generally known as intravenous infusion, was perfected and its great value in shock, hemorrhage, and exhaustion proved by the American surgeon, Rudolf Matas. In 1888, at the Charity Hospital in New Orleans, he began to give slow intravenous infusions in critical cases with striking benefit. In 1910 he evolved the continuous drip method, whereby physiological saline solution, or 5 per cent dextrose solution, were infused at the rate of 40 to 60 drops per minute over long periods of time. With this very slow method of administration toxic reactions were avoided. It became possible to sustain patients over periods of many days by this intravenous route alone, when the gastro-intestinal tract could not function.

It is only during the past decade that transfusion, hypodermoclysis and infusion have come to take their proper place in restorative therapy. Today they are so much used that "blood banks" and "shock rooms" are found in most hospitals. In the present war the treatment of shock is receiving as much consideration as the treatment of the actual wounds. Although much remains obscure concerning the fundamental mechanism of shock, it is fair to say that if it is recognized early, and these restorative measures applied promptly, it can usually be overcome.

THE SURGICAL SPECIALTIES:
OBSTETRICS AND GYNECOLOGY

Dᴜʀɪɴɢ ᴛʜᴇ last fifty years our knowledge of disease, as well as of its treatment, has grown at such a tremendous rate that no one mind can pretend to encompass it all. This is nowhere more evident than in certain branches of surgery, where accurate diagnosis depends not only upon extensive clinical experience of a special kind but upon familiarity with a variety of special instruments of precision such as the laryngoscope, and where the surgical procedures required in treatment are so varied that an adequate experience with them can be acquired only by the surgeons who limit their work to the special field in question.

Thus a whole group of surgical specialties have come into existence, and have been recognized by acceptance as part of the organized medical effort in leading medical schools and hospitals. Included are obstetrics and gynecology (usually grouped together), genito-urinary surgery, orthopedic surgery, neurological surgery, thoracic surgery, ophthalmology and otolaryngology. We shall deal in turn with the history of each of these surgical specialties, beginning with obstetrics and gynecology.

Obstetrics is the oldest surgical specialty, having developed long before the 19th Century. But the obstetrics of those distant times was for the most part done neither by surgeons nor by men; it was done by women who were called midwives. They were ignorant of both anatomy and physiology, and the folklore upon

which they based their practice often did more harm than good
to mother and child. In desperate cases, when the midwife had
failed to deliver the child, a physician was often called in. Thus
the great Renaissance physicians, Ambroise Paré and William
Harvey, both wrote on clinical obstetrics, although they were not
specialists in it. Paré revived and popularized podalic version as
a maneuver for difficult cases. This method of turning the baby
around within the uterus and delivering it feet first rather than
head first had been known before but its merit had not been
appreciated.

The most important advance during this period was the invention of the obstetrical forceps. These consist of two fenestrated
blades, curved to fit the child's head, which lock together and
form a handle at one end. When the mother lacks the power to
expel the child, she can be assisted with forceps. They were devised by a remarkable family of English obstetricians, the Chamberlens, who kept the design of their instruments and their
method of using them a family secret for more than 125 years.
They were probably first used by Peter Chamberlen the Elder,
a few years before the end of the 16th Century. When the last of
the Chamberlens, Hugh Junior, died in 1728, the secret had become known to a number of obstetricians both in England and
France, and the forceps soon came into general use.

A period of rapid development of obstetrics now took place,
centering in the British Isles. Midwives fell out of favor and physicians began to do a larger share of the obstetrical work, for the
forceps provided a new means of delivery the use of which required a high degree of surgical skill. Many of these obstetricians
were men of learning, devoted to anatomy, which was the basis
of surgery in the 18th Century. A landmark in this aspect of obstetrics was reached when William Hunter published his great
classic, *The Anatomy of the Human Gravid Uterus*, in 1774.

The teaching of obstetrics was now taken up in the medical
schools. The first professorship was established at Edinburgh in
1726, and other universities soon followed suit. Many special ob-

stetrical hospitals were founded in Britain during the last half of the 18th Century. The famous Rotunda Hospital in Dublin was established in 1745, and in London the Lying-In Wards of the Middlesex Hospital were opened in 1747, the British Lying-In Hospital in 1749, the City of London Lying-In Hospital in 1750, and the General Lying-In Hospital (now Queen Charlotte's Hospital) in 1752.

In Colonial America the trend toward transference of obstetrical practice from midwives to specially trained physicians followed the British tradition. Most of the better trained American physicians of the period got part of their training in Britain and it was but natural that they should bring back an interest in the new art of obstetrics. The New York Lying-In Hospital was founded in 1791, the Lying-In Wards of the Pennsylvania Hospital were opened in 1803, and the Boston Lying-In Hospital in 1832. The most distinguished American obstetrician of colonial times was Samuel Bard, who was appointed as the second lecturer in Midwifery in King's College, New York, in 1770. His *Compendium to the Theory and Practice of Midwifery* (1807) was the first work on the subject by an American. In 1808 the title of Bard's position was changed from Lecturer in Midwifery to Professor of Obstetrics and Diseases of Women and Children, a change indicative of the assumption of the midwife's role by the specially trained physician.

But before the obstetricians could take their part in the development of modern scientific medicine they had to conquer the same two fundamental problems that held back the surgeons—pain and infection. Until these two specters were banished they could not intervene with safety when nature failed. The obstetricians did succeed in overcoming them—and curiously enough they did it for the most part independently of the surgeons.

In a great measure the credit for overcoming the pain of childbirth is due to the efforts of the Edinburgh professor of obstetrics, James Y. Simpson. In January, 1847, less than three months after Morton had established the value of ether in surgery, Simpson began to use it in his obstetrical cases in Edinburgh. From then onward he was an ardent champion of anaesthesia for childbirth. He was not satisfied that ether was the ideal anaesthetic, however, and soon began to search for something better. Night after night, when his busy professional day was finished, at great personal risk, he would inhale the vapors, one after another, of all the likely drugs which he could obtain. Having failed with the commoner varieties, he tried out the rarer chemicals, but for some time without success. On November 4th, 1847, he tried chloroform, which had been invented by von Liebig as long ago as 1831, but had remained a chemical curiosity. Professor Miller, Simpson's colleague, tells of the evening when Dr. Simpson "with his two friends and assistants, Drs. Keith and Duncan, sat down to their hazardous work in Dr. Simpson's dining room. . . . It occurred to Dr. Simpson to try . . . a small bottle of chloroform. . . . Immediately an unwonted hilarity seized the party—they became bright-eyed, very happy, and very loquacious—expatiating on the delicious aroma of the new fluid. . . . But suddenly there was talk of sounds being heard like those of cotton mills louder and louder; a moment more, then all was quiet—and then crash! On awakening Dr. Simpson's first perception was mental— 'This is far stronger and better than ether,' he said to himself. His second was to note that he was prostrate on the floor and that among the friends about him there was both confusion and alarm."

Six days later Simpson had already used the new substance in several cases and had convinced himself of the superiority and harmlessness of chloroform. This was unfortunate from a scientific standpoint, for he was wrong. But it was certainly fortunate from the viewpoint of propaganda for obstetrical anaesthesia as such, apart from any special anaesthetic agent. Simpson met with great opposition to the use of anaesthesia in obstetrics and he made a brave fight for it.

The opposition was on medical, moral and religious grounds.

First, his critics said that the use of chloroform in childbirth would result in an increased maternal and infantile death rate, and they prophesied hemorrhages, convulsions, pneumonia and palsies. Simpson soon showed, however, that chloroform anaesthesia actually produced a decrease in the mortality of the mothers and the children. The critics then put forward the astonishing argument that pain itself is beneficial. Pain in childbirth was, they said, "a desirable, salutary, and conservative manifestation of life force." Here again Simpson was able to show statistically that pain is a potent contributing cause of shock, and that shock often leads to death. By preventing pain lives were saved.

Simpson was a fortunate champion for anaesthesia in obstetrics because he was personally popular in Britain, and loved argument, into which he threw himself with great vigor and literary skill. His fight was won when Queen Victoria, in 1853, took chloroform for the birth of her seventh child. In 1866 Simpson was made a baronet.

Chloroform has long since been shown to be a dangerous anaesthetic and its place in obstetrics has been taken, in America at least, by a variety of agents. The problem of anaesthesia in childbirth is rather different from that in general surgery. The obstetrician wants in most uncomplicated deliveries only a relatively light depth of anaesthesia, sometimes over a prolonged period, so that the normal contractions of the uterus and the well-being of the baby shall not be too much interfered with.

In America perhaps the most popular form of obstetrical anaesthesia is a combination of several anaesthetic agents. The first part of labor is carried on under small doses of one of the barbital compounds or scopolamine. These are sedatives which dull pain and induce sleep. When the labor pains become more violent, inhalations of nitrous oxide and oxygen, sometimes supplemented with a little ether during the actual delivery of the child, are often given. Many variations of this method are used with success by different obstetricians. Certain it is that because of the skill of modern anaesthetists the prospective mother today need have no fear of the pain that has been the terror of motherhood since time immemorial.

Infection contracted during childbirth, the so-called puerperal fever, became a great peril to mothers as soon as the development of operative methods of aiding delivery, such as version and forceps, made it necessary to introduce fingers and instruments into the birth canal. No sooner had special lying-in wards and hospitals been established than epidemics of puerperal fever began to sweep through them. Alexander Gordon, of Aberdeen, Scotland, was the first to make an important contribution regarding its cause. As a result of his experience with an epidemic in Aberdeen in 1793, he published a treatise in which he pointed out that the disease "seized upon such women only as were visited by or delivered by a practitioner, or taken care of by nurses who had previously attended patients affected with the disease." He included statistics to prove his point, and added that it was a disagreeable declaration for him to make that he himself had been the means of carrying infection to a great number of women.

The same point of view was vigorously put forward in 1843 by Oliver Wendell Holmes of Boston in his famous essay, *On the Contagiousness of Puerperal Fever*. It stirred up violent opposition from his colleagues. They argued that the transmission of the disease by themselves was very improbable, that a doctor who had had a series of consecutive cases of puerperal fever was merely "unlucky." Holmes brought to light the fact that in the practice of one physician sixteen fatal cases of puerperal fever had occurred during one month, and he showed by statistical analysis that there was not one chance in a million million millions that such a series should occur on the basis of chance alone. Holmes wrote: "the facts shall reach the public ear: the pestilence carrier of the lying-in chamber must look to God for pardon, for man will never forgive him," and went on to point the way to remedy this deplorable state of affairs. He advocated that no doctor should attend a woman in childbirth if he had recently had a patient with puerperal fever, or if he had attended post-mortem examinations of such cases. He extended these recommendations to include the nurses, and advised washing and change of clothes both for them and for the physicians.

Holmes's skillful polemic unfortunately made little impression on obstetrical practice. It remained for a Hungarian obstetrician, Ignaz Philipp Semmelweis, to prove the contagiousness of puerperal fever in a practical clinical experiment that could not be ignored. Working in the Allgemeines Krankenhaus in Vienna, he had noticed that the mortality from puerperal fever in the First Maternity Division greatly exceeded that in the Second Maternity Division. The First Division was used for the instruction of students, who came unwashed to the wards from the autopsy room, the Second for the instruction of the midwives who did not attend autopsies. It was not, however, until 1847, when he read the post-mortem report on the body of a colleague who had died of blood-poisoning contracted from a wound sustained while performing an autopsy, that the light suddenly dawned on Semmelweis. The appearances in his colleague's body were the same as those in the bodies of the dead mothers from the First Division. Semmelweiss realized that puerperal fever was a form of blood-poisoning carried to the mothers from the autopsy room by the physicians and students who delivered them.

He proved the truth of this theory by insisting on careful disinfection of the hands of all the physicians and students on the First Division by scrubbing with soap and water and rinsing in chlorine water. The mortality from sepsis promptly fell strikingly. In April, before disinfection of the hands was begun, it was 18 per cent. In July, after it was instituted, it was only one per cent.

Semmelweiss' discovery was at first ridiculed by most of his colleagues. In 1849 he lost his post in Vienna on the grounds that he had been associated with the Rebellion of 1848. He went then to the St. Rochus Hospital in Pest where during the next six years he again demonstrated the truth of his theory of the cause of puerperal sepsis. He disinfected not only the attendants' hands but instruments, syringes, dressings, and even bed pans, with the result that he lost only eight in a thousand of his patients. In 1856 he was given the professorship in the University Hospital at Pest, where his methods were equally successful in stamping out sepsis.

During all these years, however, he had made but two converts among all his colleagues in Europe. He had published nothing, being content to talk of his work. Finally, in 1861, he published his great classic *The Aetiology, Concept, and Prophylaxis of Childbirth Fever,* in which the facts about the causes and means of preventing puerperal sepsis were presented with striking clarity. It is an unfortunate fact, however, that this book made little impression on obstetricians throughout the world. Semmelweiss' life ended tragically in 1865. He developed sepsis and meningitis from a wound in his hand, became insane, and died a victim of the same disease that he had done so much to clarify.

It was not until Lister's methods of preventing wound infection with carbolic acid were taken up and used successfully by continental surgeons that the obstetricians began to give serious attention to the prevention of puerperal sepsis. In 1870, Professor Asger S. Stadfeldt, Director of the University Lying-in Hospital in Copenhagen, began to use Lister's carbolic acid technique for obstetrical deliveries. Ten years later he was able to report that the puerperal mortality had been reduced from 1 in 14 to 1 in 116.

Various forms of antiseptic technique for obstetrical delivery were shortly developed in lying-in hospitals all over the world, with a similar sharp decrease in the incidence of puerperal sepsis. Bichloride of mercury solution became more popular than carbolic acid. The efficacy of bichloride solution was well shown by the experience at the New York Maternity Hospital on Blackwell's Island. About 25 per cent of the women delivered there had been dying from puerperal sepsis when, in 1883, J. Henry Garrigues took charge of the service and introduced sweeping changes. He instituted a strict antiseptic regime, employing soap and water and a 1:2000 bichloride of mercury solution to disinfect the

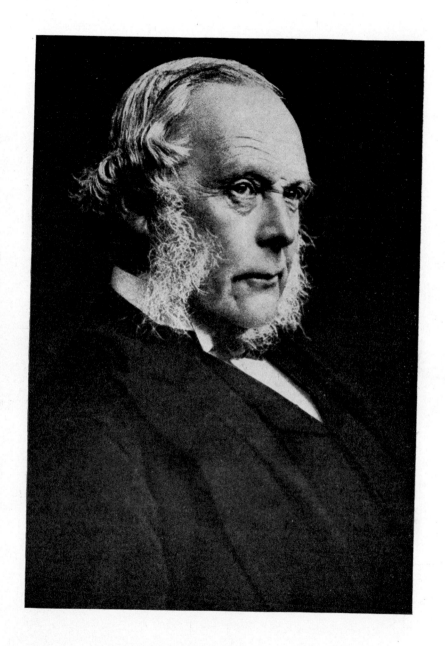

Lord Lister

Despite lack of recognition in his own country, and indeed almost everywhere except in Germany, Lister maintained a serene and lofty attitude which is well shown in his face in this photograph.

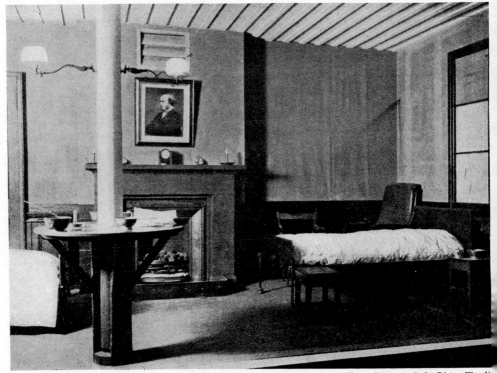

(From *Lister and the Lister Ward*)

Portion of the Lister Ward in the Glasgow Royal Infirmary
Re-erected in the Wellcome Historial Medical Museum

beds, floors, the hands of the attendants, and the patient's vulva and vagina before any manipulation was done. He forbade the patients to have any contact with visitors, or with attendants or students from other wards or the dead house. In three months the mortality rate dropped to zero.

Even after this striking experience the infectious nature of puerperal sepsis was not generally accepted in New York until a serious epidemic in private practice during the following year led to a memorable debate before the New York Academy of Medicine. In this debate the truth was presented so vigorously that the majority were compelled to accept it.

Puerperal sepsis is infrequent today, but it would be wrong to give the impression that it has been entirely eliminated. This ideal has been attained in some hospitals where the highest standard of aseptic technique is practised, but it has not been reached in all. But now that the new sulfonamide drugs have proved so effective in combatting puerperal infection the danger from it is slight. Everything considered it is certainly far safer today for a woman to have her baby in a good hospital than to have it at home.

In the latter part of the 19th Century important advances in the technique of delivery were made. The Parisian obstetrician, Étienne Tarnier, chief at the famed Maternité Hospital, introduced a new type of forceps, which he called the axis traction forceps, to facilitate difficult forceps operating. Friedrich W. Scanzoni, Professor of Obstetrics at Würzburg, also contributed an important maneuver in forceps operating which today bears his name.

Caesarian section, that is, the opening of the uterus and delivery of the child through an abdominal incision, had been occasionally done in desperate cases where all other methods had failed for several centuries, but its mortality rate had been frightful. Incidentally, the operation acquired its name not because Julius Caesar was born in this way but because Roman law or the *lex Caesarea* ordered that the child be removed in this manner from every undelivered mother who died near the end of pregnancy. In 1882, Max Saenger, a Prague obstetrician, made fundamentally important improvements in the technique of the operation, including the use of sutures to close the incision in the uterus. For the first time Caesarian section became safe enough to justify its elective use in certain cases where the pelvic bones of the mother were so deformed that delivery of the child was impossible.

The subject of maternal mortality has been much discussed in the lay press during recent years, and the medical profession has not always been treated kindly. Before drawing any conclusions it is only fair to point out what has been accomplished since physicians began to take over obstetrics from the uneducated midwives. The following table is illuminating:

AVERAGE NUMBER OF WOMEN DYING IN CHILDBIRTH

IN LONDON

In 1680	1 in every	44 delivered
In 1720	1 in every	69 delivered
In 1760	1 in every	77 delivered
In 1800	1 in every	110 delivered

IN ENGLAND AND WALES

In 1840	1 in every	168 delivered
In 1880	1 in every	217 delivered
In 1920	1 in every	231 delivered

These figures make it clear that obstetricians have done a great deal to make child-bearing safer. What troubles us today is that a point seems to have been reached where the improvement is not continuing. For example, in England and Wales, where these data have been recorded with great accuracy, the maternal mortality rate has not been lowered since about 1905. About two-thirds of these deaths are due to puerperal sepsis, and the other third to hemorrhages and other obstetrical accidents. The sulfonamides will of course lower the death rate due to sepsis. But all authorities agree that the most important factor in lowering maternal mortality is proper care of the mother, by a competent obstetrician, during her pregnancy, *before* the baby is born. The public must be educated to realize the necessity for such prenatal care, and to make social provisions that make it available to every prospective mother who cannot afford it.

It has frequently been pointed out that the United States lags behind most of the other nations of the world as to safety in childbirth. The comparisons that have been made have not always been fair, because the methods of computing maternal mortality vary so much in different countries. It is clear enough, however, that the maternal mortality in the United States is higher than it is in most European countries. And it is also apparent that there has been no significant reduction in this mortality during the last 20 years. Authorities agree that this high mortality is due to the too frequent use of forceps and Caesarian section in difficult cases. The latter operation, in particular, is such an easy way out of trouble for the obstetrician that it has been done in as many as 2.5 per cent of the deliveries in some series of cases, with a mortality of as much as 4.1 per cent. This is too much of a risk for a mother to take unnecessarily.

There is of course only one answer to this problem. Better training in obstetrics must be provided for the rank and file of physicians who deliver the great majority of babies. There are some 5,000 graduates of medicine in this country every year and there are only 287 hospital residencies offering a minimum of one year's post-graduate training in obstetrics. This means that only a small proportion of physicians can obtain adequate obstetrical training. The others have no hospital training at all in obstetrics, or at best only the sketchy one or two months' training received as part of a so-called rotating interneship. In obstetrics, as in most other fields of medicine, training and experience pay large dividends in terms of lives saved. Specialization is necessary and inevitable.

Gynecology, or that branch of surgery dealing with female genital disease other than that concerned with childbirth, is a relatively young specialty. Although McDowell performed the first major gynecological operation in 1809, when he removed an ovarian tumor, it was long before surgeons began to specialize in this operation and in the diseases of women. In America, Washington L. Atlee of Philadelphia, and his brother, John L. Atlee of Lancaster, Pa., and in England, Charles Clay of Manchester, began to remove ovarian tumors despite strong criticism, in the 1840's. After these pioneers, Spencer Wells of London became the great ovariotomist of his time, performing one thousand such operations between 1858 and 1880. These operations were done without benefit of antisepsis, and about one-third of the patients died.

But gynecology consists of much more than the removal of ovaries, which by the way was much overdone in the beginning, and the latter half of the 19th Century saw many important contributions to it. The majority were made by Americans. The same Washington L. Atlee who did so much to establish the value of ovariotomy, was the first (1847) to classify properly myomas of the uterus (the common benign uterine tumor) and to advocate their surgical removal. James Marion Sims, an Alabama surgeon, in 1852 worked out a successful method of treating fistula between the bladder and vagina. Becoming vitally interested in gynecology, he came to New York in 1853, and two years later obtained support from a large group of prominent New York citizens for the establishment of The Women's Hospital. This hospital became the center for the development of the new specialty, and many distinguished gynecologists were trained there. The man who was the dominant and the most productive figure in the hospital during these early years was not Sims, but a fellow Southerner, Thomas A. Emmet. Emmet devised several valuable gynecological operations, but perhaps his most noteworthy contribution was his recognition, in 1862, of the importance as a cause of uterine disease of the lacerations sustained in childbirth and the necessity for the prophylactic repair of such lacerations.

When antiseptic methods began to make abdominal operations relatively safe in the '70's, improved methods for the removal of the diseased uterus were worked out. Previously the operation (hysterectomy) had been done only rarely, usually for large my-omas. The technique employed had been to open the abdomen and lift the tumor out to the surface of the wound. The ovarian arteries were then ligated, and the neck of the uterus was trans-fixed with a pin. A strong ligature was then placed around the uterus below the pin and the tumor cut off, leaving the uterine stump in the open wound. This crude operation had a high mor-tality from sepsis and hemorrhage, and it was perfectly futile in cancer of the uterus, which accounts for about one-quarter of all cancer in women. To afford any chance of cure in this grim dis-ease, the entire uterus had to be removed. This had been at-tempted in a few cases but had always ended in disaster.

In this specialty, as in general surgery, German surgeons showed the way. Wilhelm A. Freund, professor of gynecology at Breslau, was the first to devise a rational plan for the removal of the entire uterus in a case of cancer. He carried it out successfully in January, 1878, employing Lister's carbolic technique, and tak-ing two hours for the operation. Adequate exposure of the pelvis was obtained by a lower abdominal incision, and the bowel held up out of the way with towel pads. The uterus was then freed from its attachments by careful dissection and completely removed. The ligatures were led out through the vagina to provide drainage. The cancer, on microscopical study, proved to be the glandular kind that occurs in the body of the uterus. Freund later reported that his patient was still alive and well in 1904.

Unfortunately most uterine cancers develop in the neck, or so-called cervix, of the uterus. It was soon found that even total hysterectomy, as carried out by Freund, was not often successful in curing this form of the disease. About 1900, Ernst Wertheim, professor of gynecology at Vienna, began to do the most radical operation possible, removing not only the entire uterus but dis-secting out the ureters and excising much of the lymph node bear-ing tissue in the pelvis to which cervical cancer spreads. During the early years of this century Wertheim was chiefly responsible for popularizing this hazardous procedure among gynecologists, and for reducing its mortality to a low point of about fifteen per cent. The difficulty with this method of treatment is that it can be used in only a small proportion of the patients that come for treatment, the disease being too far advanced in the remainder.

The next step in the battle against uterine cancer was the introduction of radium. A New York surgeon, Robert Abbe, was the first to use it in cancer of the cervix. In 1903 he purchased 150 milligrams of radium barium chloride, at a cost of $400, from the Curie laboratory in Paris. With this he carried out experiments to determine its effects on germinating seeds, ants, trout, polywogs, and mice, and began to treat a variety of human tumors. In 1905 he reported his result with it in a case of cancer of the cervix. Although these pioneer attempts of Abbe's were interesting, he failed to make any contributions of importance to the clinical development of radiotherapy during the succeeding decade, perhaps because he had no opportunity to organize his work properly. He died in 1928 from anemia, probably due to his prolonged exposure to radiation.

The radiation treatment of cervical cancer developed largely in French and German clinics between 1910 and 1915. Radium won recognition when Krönig and Gauss of Freiburg, Bumm of Berlin, and Döderlein of Munich reported their results with it at the fifteenth congress of the German Gynecological Society in Halle in 1913. They showed that large doses of the penetrating gamma rays from heavily filtered mesothorium produced remarkable cures. Systematic studies of the radiation treatment of cancer of the cervix were shortly begun in many gynecological clinics throughout the world. Although interrupted by the First World War, these studies eventually yielded clear indications of the superiority of radiation treatment for this form of cancer.

The League of Nations has recently collected the results of the radiation treatment of cervical cancer in the leading clinics of the world. In several of them approximately 35 per cent of the cases remained cured five years after their treatment had been given. This is truly one of the miracles of modern medicine.

When we look back over these accomplishments of the gynecologists, one interesting fact stands out. It is that this progress in the treatment of gynecological diseases was made largely on a purely empirical basis, for our knowledge of the fundamental physiology of the female reproductive system has been gained only very recently. Until the discovery of the human ovum in 1832, menstruation was not thought to be associated with ovulation or with the reproductive process. It was only when the 19th Century ovariotomists began to remove ovaries by the wholesale that the profound systemic effects of ovarian secretion began to be known. It was not until 1875 that Oscar Hertwig, professor of anatomy and embryology at Jena, while working with sea-urchin eggs, made the fundamental discovery that fertilization consists in the penetration of the egg of the female by the male sperm, the nuclei of the two uniting to form the nucleus of the fertilized ovum. This discovery is, of course, the basis of all modern studies of heredity.

Our modern concept of the physiology of the menstrual cycle has been developed from studies made in 1903 by Ludwig Fraenkel, a gynecologist at Breslau. Working with rabbits, he showed that a structure made up of ovarian cells of a special type, the corpus luteum cells, which develop from the ovarian follicle after the ovum has been discharged, exercises an important control over the menstrual cycle. This discovery marked the beginning of an era of intense research in this field of medicine, research from which our modern knowledge of the ovarian hormones has developed. Several different hormones have been found to be concerned in the reproductive process. The most important of these, the ovarian follicle hormone, was extracted from hog ovaries in 1923 by Edgar Allen, an anatomist, and Edward A. Doisy, a chemist, working together at Washington University School of Medicine in St. Louis. They carried out fundamentally important studies of the physiological effects of the hormone, and in 1929 Doisy succeeded in isolating it in pure crystalline form. It was now possible to undertake the study of the chemical structure of the hormone. This was finally determined in 1935 as the result of the combined efforts of English, German and American chemists. In 1936 American chemists made the hormone synthetically from ergosterol.

. The corpus luteum hormone was extracted in 1929 by George W. Corner and Willard M. Allen of the University of Rochester School of Medicine, and its physiological effects determined. Two years later this hormone was isolated in pure crystalline form by Fels and Slotta of Breslau. By 1934 several groups of chemists had independently determined its chemical structure.

Another phase of hormone study, namely that concerned with the role that the pituitary gland plays in the reproductive process, was opened up in 1920 when Herbert Evans and Joseph Long of the University of California showed that subcutaneous injections of pituitary extract in young rats caused acceleration of the growth rate and sexual maturity. In 1927 Philip E. Smith, at Stanford University, worked out a method of removing the pituitary gland from the rat. By means of this experimental method a great deal has been learned about the governing influence of the pituitary over ovarian function. A variety of extracts of pituitary hormone have been made, but their chemical structure has not yet been determined.

All of these hormones are now being studied intensely, and it is obvious that much useful knowledge will come from this work. For example, it has been found that the ovarian follicle hormone when injected into male mice will induce cancer of the breast. What bearing this fact has upon the cause of breast cancer in women we do not yet know, but it is entirely possible that it is one of the keys to the etiology of this formidable disease.

GENITO-URINARY SURGERY

SINCE TIME immemorial there have been surgeons who specialized in the operation of "cutting for stone," that is, removing calculi from the bladder by opening the organ, usually through the perineum. This operation appears to have been done by the ancient Hindus and Persians, and was probably brought to Greece at the time of Alexander's campaigns. In medieval and renaissance times, it was the most frequently performed major surgical procedure, excepting, of course, amputation. During the 17th and 18th Centuries a family of French specialists in cutting for stone, the Collots, improved the operation considerably, and retained almost a monopoly of it in France. They might be regarded as the first specialists in genito-urinary surgery, although their repertoire consisted of only one operation.

In England the great lithotomist of the period was William Cheselden, surgeon to St. Thomas' Hospital in London from 1718 to 1752. He brought the operation to the highest stage of perfection that it could attain in those pre-anaesthetic, pre-antiseptic days. His skill may be judged by the fact that he performed it—difficult as it was—in as little as 54 seconds. The operation, even when skillfully performed, had a considerable mortality. Thus Morand, Cheselden's Parisian pupil, reported that among a total of 812 patients operated upon at the Hôtel Dieu and the Charité, there were 255 deaths, and that many of those who survived were left with urinary fistulas.

The next advance in dealing with bladder stone was the invention, in 1822, by Jean Civale, a young Parisian surgeon, of an ingenious instrument for crushing the stone within the bladder. The lithotrite, as it was called, was inserted through the natural urinary passage, the urethra, and grasped and broke up the stone, the fragments of which were then washed out of the bladder. This procedure was often successful with scarcely any mortality. Civale's invention gained for him a special service for genito-urinary cases at the Necker Hospital in Paris. This service became a famous center for the study of genito-urinary problems, and during the following century a long line of distinguished French genito-urinary surgeons who were trained there made many important contributions to their specialty. The lithotrite was perfected in 1878 by Henry Bigelow, the dean of Boston surgery during the last half of the 19th Century. Oliver Wendell Holmes, who was ever ready with a name, baptised Bigelow's improved method "litholapaxy."

This brings us to the modern or cystoscopic period of genito-urinary surgery. Before the cystoscope, diagnosis of disease of the urinary tract rested upon clinical symptoms and external palpation alone. The surgeon was often uncertain and dared not operate. The cystoscope, and all the methods of studying the condition of the bladder, ureters, and kidneys which it has made possible, transformed diagnosis and opened up a whole new field of therapy. The cystoscope was invented by an ingenious Viennese urologist, Max Nitze. By 1876, when he first began to work on his idea of developing an instrument for viewing the interior of hollow cavities like the bladder and the nose, an urgent need for a cystoscope had developed. Anaesthesia and antiseptis had made it possible to open the bladder above the pubis and to remove tumors or stones from it, but such procedures could not of course be attempted without making sure of the diagnosis. Nitze's first cystoscope was a hollow tube equipped with a system of lenses for magnifying the image, and had a platinum wire loop on its tip which provided illumination when heated white-hot with a galvanic current. It was kept from burning the bladder by irrigation with a stream of cold water. It could be inserted into the bladder through the urethra without undue difficulty. When Edison invented the electric light in 1879, the Viennese cystoscope makers quickly adapted it for use in the cystoscope, providing it with adequate illumination for the first time.

Nitze himself, and many other urologists, continued to improve the cystoscope so that by the '90's it was possible to inspect all portions of the bladder with it, and to carry out all sorts of minor operations upon the interior of the bladder with small cutting, clamping, and cauterizing instruments inserted through it. Most important of all was the development of the method of catheterizing the ureters through the cystoscope. The ureters, which conduct the urine from the kidneys, open into the base of the bladder through two tiny openings. To study the relative function and condition of the two kidneys, it was necessary to insert separate catheters into these openings. Alexander Brenner, a 29-year old Viennese urologist, devised a special cystoscope for this purpose and succeeded in catheterizing the ureters in the female in 1888. An American, James Brown, chief of the genito-urinary dispensary at Johns Hopkins, improved Brenner's apparatus and accomplished the more difficult task of catheterizing the ureters in the male in 1893.

Now that it was possible to study the urine from each kidney separately, various important tests to determine the condition of the individual kidney were developed. Infection was detected by finding numbers of pus cells or leucocytes in the urine. Cultures were made, revealing the bacteria responsible for the infection. An ingenious dye test of kidney function was worked out at Johns Hopkins University. The professor of chemistry, Ira Remsen, discovered a new purple dye, *phenol-sulphone-phthalein*, in 1884. His colleague, the pharmacologist John J. Abel, found that it was eliminated largely by the kidneys, and Drs. Leonard G. Rowntree and John T. Geraghty in 1910 showed that the excretion was diminished when the kidney was damaged by disease. In 1906 Fritz Voelcker and Alexander von Lichtenberg of Heidelberg discovered that a colloidal solution of silver injected up the ureter would give, on x-ray examination, an image of the course of the ureter and the contour of the cavities (calyces) within the kidney. They called their method of examination "pyelography." When perfected a few years later by the substitution of sodium iodide for silver solutions it provided further valuable evidence of the condition of the kidney.

With these modern methods of examination the urological surgeon had means of obtaining information about the condition of bladder, ureters, and kidneys that enabled him in almost every instance to make a definite diagnosis. Armed with a reliable diagnosis he could attack genito-urinary disease surgically.

This attack had begun, as a matter of fact, even a few years before the cystoscope was invented. The pioneer in kidney surgery was Gustav Simon, professor of surgery at Heidelberg. In 1869 he successfully removed a normal kidney in a woman who had had a ureter cut during a uterine operation. The following year he removed a cystic kidney, and in 1871 a kidney containing stones. His book on kidney surgery, published in two parts in 1871 and 1876, was the first classic treatise on the subject. With the perfection of cystoscopic methods for study of the kidneys, operations for many types of kidney disease began to be done. Dr. Halsted, in 1893, was the first to remove a kidney in a male after it had been proved by urethral catheterization to be badly infected. In tuberculosis of the kidney, nephrectomy was found to offer a good chance of cure. Stones were removed from the kidney and its function restored. Cancers of the kidney were for the first time attacked with some hope of success by removal of the kidney and the blood vessels leading to it.

Bladder surgery also developed quickly during this same period. In the early 1870's both French and German surgeons began to open the bladder through the abdominal wall above the pubis, and to remove stones and tumors from it. In the 1880's the distinguished chief of the genito-urinary service at the Necker Hospital in Paris, Joseph C. F. Guyon, did more than anyone else to popularize this method of opening the bladder, which time has proved to be the best one. He was also one of the foremost early cystoscopists. His pupil and successor at the Necker, Joachim Albarran, became particularly interested in bladder cancer and from his experience with a large number of cases, published in 1892 the first really comprehensive treatise on this disease. It was shown that surgical excision can cure this kind of cancer when it develops in the portion of the bladder that can be resected. Unfortunately, only about one-fourth of these tumors are so situated.

During recent years, two new methods of treating bladder tumors have been developed. In 1908 Edwin Beer of New York worked out a technique for burning these tumors off with an electric sparking apparatus used through the cystoscope (fulguration). A few years later radium was first used for bladder cancer. This method of treatment has been greatly improved since it was introduced, and is now a useful resource for the urological surgeon. Roentgen rays, too, have been found helpful. Unfortunately, none of these methods gives a satisfactory percentage of cures.

But the genito-urinary surgeon is more often called upon to deal with enlargement of the prostate gland than for any other disease. The prostate is a small accessory sexual gland surrounding the urethra just below the bladder. For reasons which we do not as yet understand, the prostate becomes enlarged in older men. Approximately one man in five past the age of 50 has enlargement of the gland, causing some degree of obstruction to urination. In the more common benign form of prostatic enlargement, rounded masses of the hypertrophic glandular tissue develop. They compress the urethra and project into the bladder, preventing complete emptying of the organ. As a result of the urinary backpressure, the kidneys may eventually be damaged to such an extent that death results.

Until about fifty years ago sufferers from this condition could get no relief except that provided by repeated catheterization with resultant bladder infection, or by a permanent bladder fistula—miserable alternatives. It was in the early 1880's that the operation of opening the bladder and excising the hypertrophied prostatic tissue first began to be done. The first procedures of this kind were incidental to operations for the removal of bladder stones, and consisted merely of cutting out the masses of prostatic tissue that were causing obvious obstruction. Arthur F. McGill, surgeon to the Leeds Royal Infirmary, was the first to realize the usefulness of prostatectomy as a separate elective procedure. He successfully carried out three of these operations during 1887, opening the bladder suprapubically and excising as much as he could of the hypertrophic prostatic tissue. His success soon led to general acceptance of the operation in his own country and in America and Germany. By 1902, when the Basel urologists, Auguste Socin and Emil Burckhardt, published their excellent monograph on prostatic disease, they were able to collect reports of a total of 109 operations, with a mortality of 30 per cent.

Since then the technique of this operation has been considerably improved and its mortality greatly reduced. Under favorable circumstances it does not today exceed five per cent. Undoubtedly the most important factor in making this operation safer has been the careful study of kidney function before operation, and the adoption of a period of preliminary bladder drainage to permit the kidneys to regain their function whenever there are evidences that they have been damaged.

In recent years a relatively simple method of relieving urinary obstruction caused by certain forms of prostatic hypertrophy has been revived. This is the so-called "punch" method. The instrument is a tube with a cutting arrangement that can be inserted through the urethra to slice out a channel through the obstructing prostatic tissue. In a limited number of cases this method has been shown to be advantageous.

Unfortunately, in a considerable proportion of men who develop symptoms of prostatic obstruction, it is found to be due to cancer. This subtle disease causes about one fifth of all deaths from cancer in men. In 1869 Theodor Billroth, while he was still professor of surgery at Zurich, was probably the first to attempt to excise prostatic cancer radically, via the perineal route. The operative attack has been carried to its probably ultimate surgical limits by Hugh Young, the distinguished chief of the Brady Urological Institute at Johns Hopkins, who in 1904 began to do as radical a resection as possible. It must be admitted, however, that even this thoroughly radical operation has little chance of succeeding except in small, early prostatic cancers. Unfortunately, the disease is far advanced in most patients when they first come for treatment. Recently radium and x-rays have been used in various forms, but none of these methods of treatment has had much success. Prostatic cancer remains one of the important unsolved problems of modern medicine. Fortunately, there are today good leads for research regarding its etiology. It has been known for a long time that the growth of the prostate is controlled by the sex hormones, and the recent advances in the chemistry of these hormones have paved the way for study of their relationship to prostatic tumors.

In most of the larger hospitals in America, at least, genito-urinary surgery is today a separate clinical service. The facilities for training genito-urinary specialists cannot be regarded as adequate, however, and there is a special need of funds and organization to carry on fundamental research such as that concerned with prostatic cancer.

ORTHOPAEDICS

THE WORD orthopaedic was compounded in 1741 by the Parisian physician Nicolas André from the Greek roots *orthos,* meaning straight, and *pais,* meaning child. He used it in a treatise on skeletal deformities which he attributed to muscle inbalances during childhood. The word has survived, while André's theory has long since been discarded. Today the word has a quite different meaning. Orthopaedics is the branch of medicine that deals with diseases and injuries of bones and joints, including deformities, both congenital and acquired, fractures, and dislocations. The orthopaedist is a surgeon rather than a physician prescribing corrective exercises as André had intended.

Nevertheless, the beginning of orthopaedics as a specialty, and the establishment of the first orthopaedic hospitals can be traced back to the interest of the 18th Century French humanitarians in crippled and deformed children. Jacques Mathieu Delpech, professor of surgery at Montpellier, was the real founder of the specialty. In 1828 Delpech published a treatise entitled *Orthomorphy,* which is the earliest comprehensive discussion of bone and joint deformities. He also planned and built a charming orthopaedic hospital in the country between Montpellier and Toulouse. A contemporary of his, Johann Georg von Heine, an instrument and brace maker to the faculty of the University of Würzburg, founded an orthopaedic institute in that city in 1816 which had a leading role in the development of the specialty in Germany. Heine's nephew, Bernard Heine, graduated in medi-

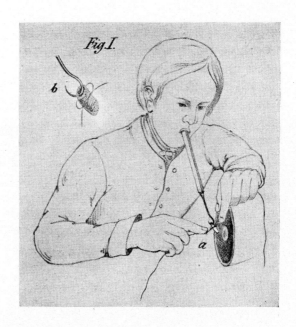

Fig. I.

The Old Methods of Hemostasis

The lithograph shows a surgeon, who is apparently short-handed, doing an amputation. He has hooked up a blood vessel with a tenaculum, and is tying it while he holds the end of the instrument in his mouth (from Günther's Lehre von den blutigen Operationen am menschlichen Körper, Leipzig, 1859, Vol. 1, Plate 5). Halsted stated that until about 1890 the tenaculum was a favorite instrument in America for checking hemorrhage, especially with some of the senior surgeons. Its only rivals were the fenestrated, mouse-toothed, spring forceps, shown below. These were the only artery clamps that most New York hospitals possessed in 1880.

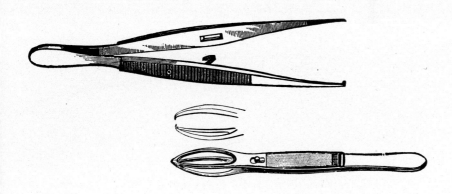

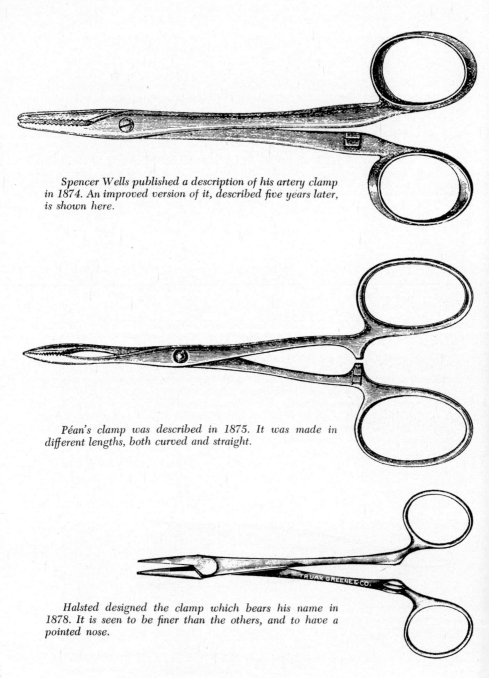

Spencer Wells published a description of his artery clamp in 1874. An improved version of it, described five years later, is shown here.

Péan's clamp was described in 1875. It was made in different lengths, both curved and straight.

Halsted designed the clamp which bears his name in 1878. It is seen to be finer than the others, and to have a pointed nose.

The Evolution of the Hemostatic Clamp

cine from Würzburg, and became its first professor of orthopaedics in 1838. In England, the first orthopaedic hospital was
founded at Birmingham in 1817. William John Little, an eminent
orthopaedic surgeon who himself had a clubfoot, founded the
Orthopaedic Institute of London in 1837. Subsequently called the
Royal Orthopaedic Hospital, it became the leading British institution for the care of the crippled poor. In America two pioneer
orthopaedic surgeons both established special orthopaedic clinics
in the same year, 1861. Lewis A. Sayre of New York organized a
clinic at Bellevue Hospital, and Buckminster Brown of Boston
opened a small private hospital, the Samaritan Hospital. Two
special orthopaedic hospitals were shortly founded in New York,
the Hospital for the Ruptured and Crippled in 1863, and the New
York Orthopaedic Dispensary and Hospital in 1866.

These special hospitals and clinics made possible the tremendous growth of our knowledge of bone and joint diseases that
took place in the last half of the 19th Century. As a result of the
correlation of clinical findings and the new microscopical pathology, a great many new diseases of bones and joints were identified
and described. We have not space here even to list them.

But progress was not limited to the description of new diseases. For the first time experimental methods began to throw
light upon the complex mechanism of bone growth and repair. In
this work two men took an outstanding part. The first was
Louis X.-E.-L. Ollier. Trained at Montpellier and Paris, Ollier began the experimental study of bone growth early in his career.
He became professor of surgery at Lyon in 1859, and eleven years
later published a two-volume work, *A Clinical and Experimental
Treatise on the Regeneration of Bone and the Artificial Production of Osseous Tissue*, which gave us, in the words of an eminent
present-day orthopaedic surgeon, "the clearest conception of the
processes of bone growth and repair which we possess." Ollier asserted that bone grew chiefly from the periosteum, the fibrous
envelope that surrounds it.

A little later Sir William MacEwen, professor of surgery at

the University of Glasgow, showed that the periosteum is by no means the sole source of new bone. In a series of experiments done upon dogs, he proved that bone can develop from grafts of bone chips from which the periosteum has been entirely removed. In 1880, in the case of a boy whose humerus had been almost entirely removed for osteomyelitis, leaving him with a flail arm, MacEwen removed a series of wedges from the tibia and implanted them in a row in a furrow in the arm muscles. The grafts lived and provided a useful humerus, which doubled in length as the boy grew up. This was the beginning of modern bone-grafting methods, which orthopaedic surgeons today use in treating a variety of bone diseases.

The rapid development of modern surgery in the 1880's was shared by the orthopaedic surgeons, who now began to operate upon all sorts of conditions which hitherto they had treated only by external means. Muscles and tendons were transplanted, shortened, lengthened, and re-arranged in a variety of ways to overcome deformities and paralyses. It was, as a matter of fact, on May 15, 1880, that Karl Nicoladoni, professor of surgery at Innsbruck, carried out the first operation of this kind. He cut the tendons of the peroneal muscles, which arise from the side of the leg, and sutured them to the cut end of the Achilles tendon or heel cord, in the case of a boy aged 16 whose posterior leg muscles, from which the Achilles tendon springs, had been paralyzed by infantile paralysis. A great many ingenious technical procedures have been devised during the last generation to make this tendon-muscle surgery more effective. Today even the slender tendons of the hands and fingers can be successfully dealt with.

A variety of operations upon bones and joints were also developed in the new surgical era. In 1873, Billroth performed the first operative correction of the knock-knee deformity so frequently caused by rickets. He chiseled part way through the tibia just below the knee, broke the bone across, and straightened it. In 1877, MacEwen devised a much better operation in which the lower femur rather than the tibia was straightened. This procedure soon gained wide favor and the principle upon which it was based was applied to the correction of various other bone deformities.

Another operation which came to be done frequently was the excision of tuberculous joints. It had been successfully carried out in a series of cases in the 1820's by James Syme, the famous Edinburgh surgeon. The great French orthopaedic surgeon, Ollier, of whose work we have spoken above, perfected this operation in the last years of the 19th Century and published a monumental work in three volumes on it.

Such a resection of a joint usually resulted in a stiff joint. In an effort to prevent ankylosis and to obtain a movable joint surgeons have interposed a variety of substances such as the patient's own fat or fascia, and metal plates of various kinds, between the cut ends of the bones. This operation of *arthroplasty* has not had great success. The converse operation, *arthrodesis*, which has for its purpose the permanent fusion of a joint, is a simpler and more generally successful procedure. It was devised in 1878 by Edward Albert, professor of surgery at Vienna, for the purpose of stabilizing paralyzed joints which would otherwise have to be fixed with braces. Russell Hibbs at the New York Orthopaedic Hospital adapted this operation to the treatment of tuberculous joints, particularly the spine, in 1911. Hibb's spinal fusion has since become a standard procedure for several other conditions, and is one of the most useful of modern orthopaedic operations.

But it is in the treatment of fractures that we see the technical skill and wisdom of the orthopaedic surgeon most frequently displayed today. In former times fractured limbs were roughly manipulated and fixed in crude wooden splints. Hugh Owen Thomas of Liverpool began what we might call the modern epoch in fracture therapy in the latter half of the 19th Century. Thomas was descended from a long line of Welsh bone-setters, but he had in addition been soundly trained in medicine and surgery at Edinburgh, London, and Paris. He set up in practice in Liverpool, first with his father, and then independently, near the docks where there was an abundance of orthopaedic work among the poor. Thomas was not only a learned physician with a thorough knowledge of disease, but a skilled mechanic as well. He devised and himself made the ingenious splints for which he became famous, and which today still bear his name. These were no cumbersome affairs of wood, but skillfully designed and accurately fitted appliances of iron and leather. The fundamental principle of Thomas' art was rest for the diseased or injured limb. With his ingenious splints, he often succeeded in keeping the limb at rest while the patient continued up and about, an important point for the poor who were his patients. His devotion to them was such that he worked from dawn until late at night over them every day of the week without ever a holiday, and died prematurely in 1891 at the age of 57.

His work was carried on by his nephew, Robert Jones, whom he took into his house in Liverpool as a youth and whose training he guided into maturity. Practising among the same poor dockworkers Jones became more famous than his uncle. It was he who, early in this century, introduced the modern practice of the immediate reduction of fractures under an anaesthetic. This makes possible much more accurate re-alignment of the broken bone, and decreases the damage to the surrounding muscles and other soft tissues. When the First World War came his government gave him a free hand as director of the orthopaedic services in the British Army with the rank of Major General, and knighted him. Jones instituted improvements in the handling of fractures on the battlefield that were of tremendous importance. His plan was to apply protective splints to the limb whenever possible before moving the patient to the casualty clearing station—to "splint 'em where they lie." For compound fractures of the thigh, for instance, the so-called Thomas hip splint was applied. Under this plan, the mortality for this injury in the British Army was reduced

from 80 per cent to 15 per cent. Jones's methods were enthusiastically adopted by American orthopaedists, with the result that the
toll of preventable deformities was less in percentage in the
American Army than in any of the other armies.

After the war the need for special orthopaedic clinics to do
the reconstructive surgery of bones and joints to fit the injured
for civil life was obvious. Orthopaedic surgery in general was
greatly stimulated. The lessons learned in the war were also applied to civilian injuries. Fracture services were organized in general hospitals where specialists in fracture work could control the
whole course of the patient's treatment and convalescence. The
first fracture services of this kind were organized at the Ancoats
Hospital in Manchester, England in 1914, and at the Massachusetts General Hospital in 1917. Today a number of general hospitals both in Great Britain and the United States have such fracture services. A comparison made in 1935 by the British Medical
Association of the results of the treatment of fractures on these
special services with those obtained in general hospitals showed
clearly the advantages of this kind of specialization.

The modern treatment of fractures is facilitated by several
technical procedures, concerning the history of which we must
make some mention. The first of these is the use of plaster of Paris
bandages to make casts. The method was devised by a Dutch
army medical officer, A. Mathijssen, in May, 1852. It was one of
the great surgical inventions, for it made it possible to prepare
quickly and simply, perfectly fitting, light-weight supports for
fractured or injured limbs. The cumbersome and ill-fitting wooden
and metal braces and splints were no longer necessary. Plaster of
Paris, which is anhydrous calcium sulphate or so-called gypsum,
had been used to make casts before Mathijssen's time. It was
poured into a mold around the limb and trimmed down while
hardening. But this method was so messy and so complex that it
was not practical. Mathijssen's idea of spreading the plaster on a
roller bandage, moistening it, and wrapping the limb with it, was

a stroke of genius. As the plaster crystallized within the meshes of the cloth, it formed a stronger and lighter cast than could be made by any other method.

Plaster of Paris bandages were soon used in orthopaedic clinics all over the world. Lewis A. Sayre, the pioneer New York orthopaedic surgeon, in 1874 used plaster bandages to make a snugly fitting jacket encircling the whole trunk, while the patient was suspended by overhead slings around the head and shoulders. This straightened and immobilized the spine, and by providing rest for the diseased tissues, aided their recovery. It was an important therapeutic method. Today, plaster casts are used for providing support and immobilization in a great variety of orthopaedic conditions. They are an almost indispensable surgical aid.

Another indispensable aid to the orthopaedist is the x-ray machine, for with it we can see the bones with which we work. Röntgen himself was, of course, the first to do this, for in studying the penetration of the rays that he discovered on November 8, 1895, he found that the bones of his own hand were opaque. In his first report on his discovery he included an x-ray picture of the bones of a hand. By January, 1896, several German surgeons had made x-ray photographs of fractured and diseased bones. In February and March similar pictures were made in England, France and the United States.

In March, 1896, an American, an Austrian, and a German simultaneously discovered that x-ray photographs could be taken stereoscopically, enabling the observer to view the fragments of a broken bone in perspective and to establish their relative position in all planes. The surgeon could now be certain that a fracture was satisfactorily set, and he could follow the whole process of bone repair.

Another important modern development in the treatment of fractures is open reduction, that is, operative exposure and correction of the malposition of the fragments. As long ago as 1827, J. H. Rodgers of New York wired together the ends of a fractured humerus that had failed to unite. In 1861, E. S. Cooper, of San

Francisco, wired together a fractured knee-cap. Lister did a similar operation with his carbolic acid technique in 1877. A French naval surgeon, L.-J.-B. Bérenger-Féraud, wrote an interesting book in 1870 advocating wiring fractures of the long bones. A good deal of wiring was done during the next decade without much success.

The first real progress came with the use of metal screws to hold the fragments together. This method was first employed successfully by Albin Lambotte, an Antwerp surgeon, in 1888, and by William Arbuthnot Lane, surgeon to Guy's Hospital in London in 1894. It was Lane who persisted in his efforts to fix difficult fractures in position by internal mechanical means, until eventually he worked out a method of employing metal plates, fixed with long screws through the bones, which is generally accepted today. The wires, bands, and pegs of various types that had been used by Lane's predecessors were not satisfactory because they worked loose and acted as irritating foreign bodies. The metal plates firmly screwed down to the ends of the broken bone, on the other hand, held them solidly together and favored bony union. Lane also worked out a specially rigorous aseptic technique for open operations on bones, which required that all of the manipulations in the wound be carried out with instruments. Infection is especially to be feared in operations of this kind, for bone infections are notoriously chronic and serious. Lane was knighted for his accomplishments, and today he and his pupils have the satisfaction of seeing their methods widely used in fracture clinics.

A final word might be said about the modern non-operative methods of reducing fractures of the long bones. Under certain conditions, as for instance when the fracture is oblique, the fragments must be held in proper position by some sort of continued traction on the limb. Otherwise they slip past each other and a shortened limb results. During the last half of the 19th Century this was generally obtained by adhesive plaster fixed to the skin, said to have been first suggested by Samuel D. Gross, the famous

Philadelphia surgeon. This form of traction was used in an apparatus devised by Gordon Buck of New York in 1860, which soon gained wide popularity and has since been known to surgeons as "Buck's extension."

But this kind of traction was sometimes inadequate. Direct traction on the bone itself was first carried out by a distinguished Italian surgeon, Alessandro Codivilla, professor of orthopaedic surgery at the University of Bologna, and director of the Rizzoli Institute, one of the most noted orthopaedic clinics in the world. In 1904 he described a method of driving a steel pin through the calcaneus or heel bone to obtain adequate traction in cases where he had fractured the bones of the leg in order to lengthen the limb. In 1911 this idea was utilized to provide skeletal traction in difficult fracture cases by Fritz Steinmann, professor of surgery at Bern, Switzerland. Various modifications of this method of providing skeletal traction are widely used today, and have proved of great value where adequate traction can be obtained in no other way.

For the benefit of the layman who reads this chapter we should include a few words about osteopathy and chiropractic, the popular forms of medical quackery in the United States today. It is a curious fact that quackery has often based its theory upon presumed disorders of the bones. Until recent times there was in the British Isles a cult of bone-setters. These were for the most part men without any kind of education, who manipulated not only fractures but all sorts of conditions. Some of them were clever in their management of sprains and broken bones, but on the whole they did more harm than good, for they had no fundamental understanding of the diseases which they attempted to treat. Their greatest hold on the public was their occasional success with locked knee joints, which are due to tearing and displacement of the cartilages of the knee. The bone-setters learned that by twisting the knee in a certain way they could often restore its motion. The condition soon recurred in most patients, but the bone-setters were glad to manipulate again. When Thomas Annandale, professor of surgery at Edinburgh, in 1879 opened the knee joint and removed the loose cartilages, he solved the problem and put the bone-setters almost out of business as far as the knee was concerned.

The last important publicity the bone-setters got was the publication in 1871 of their so-called secret methods of manipulation by an English surgeon, Wharton Hood, who had become interested by the success of the celebrated London bone-setter Richard Hutton. Hood showed that their methods were not based upon any understanding of the anatomy of the conditions which they attempted to deal with, and that they consisted merely of the simplest kind of manipulations, which they applied indiscriminately to all patients. Most of their successes were like that described by Homans. A gentleman, while taking the waters at Harrogate for pain and stiffness of the shoulder, was cured by a cow. For in trying to escape the animal he leaped a ditch, throwing his stiff arm up as he did so, and thus regaining full motion of his shoulder.

It was shortly after Hood's book was published that osteopathy and chiropractic made their appearance in America. Andrew Still, an itinerant inventor of farm machinery and free lance doctor among the Shawnee Indians in Kansas, in his own words "flung to the breeze the banner of osteopathy" on June 22, 1874. The *divine* revelation of the theory of osteopathy, for so Still regarded it, was simply "that the mechanical displacement of the vertebrae constitutes most of the lesions causing disease." Still was such a successful salesman that by 1908, when he was at his prime, he could claim some 4,000 graduates from his school of osteopathy.

Chiropractic is merely a jazzed-up version of the osteopathic theory. It was devised by one D. W. Palmer, a magnetic healer, of Davenport, Iowa, about 1894. It attributes all diseases to abnormal pressure on the nerves as they emerge from the spinal column, due to "subluxations" of the vertebrae. Chiropractic has been almost as successful as osteopathy, and although chiropractors are looked down upon by osteopaths as interlopers, it is clear that there is not much to choose between their respective manipulations.

The truth is, of course, that careful studies of the spine in countless thousands of dissections and autopsies done by physicians trained in the best scientific knowledge of modern medicine have failed to reveal the existence of any displacements or "subluxations" of the vertebrae pressing upon the spinal nerves. At the same time we know the causal mechanism of many diseases to be something quite different, and in certain diseases have brought it under control by operation, drugs, or other treatments. In the light of these simple facts it is difficult to understand how any intelligent man can place his life in the *hands* of one of these manipulators. Our legislators in some states have granted the legal right to chiropractors and osteopaths to assume the full responsibility of the practice of medicine. In such states a chiropractor, for instance, is permitted to treat diphtheria by manipulation. This may be called freedom but it is certainly not common sense. Not only is the poor victim's life endangered thereby, but, since the disease is contagious, the lives of others are threatened as well. In a truly democratic society one individual should not be permitted to endanger the lives of his fellow citizens in this manner.

NEUROSURGERY

THE SPECIALTY of neurosurgery was born at the turn of the present century, and is unique in that it was largely the creation of two individuals, an Englishman and an American. Sir Victor Horsley laid its foundations, and Harvey Cushing built the edifice of special technique and knowledge that today stands as one of the notable achievements of modern surgery. Neurosurgery is concerned very largely with lesions within the cranium and the spinal canal that can be attacked surgically—new growths, certain types of inflammation, and injuries. The neurosurgeon also treats lesions of the peripheral nerves, but these operations do not form a great part of his work.

Within the brain and from the fibrous envelopes that enclose it, the meninges, there arises a variety of tumors. These constitute less than one per cent of all new growths, yet until the modern neurosurgical attack they were inevitably fatal, for there is no method of treatment except removal that offers hope of cure.

Before any operations to remove these tumors could be attempted, it was necessary to know the clinical signs and the pathological nature of these tumors, as well as how to localize their position in the brain so that the opening in the skull could be made at the right place. The first steps in the localization of brain function had already been made in Germany by Gustav Theodor Fritsch and Eduard Hitzig. In 1870, they had shown by experiments on dogs that local bodily movements and convulsions

319

could be produced by electrical stimulation of definite areas in the brain. Subsequent progress in the localization of cerebral function was made largely by the British. Sir David Ferrier, the London physiologist, between 1872 and 1876 carried out extensive experiments in which he charted the areas of brain function in birds, frogs, fishes and mammals. John Hughlings Jackson of Yorkshire, generally regarded as the "father of neurology," did more than anyone else to apply these new facts in the clinical study of diseases of the brain.

By 1884 enough knowledge about brain tumors had been accumulated in England to make possible the first clinical localization and removal of such a growth. The patient was a man of 25 who had developed twitchings and weakness of the left arm and leg, vomiting and headache. Alexander Hughes Bennett, physician to the Hospital for Epilepsy and Paralysis in London, decided that he had a tumor in the region of the right fissure of Rolando. He persuaded Rickman Godlee, Lister's assistant, to attempt to remove it. On November 3, 1884, Godlee opened the skull with a trephine at the point Bennett had indicated and found a glioma within the substance of the brain cortex. He enucleated it by blunt dissection. The patient survived the operation and his symptoms were relieved, but unfortunately the wound became infected and he died a month later of meningitis. It is of interest to note that Bennett, who correctly diagnosed the site and nature of this lesion, was stimulated to study brain tumors through the fact that his father, a distinguished Edinburgh pathologist, had died from one.

Already at this date the man who was to lay the foundation of neurosurgery was at work—Victor Horsley. Horsley's career is one of the best examples in the history of surgery of the value of experimental work on animals as a preparation for clinical surgery. In 1884, three years after he had completed his term as house-surgeon, he began, with Professor Schäfer at University College, London, a series of experiments on monkeys, to study cerebral localization. In the course of these experiments, which required several years, he not only added important new knowledge to the subject of brain physiology, but he worked out a method of opening the skull and spinal cord safely.

When he was offered, in 1886, the appointment as surgeon to the National Hospital for the Paralyzed and Epileptic at Queen's Square in London, where he could hope to attack brain lesions in human beings, he was ready for it. He did his first brain case at Queen's Square on May 25, 1886, but it was not until September 23rd of the same year that he operated on a brain tumor. It was his fourth case. The patient was completely paralyzed on his left side and semi-comatose. Horsley correctly diagnosed a glioma of the right hemisphere and removed it. The patient survived the operation, his paralysis improved, and his mind cleared, although he died six months later with recurrence of the growth. This was the first operation for brain tumor from which the patient survived. By the end of 1886, Horsley had done ten operations on the brain with but one operative death, a hitherto undreamed of accomplishment.

Shortly afterward Horsley made another landmark in surgery —the first successful removal of a tumor of the spinal canal. On June 9, 1887, he removed a subdural endothelemia at the level of the fourth dorsal vertebra. The patient, an army officer, was entirely relieved of his pain and paralysis and lived in the best of health for many years afterward.

These triumphs were not accidental but the direct result of the new technique for neurosurgery that Horsley had worked out. It included three important innovations: (1) good asepsis; (2) making a large, semi-lunar flap of the scalp, rather than a cruciform incision; (3) the use of wax on the cut edges of bone to control hemorrhage.

While Horsley was working out the technique of operating on the brain in London, an Edinburgh physician and pathologist, Byrom Bramwell, had been studying the clinical and pathological features of brain tumors. In 1888 Bramwell published the results in a monograph which, as the first comprehensive work on brain tumors, has become a classic. He described the headaches, vomiting, eye symptoms, and paralyses caused by these growths with such clarity and accuracy that his book can still be read with profit today.

By 1889 Horsley had done a total of 44 operations on the brain with only ten deaths, and a total of 19 on the spinal cord with only one death. Although this was an unequalled record, Horsley's London colleagues remained unenthusiastic over the prospects of neurosurgery and never gave him their full sympathy. He persevered, however, until the specialty that he had founded was taken up on the other side of the Atlantic.

Horsley had many other compensations and interests. In 1887 he married Rosamond Bramwell, daughter of the distinguished Scot who wrote the classic work on brain tumors that we have mentioned above. Horsley was, as Cushing has put it, "a man of superhuman standards." He threw himself into the fight for woman suffrage and for temperance. When the First World War came, he would not remain idle, and asked to be assigned to active military duty. He was sent to Egypt, where in 1916, at the age of 59, he died of heat-stroke.

After the beginning that Horsley had made, surgeons elsewhere began to attempt occasional brain operations. Some of them made important contributions to the technique of opening the skull. Horsley and his predecessors had used the trephine, or burr, with which they drilled one or more holes and enlarged them with a chisel. This method did not give adequate exposure of the brain. A German surgeon, Wilhelm Wagner, in 1889 first attempted to provide proper exposure by cutting and turning down a flap of bone. He cut the flap with mallet and chisel, a dangerous and awkward method. A French surgeon, J. Toison, of Lille, in 1891 suggested the modern method of cutting the bone flap. He bored a series of primary trephine openings and then cut the intervening bone with a chain saw, cutting from within outward. In 1894 a young Italian surgeon, Leonardo Gigli, introduced the flexible wire saw in surgery. In 1898 he utilized it for cutting a bone flap from the skull. Opening the skull then became relatively safe and easy.

Nevertheless, neurosurgery made but little progress. Its status at the turn of the century has been well summed up by Harvey Cushing, the man who is largely responsible for its great advance since then. Cushing found in reviewing the records of the Johns Hopkins Hospital in 1901 that the diagnosis of brain tumor had been made only 32 times in the 36,000 patients admitted during the preceding decade. Thirteen of these 32 patients had been transferred to the surgical wards, where two of them had been operated upon, both with fatal results.

At the time he reviewed this distressing record, Harvey Cushing was a soundly trained young surgeon of 31, just returned from a year's work in the laboratory of physiology at Bern, Switzerland. There he had worked on the problem of intracranial pressure, and had become deeply interested in the experimental pathology of the nervous system. He determined to devote himself to neurosurgery. At Johns Hopkins, on his return from abroad, he was given the opportunity. There, during the next twelve years, he developed the method of precise localizing diagnosis for brain tumors and worked out the highly specialized technique for operating upon the brain that has led to the miracles performed by the neurosurgeons today. In order that he might assume personal responsibility for the diagnosis in his patients, he studied neurology, and with infinite care took the history and examined each patient himself. The general principles of surgical technique that formed the basis of Cushing's methods were those of his great chief, Halsted. They included meticulous hemostasis, painstaking care and gentleness in the handling of tissues, and the use of layers of interrupted sutures of fine silk in closing the wound.

Cushing applied these principles to brain surgery with great skill. He controlled bleeding from the scalp by placing a tourniquet around it. For tumors of the sub-occipital region he devised the so-called cross-bow incision which has been the standard one

ever since. When he had the tumor exposed he shelled it out of
its bed by the gentle use of cotton pledgets, instead of plunging
the fingers into the brain and digging it out as his predecessors
had done. By such crude methods they had lost the great majority
of their patients from hemorrhage. Cushing not only minimized
bleeding by his gentle manipulation, but he devised important
methods for checking it. These included the use of small pieces
of fresh muscle which he placed over oozing surfaces, tiny silver
wire clips with which small vessels were clamped, and electro-
surgical methods which coagulated bleeding vessels.

By all of these methods he avoided operative shock, and he
was able to carry out his hazardous procedures in one stage instead of several stages as his predecessors had been accustomed
to do. He introduced the practice of keeping a running record of
the patient's blood pressure during the whole course of the operation in order to detect the development of shock—a practice
which has since been adopted in all types of surgery. An amusing
anecdote is told of Cushing's trials in the early days when he was
introducing the blood pressure apparatus to the operating room.
At a crucial point during one of his operations the patient showed
signs of collapse and he ordered one of the nurses to get the blood
pressure machine and find out what the pressure was. It was the
custom to apply the apparatus to the patient's leg in those days.
There was a long delay during which Cushing, absorbed as he
was with difficulties in the operative field, had no time to pay attention to anything else. Finally, he felt some encumbrance on
one of his own legs and looking down found that the eager nurse
had applied the apparatus to his leg rather than to the patient's.

In 1912 Cushing was called to Harvard as Mosley professor of
surgery, and surgeon-in-chief to the Peter Bent Brigham Hospital.
There his clinic for neurosurgery became world famous. He perfected his methods, accumulated a great mass of data concerning brain tumors, and trained a succession of young men who carried his teachings abroad and established neurosurgery as a
specialty in the chief centers of medical education everywhere.

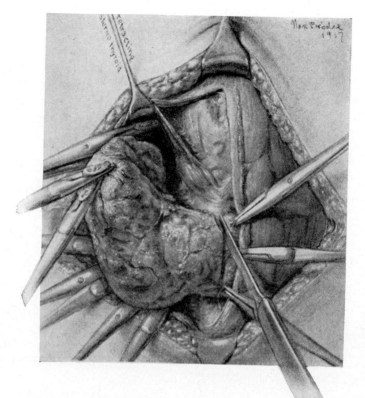

(The Operative Story of Goitre, *Johns Hopkins Hosp. Rep.*, 19:71, 1920)

The Modern Method of Hemostasis

An illustration from Halsted's description of his technique for operating for exophthalmic goitre shows how hemorrhage can be controlled by the use of many fine hemostatic clamps, even in an excessively vascular organ such as this.

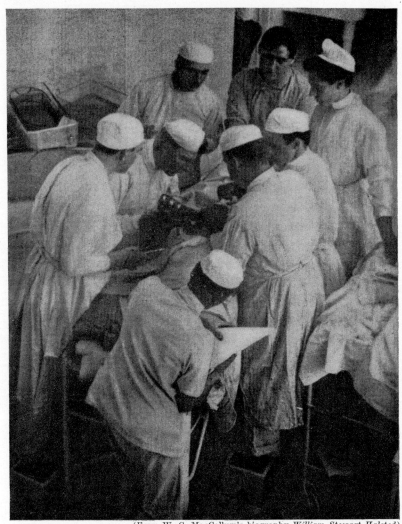

(From W. G. MacCallum's biography *William Stewart Halsted*)

Halsted Operating in 1904

Assisted by Finney, Cushing, Young, Mitchell, Clopton, and Miss Crawford.

When he retired from Harvard in 1932, at the age of 63, he summarized his life's work in a monograph entitled, *Intracranial Tumors. Notes Upon a Series of Two Thousand Verified Cases with Surgical Mortality Percentages Pertaining Thereto.* During the last three years (1928–1931) that he worked, his mortality was only 8.7 per cent for a total of 635 operations. These results stand today unequalled by those of any other neurosurgeon.

Cushing wrote a long series of articles and monographs on special forms of brain tumors, each of which was a classic, and marked an important advance in the subject. The first of these, a chapter on *Surgery of the Head,* in Keen's *System of Surgery,* appeared in 1908. In 1917 he published *Tumors of the Nervus Acusticus.* His work was interrupted by the war, during which he spent two years in France, where he developed a method of handling gunshot wounds of the skull and brain. Consequently his next book did not appear until 1926, when he and Percival Bailey presented their *Classification of the Tumors of the Glioma Group on a Histogenetic Basis.* This was the first attempt to classify this largest group of brain tumors properly. In 1928 his monograph, *Tumors Arising from the Bloodvessels of the Brain,* appeared. His final book, *Meningionias,* was published in 1938.

Like Horsley, Harvey Cushing was a man of wide interests. Through his neurosurgery he did more than anyone else in his generation to further specialization in surgery, for he proved so strikingly how it paid in improved results. He was a strong influence for the elevation of standards of surgical teaching, and for the Halstedian type of surgery. As an essayist and medical historian, he won wide recognition, his biography of Sir William Osler having become the best known medical biography of our time. He died in 1939 at the age of 70, honored throughout the world.

THORACIC SURGERY

Thoracic surgery is the youngest of all the surgical specialties. It is so young that the surgeons who today concentrate their efforts on diseases of the chest are the first generation of thoracic surgeons, the men who originally did the daring surgical feats that have earned recognition for their specialty. They are perhaps the only real pioneers in surgery that the present day medical student can view in person. And if he sees one of them in action, removing a lung or a mediastinal tumor, with the great cavity of the chest opened wide and the heart and great vessels beating away in plain view, he may well regard the thoracic surgeon as unbelievably bold. For this is the most spectacular of all modern surgery.

In 1896, Stephen Paget, son of the eminent Victorian surgeon, Sir James Paget, and distinguished biographer of his father, of John Hunter, and of Victor Horsley, published a scholarly book: *The Surgery of the Chest.* This was the first work devoted to this subject in English, and the most comprehensive so far attempted in any language. We might well take Stephen Paget's work as a signpost marking the beginning of the specialty of chest surgery, for when he wrote it he and several of his Continental contemporaries had but recently discovered that they could, under certain conditions, open the chest with relative impunity. New hope was born for empyema, lung abscess, and bronchiectasis. To make clear what now developed, we must discuss these several diseases separately.

Empyema is an accumulation of pus in the thorax or in the pleural cavity which is formed by the thin envelope of tissue surrounding the lung and lining the inside of the chest wall. Empyema usually follows pneumonia. Unless the pus is evacuated adequately it compresses the lung more and more and leads to complications which are eventually fatal. Until the 1880's surgeons dared not open the chest to provide free drainage. They aspirated it with a large bore needle again and again, usually without avail. Thus in a series of 48 patients to which Paget refers, only six were cured by this method of treatment.

When the adoption of Lister's antiseptic methods led to the great expansion of surgery in the 1870's and '80's, a number of German surgeons found that wide incision through the chest wall, preferably with excision of a portion of a rib to give free drainage, improved the results in empyema. In 1891, Franz Koenig, professor of surgery at Göttingen, was able to report 66 cures in a series of 76 cases treated for the most part by wide incision. This method was soon taken up both in France and England, Paget himself using it in London. It gradually became the standard method of treating empyema all over the world. Yet the disease continued to be one of the most serious confronting the surgeon. In most clinics the mortality ranged between 20 and 30 per cent.

The next important advance in the treatment of empyema came during the First World War, when the great influenza epidemic of 1918 swept through the army camps, where millions of men were crowded together. Countless cases of empyema resulted. Most of these were of a special type, being due to the streptococcus rather than the pneumococcus. In these streptococcus infections a massive effusion into the pleural cavity often occurs early in the course of the pneumonia. It was soon found that the usual surgical method of prompt open drainage of the pleural cavity in these cases gave disastrous results. In some American camps the mortality was over 70 per cent, and the replies to the Surgeon General's questionnaire in February, 1918, showed that the average mortality in all camps was 30.2 per cent.

It was at this time that a classical experimental and clinical study of the problem of empyema was made by Evarts A. Graham, professor of surgery at Washington University School of Medicine at St. Louis, and member of the Empyema Commission of the U. S. Army. Graham succeeded in producing streptococcus empyema experimentally in dogs. In one series of these animals he performed early open drainage of the pleural cavity, while in another series no operation was done. Most of the former series died while most of the latter series recovered. Graham showed that the principal reason why operation caused death was the altered air pressure relationships in the chest which it produced. In the act of respiration, the lungs are filled with air as a result of expansion of the thorax and lowering of the diaphragm. A slight negative pressure results within the pleural cavity. The chest is, of course, divided into two halves by the mediastinum, which is a more or less flexible partition, able to deviate toward either side. Now when a drainage opening is made into one pleural cavity it at once fills with air due to the negative pressure within it. The mediastinum, as yet a flexible partition in the early stage of the empyema, bulges toward the uninvolved side, compressing the opposite lung to the point where fatal interference with breathing may result.

Applying these experimental findings to human beings, Graham and his associates stopped the practice of early open drainage in empyema and brought about an almost miraculous improvement in the results. At Camp Lee, Virginia, where the Empyema Commission did its work, this new principle of treatment brought the mortality for empyema down from 48 per cent to 4.3 per cent. Drainage later in the course of the disease, when the mediastinum had become stiffened by the inflammatory process, and the empyema cavity walled off by pleural adhesions, was often necessary, and was performed at this stage without much hazard. Frequent washing out of the empyema cavity with Dakin's Solution (neutral sodium hypochlorite) was also found to be of great value.

A recently adopted method of avoiding the compressive effect upon the lung of a drainage opening into the pleural cavity depends upon the principle of so-called closed drainage. This consists simply of making the connection between the drainage tube and the chest wall air-tight, and placing the lower end of the drainage tube below the surface of the water in a large bottle well below the level of the wound. The water in the bottle acts as a simple one-way valve. As long ago as 1876 this kind of drainage, by means of a small rubber tube inserted through a trocar, was adopted by both C. Hewitt, a London surgeon, and by G. Bülau, a surgeon in Hamburg. It was used for many years in Hamburg without gaining much popularity elsewhere, because of the fact that the thick pus and fibrin often filling empyema cavities clogged the small drainage tube. In recent years the advantage of using a drainage tube of large caliber that will provide free drainage has become apparent to all, and with this provision the use of the closed method for a short period of time after operation in the early stages of empyema has become practical and desirable. It is generally adopted in American clinics today.

Another disease of the thorax, bronchiectasis, has been successfully attacked by surgery within recent years. In bronchiectasis the terminal bronchi, because of infection or congenital anatomical defects, become dilated and filled with pus. The disease involves chiefly the lower lobes of the lung, a fact which suggested to the surgeons of fifty years ago who first began to operate upon the lung itself, that excision of the diseased lobes might achieve cure. Here, as with so many other technically difficult surgical problems, experimental work on animals showed the way.

In 1881, Themistokles Gluck, a young Berlin surgeon who in later life became world famous for his skill in excising the larynx, attempted to remove one lung in dogs and rabbits. He succeeded in rabbits. Other surgeons shortly thereafter carried out successful pneumonectomies in dogs and cats. Encouraged by these results, surgeons began to attempt to remove lobes of the human lung. Lothar Heidenhain, director of the state hospital at Worms, Germany, first did this successfully in a patient with bronchiectasis in 1901. A few daring surgeons in Germany and in America then took up the operation, but it proved to be so hazardous, having a mortality of over 50 per cent, that only the most desperately ill would consent to it, and the numbers of operations were few. Among the early leaders in this surgical attack on bronchiectasis Howard Lilienthal of New York might be mentioned. By 1925 he had done lobectomy in 34 cases, with a mortality of 61 per cent.

The 1920's brought essential improvements. New methods of bronchoscopic and x-ray examination simplified and made certain the diagnosis of this disease and provided larger numbers of cases for study. In 1923 Graham introduced a method whereby the diseased lobe of the lung was destroyed in stages by means of the cautery. Even with this improvement, however, the total operative hazard was considerable, and surgeons hesitated to attack the disease. The modern one-stage method of lobectomy was worked out by Harold Brunn, at the University of California. In 1928 he began to remove bronchiectatic lobes in one stage, controlling the hemorrhage from the pedicle of the lobe by constricting it with a rubber tube tourniquet, ligating the vessels and bronchi in the stump individually, and closing the stump with sutures. Norman S. Shenstone, of the University of Toronto, improved upon the method by introducing a snare type of tourniquet in 1932. The recent improvements in anaesthesia have also been of great help in these cases. All of these factors have combined to make it possible today for several American surgeons to report series of cases of bronchiectasis treated by lobectomy with an operative mortality of less than five per cent.

Abscess of the lung is another important condition where surgery has made rapid progress. Many of these abscesses are due to the aspiration of infected material from the mouth. Often they follow operations such as tonsilectomy or tooth extraction. When lung abscess develops and does not yield to medical methods of treatment, surgical drainage should be instituted at once. It has given excellent results when employed before the development of complications.

The thoracic surgeon has also been able to make valuable contributions to the treatment of pulmonary tuberculosis. The first surgical effort of this kind was, however, a tragic one. At a time when surgeons were accomplishing new miracles almost every day it was to be expected that surgical resection of the tuberculous lung would be attempted. A young Berlin surgeon, Block by name, in 1882 repeated Gluck's experimental resection of the lung in animals, and concluded that such an operation would be both easy and safe for human beings having tuberculosis of the lungs. In 1883 he attempted such an operation upon a young woman relative of his, resecting the apex of the lung on both sides. She died in a few hours, and investigation showed that she had not had pulmonary tuberculosis at all. Block was so chagrined that he (quite appropriately) shot himself. During the next few years several other European surgeons attempted to treat tuberculosis in this way, but the results were disastrous and the method was fortunately soon abandoned. The hazard of lung resection has been so reduced today, however, that this method of treatment for tuberculosis is being taken up again.

At the same time that the early futile attempts at excision were made, a new therapeutic approach was being discovered that ultimately was to prove of great value in pulmonary tuberculosis. We have told elsewhere how Forlanini, in 1882, put forward the idea of injecting air into the pleural cavity to compress the lung and put it at rest so that it could heal. Soon after, a young Swiss surgeon, Edouard de Cérenville, of Lausanne, conceived another method aimed at putting the lung at rest mechanically. He proposed to remove the ribs overlying the diseased lung, thus allowing the chest wall to collapse and obliterating the underlying tuberculous cavity. He performed the first operation of this kind in 1885. During the next decade several other surgeons took up the operation and achieved occasional successes with it. None of them, however, carried the new principle far enough to make it work well, until the internist Ludolph Brauer, of Marburg, became interested in the problem and concentrated his attention on it between 1904 and 1907. He worked out the fundamental physiology of pneumothorax and arrived at the conclusion that the more complete the collapse of the chest wall, the better the chance of cure. With this aim in mind, in 1907 he persuaded his surgical colleague, L. P. Friedrich, to attempt to remove all of the ribs in tuberculous patients. Friedrich carried out a number of such operations, but found that the procedure was so shocking, resulting in death in one out of every three patients, that it had to be modified. Ferdinand Sauerbruch, who later became the leading thoracic surgeon in Germany, and who was then a young assistant of Friedrich's at Marburg, took a large part in devising a better method of thoracoplasty. The operation was divided into stages, and the extent of the resection limited to a few inches of the posterior portion only of each rib. In recent years the operation, still further improved, has won for itself an established place in the treatment of tuberculosis. The operative mortality has fallen to below ten per cent, and the percentage of patients benefited has greatly increased.

Another surgical procedure useful in occasional cases of pulmonary tuberculosis, and one which is practically without risk, is the cutting or removal of a part of the phrenic nerve, the nerve which supplies the diaphragm. This procedure also aims at putting the diseased lung at rest. The operation was first proposed in 1911 by Ernst Stuertz of Cologne, and shortly afterwards was performed for the first time by Sauerbruch, then professor of surgery at Munich.

Of all the problems that the thoracic surgeon has to face, however, the most serious is that presented by cancer of the lung. This is a disease of which Stephen Paget had not the faintest hope of cure when he wrote 50 years ago in his classical work that surgery of the chest was then "nearly at its zenith." Yet today it can be said that cancer of the lung has been cured by removal of the lung.

This disease, modern diagnostic means have proved, is distressingly common, and appears to be increasing in frequency. According to various compilations of autopsy statistics, cancer of the lung today constitutes about 15 per cent of all cancer, while at the beginning of this century it formed only about 5 per cent of all cancer. Its presence should always be suspected when there is a persistent cough, pain in the chest, or the raising of blood or blood-streaked sputum. The disease can be diagnosed accurately in about 75 per cent of the cases by bronchoscopic and x-ray examination.

As with most other forms of cancer, surgical excision, if it is to have a chance of success, must be radical. Since most cancers arise in the central part of the lung, removal of the whole of the lung containing the tumor, or total pneumonectomy, is usually required, rather than removal of only one lobe. This formidable operation was first successfully carried out on a human being in 1931 by Rudolph Nissen, Sauerbruch's successor, at the University Clinic in Berlin. The patient was a twelve year old child with advanced bronchiectasis affecting the whole of one lung. The first successful total pneumonectomy for cancer was done by Graham on April 7, 1933. His patient was a physician, who was still well five years afterwards.

Unfortunately there are not many such cases on record. A good many total pneumonectomies for cancer have been successfully carried out since Graham's first triumph, but very few of the patients have survived longer than a year. The main reason for this lack of success is the fact that in the great majority of patients diagnosis is so long delayed that when the thoracic surgeon finally sees the patient the disease is too far advanced for removal. Only ten or fifteen per cent of the cases are really operable. Here, as in so many other forms of internal cancer, surgery is helpless without better methods of early diagnosis. We have

to depend today upon clinical signs alone, and these are not sufficiently striking, in most cases, to call attention to the disease in
its early stage.

X-rays and radium have as yet given no indication of being
of much value in lung cancer. Thus the only hope of cure rests
in the last analysis upon the thoracic surgeon. This disease is one
of the great unsolved problems of modern medicine, and a harsh
challenge to surgical skill.

We have no space here to write in detail of other daring feats
of the thoracic surgeons, such as the surgery of the heart and its
great vessels. Ambroise Paré long ago suggested that wounds of
the heart might be sutured, but he dared not attempt it. Nor did
anyone else until in 1896, Guido Farina, an Italian surgeon, tried
to suture a dagger wound of the heart. The patient died after a
few days, however. The honor of succeeding in such a case went
to Louis Rehn, of Frankfort, who later on in the same year sutured
a stab wound of the right ventricle of the heart. Since then there
have been a great many successful operations of this kind. The
newspapers always give space to accounts of such operations, for
to the public they seem miraculous. As a matter of fact the
thoracic surgeon, during the course of some of the other operations on the lung which we have mentioned above, is often in a
more hazardous situation, and takes it as part of his day's work.

The most recent accomplishment of the thoracic surgeons is
the ligation of the patent ductus arteriosus. The ductus arteriosus is a vessel of considerable size which, during fetal life, forms
a short-circuiting communication between the pulmonary artery
and the arch of the aorta. Normally it closes after birth, but in
some instances it remains open, forming a serious handicap to
heart function which is usually eventually fatal. In August, 1938,
at the Children's Hospital in Boston, Robert E. Gross successfully
operated upon and ligated a patent ductus arteriosus in a child
aged seven and a half years. This was the first successful operation
of this kind ever done. Gross was led to attempt it because he
was urged by the child's pediatrician, John P. Hubbard, who

argued that the child had withstood a previous operation for appendicitis and was therefore strong enough to stand a more formidable procedure. They both knew that the child, like all others with a patent ductus arteriosus, had little chance of growing up if the attempt was not made. The determining factor of course was the fact that Gross was a trained thoracic surgeon. Again, specialization paid dividends. Several other surgeons have since duplicated his feat.

OTHER SURGICAL SPECIALTIES

OPHTHALMOLOGY

OPHTHALMOLOGY BEGAN with the ancient Greek, Roman, and Arabian surgeons who operated on cataracts. Their operation, called "couching" or "inclining" a cataract, consisted merely of perforating the eye with a needle and pushing the clouded lens backward into the posterior chamber of the eye out of the line of vision. It was a hazardous procedure, for sight was lost entirely in two out of every five eyes thus treated. In the 14th Century, Blind King John of Bohemia had an eye surgeon thrown into the Oder river when he failed to cure his blindness by couching.

The modern cataract operation, consisting of incision of the cornea or outer coat of the eye and extraction of the clouded lens through the pupil, was first done by the Parisian, Jacques Daviel, in 1748. By 1756 he was able to report 434 extractions with only 50 failures. Although Daviel's operation was a great advance, it was not immediately accepted, and "couching" continued to be done for a long time.

The treatment of eye diseases was largely in the hands of untrained quacks until the latter half of the 18th Century, when reputable surgeons began to take some interest in it. Georg Joseph Beer, of Vienna, gave special courses on diseases of the eye in the last years of the century, and in 1812 a professorship in ophthalmology was created for him, the first of its kind. In London, John C. Saunders founded the first Eye and Ear Infirmary in 1805. Two years later it was transformed into a hospital for eye diseases only, and came to be known as "Moorfields." In these clinics generations of ophthalmologists were trained, gaining for their specialty a recognized place in the organization of medical practice.

John Kearney Rogers and Edward Delafield, two young Americans trained at Moorfields, returned to New York and founded the New York Eye and Ear Infirmary in 1820. In Boston, the Massachusetts Charitable Eye and Ear Infirmary was founded in 1824. By the middle of the 19th Century all medical schools had established professorships of ophthalmology, and most of the larger cities had special hospitals for eye disease.

Ophthalmology now quickly developed into a complex science. In 1850 the great German physiologist, Hermann von Helmholtz, who at the age of 26 had established the first law of thermodynamics, contributed to ophthalmology its most important instrument, the ophthalmoscope. This was a silvered mirror with a central perforation and a series of changeable lenses through which the observer could study the fundus or inner surface of the patient's eye. It provided a means of observing all sorts of important changes in the optic nerve, the retina, and the blood vessels within the eye, on the basis of which diseases of the eye could be described and classified. Since the light rays from the ophthalmoscope necessarily had to pass through the lens to reach the fundus, the instrument also provided an exact means of measuring the manner in which the rays were refracted by the patient's eye. Errors of refraction could thus be accurately determined and properly corrected with glasses. Spectacles of the crudest kind had been in use since the 15th Century, but it was not until the Dutch ophthalmologist, Frans Cornelius Donders, worked out the common types of refractive errors in a monumental work accomplished between 1858 and 1864 that the fitting of glasses was put upon a scientific basis.

A method of controlling glaucoma was discovered in 1857 by

the Berlin eye surgeon, Albrecht von Graefe. Von Graefe found that the increased pressure within the eye, which is the essential feature of glaucoma, could be reduced by removing a part of the iris. Glaucoma had hitherto inevitably led to blindness. Other operative methods for controlling chronic glaucoma have been recently developed, but von Graefe's operation of iridectomy remains one of the important procedures in eye surgery.

With the development of aseptic surgical technique in the 1880's, and the introduction in 1884 of cocaine as a local anaesthetic for the eye, it became possible to carry out a great variety of operations on the eye with safety. One of the most frequently performed eye operations today is that in which the muscles which move the eyeball are shortened or re-attached at a different point on the eyeball in order to correct strabismus or squint, that condition in which the axes of vision of the two eyes assume a position relative to each other different from that required by normal physiological conditions. Many small children have strabismus, which may lead to serious difficulties of vision later on in life, unless corrected in youth.

OTOLOGY

Knowledge of diseases of the ear developed somewhat later than ophthalmology, although as we have seen, some of the earlier special hospitals dealt with the ear as well as the eye. The first special hospital for ear disease only was the Royal Ear Hospital founded in London in 1816. The first Department of Aural Surgery to be set up in a general hospital was also in London, at St. Mary's Hospital in 1851. Another important center for diseases of the ear in the British Isles was St. Mark's Ophthalmic Hospital in Dublin, founded in 1844.

Thus it happened that the foundations of modern otology were laid in Britain, early in the 19th Century. Two men were chiefly responsible. The first was Joseph Toynbee, of St. Mary's in London. He became curator of the Hunterian Museum of the Royal College of Surgeons in 1838, and devoted most of the next thirty years to the pathology of ear disease. His book, *The Diseases of the Ear*, published in 1860, did more to advance the understanding and proper classification of ear diseases than the works of all his predecessors. Among other things, Toynbee clearly showed that the great majority of ear diseases producing deafness result from preceding inflammation in the ear. Incidentally, Toynbee was deeply interested in the welfare of the working classes, then suffering from the dislocations of the industrial revolution, and he gave much time and thought to the problem of improving their living conditions.

The other important British contributor to otology was an Irishman, William Wilde, who founded the ear service at St. Mark's in Dublin. Although he kept abreast of Toynbee's pathological studies and based his understanding of ear disease on sound pathology, he was primarily a clinician, and his book *Practical Observations on Aural Surgery and the Nature and Treatment of Diseases of the Ear*, published in 1853, was the best treatise of its kind that had been written up to that time.

The means that these early 19th Century otologists had for studying ear disease were, of course, limited. In the first place they had nothing better than direct sunlight with which to inspect the ear drum, and in many individuals, because of the shape of the ear canal, a satisfactory view of the drum could not be obtained. Without this the drum could not be opened when acute inflammation of the middle ear made drainage necessary. All that Wilde and his contemporaries could do was to give calomel and opium and apply leeches to the ear.

This problem was solved by Friedrich Hofmann, a general practitioner in the little town of Burgsteinfurt, Germany. In 1841 he hit upon the idea of using a concave mirror, with a central perforation through which the observer could look, to reflect sunlight or lamp light into the ear canal. This instrument, later mounted on a head band, became the modern head mirror with which we today look into the nose and throat as well as the ear.

Adam Politzer, a young Viennese who had worked with Toynbee in London, made the next advance. Using the perforated mirror, he compared the clinical appearance of the ear drum in the living with the pathological changes in the ear found at autopsy in a large series of cases in Rokitansky's laboratory. In 1865, at the age of 30, he published his results in a monograph, entitled *The Appearance of the Illuminated Ear Drum*. Politzer's work established the clinical diagnosis and classification of disease of the middle and inner ear on a modern pathological basis. It is indeed surprising how complete his work was, and how little he missed of what we know today about the ear. He became chief of the ear clinic at Vienna and made it the leading center for the study of ear disease. His textbook, *Diseases of the Ear*, was the standard work on the ear for more than a generation. He lived an extraordinarily long and productive life—48 years elapsing between his first monograph on the ear drum and his final work, a *History of Otology*, published in 1913. He died in 1920 at the age of 85.

The diagnosis of ear disease having been put on a solid basis, it was possible for the first time to do something effective about treatment, particularly for acute earache or otitis media. This is a frequent disease of childhood in which the middle ear becomes infected by bacteria from the nose and throat, which find their way up along the Eustachian tube from the throat to the ear. Otitis media develops in association with colds or sore throats, sinusitis, and in infectious diseases like measles and scarlet fever, in which the mucous membranes of the nose and throat are irritated. The middle ear may fill up with pus which cannot find an outlet because the Eustachian tube is blocked by inflammatory swelling. Finally, perforation of the ear drum occurs. Serious complications and sequelae may develop as a result of the involvement of the mastoid cells by the acute process, or a chronic

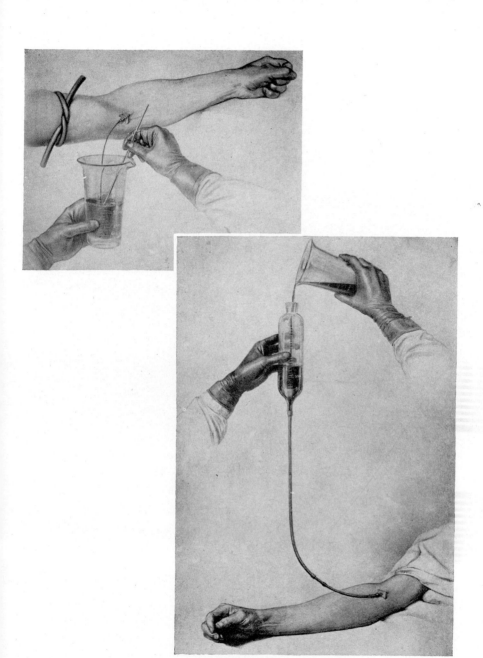

The First Practical Transfusion Method

The citrate method of transfusion as shown in Lewisohn's illustrations (from Boston Med. & Surg. J., 190:733, 1924). This was the first method for transfusion that was simple enough to be practical.

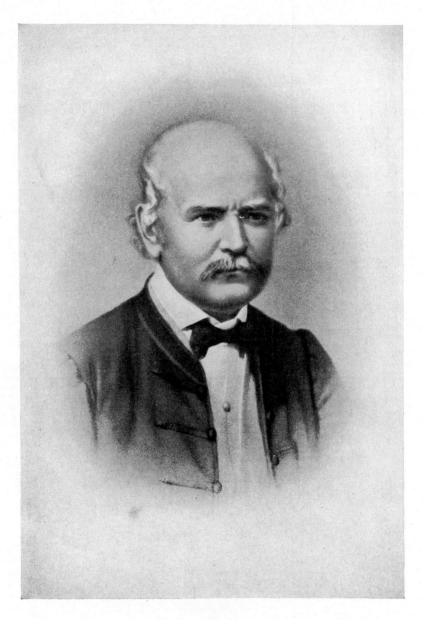

Semmelweis

He was a member of the Academic Legion of the University of Vienna which took an active part in the revolution of 1848, and he wore his uniform even on his hospital ward during the critical days when Metternich was overthrown. When the conservatives regained power Semmelweis lost his university post.

inflammatory state may ensue in which the ear discharges for months or years and partial deafness results.

Hermann Schwartze, an outstanding otological surgeon of Halle, Germany, was responsible for introducing incision of the ear drum to provide drainage in acute suppurative otitis media. This operation had been done occasionally for chronic ear disease and deafness since Astley Cooper's time, but Schwartze was the first to realize its usefulness in acute middle ear suppuration. In 1867 he wrote a classical paper on the indications for, and the value of, the operation, and it gradually came into use in the leading ear clinics.

Politzer's name is attached to another procedure that is valuable in the treatment of inflammation in the ear. This is the maneuver of opening up the Eustachian tube by means of a blast of air into the nose. By this procedure drainage of secretion from the middle ear is secured and inflammation reduced. The procedure was actually discovered by the great Italian anatomist, Antonio Valsalva. While professor of anatomy at Bologna he wrote a classic description of the anatomy of the ear, *De Aure Humana Tractatus* which appeared in 1704. He also made important observations regarding the physiology of the ear, including the phenomenon of inflation of the Eustachian tube by holding the mouth and nose closed and blowing the nose. Politzer merely devised a new method of obtaining inflation of the tube by means of a blast of air from a rubber bulb.

There is an interesting story regarding the maneuver of catheterizing the Eustachian tube, a method of treatment for ear disease that was very popular in the past century but which is not much used today. An obscure Frenchman with an interest in natural science, named Guyot, who was postmaster at Versailles, proposed to the Parisian Academy of Sciences in 1724, that a catheter might be inserted into the Eustachian tube via the mouth. That distinguished scientific body debated the proposal and finally decided that it was impractical, since Guyot had never himself practised it. In 1741 an English army surgeon, Archibald

Cleland, actually did catheterize and irrigate the Eustachian tube, but he did it with a catheter inserted through the nose, the route by which the opening of the Eustachian tube is most accessible.

Another important conquest by the otologists has been the operative attack on mastoiditis. The mastoid cells are a group of air spaces extending backward and downward from the middle ear into the mastoid process of the temporal bone. Inflammation in the middle ear may extend into these mastoid cells and produce an abscess within the mastoid. This kind of an abscess was usually fatal before the modern operation for mastoid drainage was known. The versatile Parisian surgeon, Jean-Louis Petit, was the first to realize the need of surgical drainage in the disease, and to carry it out successfully. He did the operation in several cases prior to his death in 1760, but his work was not published until 1774, and never attracted much attention. Only occasional attempts at surgical treatment were made until Schwartze, whose work on otitis media we have referred to above, realized the necessity of adequate surgical drainage of the diseased mastoid cells, and in 1873 devised an operation that achieved it. He chiseled away the outer shell of cortical bone over the mastoid, and gouged and curetted out the diseased cells. The operation done today is somewhat more radical but it remains essentially Schwartze's operation, and the great numbers of lives that it has saved must be credited to him.

During the present century important advances have been made in the understanding of deafness as a result of the development of highly accurate electrical methods of measuring acuity of hearing. In this way, a so-called audiogram for each ear is plotted by which the otologist can classify and keep track of the progress of the hearing difficulty.

RHINOLOGY AND LARYNGOLOGY

Special knowledge concerning diseases of the nose and throat developed considerably later than ophthalmology and otology.

For example, when the Manhattan Eye and Ear Hospital was founded in 1869 it lacked a nose and throat department entirely, because even at that late date no one could be found who devoted his attention specially to diseases of these organs. It was not until 1871 that a small throat department was organized in the hospital. Today many more people are treated there for nose and throat diseases than for eye or ear disease.

The lack of knowledge of diseases of the nose and throat was due primarily to two factors: first, the lack of instruments that would illuminate the interior of these hollow organs, and second, the lack of a local anaesthetic that would make it possible to manipulate instruments in them. The development of the head mirror and the laryngoscope (1858) made it possible to see into them, and the introduction of cocaine into nose and throat work solved the anaesthesia problem. Edward Jelinek, a young Viennese, began to use cocaine for this purpose in 1884, and within a few months it was adopted in many continental clinics.

Knowledge of disease in the nose and throat now grew phenomenally. The most important of the diseases that this epoch brought to light was sinusitis. Indeed, we know today that there is probably no more frequent disease afflicting those who live in the North Temperate Zone. Very few escape it, and many have sinusitis several times a year. In former times sinusitis to the layman was a "head cold that couldn't be shaken off" or "nasal catarrh." He used home or drugstore remedies and waited patiently for the disease to subside. Today something can really be done about it.

The nasal cavity is a surprisingly large space, and a very complex one, if the folds that project into it (the turbinates) and the outpouchings from it (the accessory sinuses) are taken into account. The sinuses normally contain air, and thus give lightness and bulk to the contour of the face. There are four groups of them: the maxillary antrums, situated one in each cheek; the ethmoid sinuses, a labyrinth of air cells in the roof of the nose; the frontal sinuses, situated one beneath each eyebrow; and the sphenoid sinuses, a pair of sinuses at the back of the upper part of the nasal cavity. Of all these, the antrums are by far the largest, as reference to the drawings taken from Emil Zuckerkandl's classical treatise on the anatomy of the sinuses will show. All of these sinuses have small natural openings or ostia into the nose. Most of these ostia open from the dependent part of the sinuses when the patient's head is erect, an important exception being the antrum. Its regular ostium, and also an accessory ostium which is present in a considerable proportion of cases, open into the nose from near the top of the cavity (see Zuckerkandl's drawing). During a head cold the mucous membrane lining all of the sinuses is usually inflamed and secretes profusely. This secretion as a rule drains out well enough from all the sinuses except the antrum, where it tends to accumulate.

As long ago as 1804, the symptoms of antral sinusitis were fairly well described by a Parisian surgeon, J. L. Deschamps, in his book: *Diseases of the Nasal Fossae and their Sinuses.* Deschamps advocated draining the antrum by extracting one of the upper teeth whose roots often extend to the floor of this sinus. This method relieved the acute infection but often left the patient with a fistula from the mouth to the antrum, an undesirable condition. Deschamps thought that antral sinusitis was always due to diseased teeth, and this belief persisted until the revival of interest in sinusitis in the 1870's.

The first step in the development of modern rhinology was a thorough study of the normal anatomy and gross pathology of the sinuses made by Emil Zuckerkandl in the anatomy laboratories of the University of Vienna. Zuckerkandl had been trained not only by the distinguished anatomist, Josef Hyrtl, but by the great pathologist, Rokitansky, so that he was able to interpret the consequences of disease as well as the normal relationships in the 300 specimens that he dissected. The first volume of his treatise appeared in 1882, and was a great stimulus to the study of sinus disease. The second volume was published ten years later.

Arthur Hartmann, professor of otolaryngology at Berlin, had

also become interested in sinus disease at this same period. In 1882 he published the first accurate clinical description of acute sinusitis, emphasizing the nasal discharge and obstruction to breathing, and the pain in the forehead caused by the accumulation of secretion in the antrum and frontal sinuses. Two years later he devised a small curved cannula that he was able to insert into the antrum through its ostium, and wash out the accumulation of pus. Washing out the antrum brought prompt relief, and a few treatments of this kind usually cleared up the attack. Three years later, in 1887, Johan von Mikulicz, of whom we have spoken before, described a method of making an artificial opening into the antrum through the nasal wall with a special trocar. This provided a sure means of washing out the sinus when the natural opening could not be cannulated. Further progress was made in 1889 by Friedrich Voltini, otolaryngologist at Breslau, when he discovered an important diagnostic sign of sinus disease. When a small electric light was placed within the mouth, and the outside of the face observed in a darkened room, healthy air-containing frontal sinuses and antrums transmitted the light but diseased sinuses were opaque. In 1897 Scheier found that in roentgen ray pictures diseased sinuses were also clouded, and this method of diagnosis has been widely used since.

With these means of diagnosing and treating sinusitis at hand, otolaryngologists were surprised to discover the high frequency of the disease. Their experience was shortly confirmed by the findings of the pathologists who now began for the first time to investigate the sinuses carefully at autopsy. Thus Eugene Fraenkel of Hamburg, in a careful study of this question in 1896, found that in a series of 146 routine autopsies, the sinuses were diseased in 40 per cent of the cases. The antrums were involved much more frequently than the other sinuses.

In 1899, Markus Hajek, to whose nose and throat clinic in Vienna countless foreign physicians came for training around the turn of the century, published an important monograph on sinus disease which embodied all this new information. It was the standard work on the subject for the next generation and did much to spread knowledge of sinus disease throughout the world.

In certain cases of chronic antral sinusitis, where repeated irrigation fails to clear up the infection, some sort of permanent opening between the antrum and the nose may be required. In 1893, a New Yorker, George W. Caldwell, devised the operation which has come to be the one generally used to provide such a permanent opening. It consisted of opening the antrum through its outer wall in the canine fossa of the upper jaw, curetting it out thoroughly, making a large counter opening through the wall between the sinus and the nasal cavity, and then sewing up the canine fossa opening.

Today the methods of draining infected sinuses are highly developed. The next efforts must be directed toward the prevention of sinus disease. This means research regarding the common cold, which is by far the most frequent cause of sinusitis. Very little money is available for such research, although the common cold is certainly responsible for more time lost from work than any other disease. It would seem that the largest industrial corporations might find it a good investment to establish a common fund to support research regarding colds. In the medical schools and research institutes there are many students with good ideas for such research, but no funds with which to carry it out. When compared with the relatively large sums of money raised for research regarding the comparatively infrequent disease of infantile paralysis, the money devoted to study of the common cold is ridiculously little.

We must refer, although briefly, to disease of the larynx. Modern knowledge of it began when indirect laryngoscopy made it possible to inspect the pharynx and larynx in the living. The pioneer in laryngoscopy was not a physician, but a Spanish singing teacher living in London, Manuel Garcia. Garcia's interest in phonetics led him in 1855 to devise a small mirror, which when placed against the soft palate and uvula permitted him to follow the movements of the larynx. Two years later the Viennese neurologist, Ludwig Türck, and Johann N. Czermak, professor of physiology at the University of Pest, both began to use the method clinically to examine the pharynx and larynx. These two gentlemen unfortunately became involved in a jealous feud over the priority of their discovery, but they nevertheless made important observations regarding laryngeal disease. They both published widely and demonstrated their methods abroad. Czermak's contribution was probably the more important, for it was he who first utilized the perforated concave mirror of the otologists to reflect light onto the laryngoscopic mirror in the throat, thus providing the necessary illumination. Czermak at first held the perforated mirror between his teeth. It was next mounted on a spectacle frame, and then on a head band, giving us the modern head mirror. By 1865 laryngoscopy was so well popularized that it was widely used both in Europe and America. Clinics for diseases of the throat bloomed everywhere.

Cancer of the throat, the most serious problem the laryngologist has to face, could now be diagnosed and attacked. Billroth, at Vienna, was the first to resect the larynx for cancer successfully, in 1873. During the next ten years a score of such operations were done, mostly by German surgeons. In 1886 Crown Prince Frederick of Germany developed persistent hoarseness, and was found to have laryngeal cancer. He refused to permit removal of his larynx, perhaps wisely, for about half of the patients on whom the operation had been done had succumbed to it and none had been permanently cured. He wished to live at least long enough to become emperor and combat the "blood and iron" imperialism of Bismarck, whom he bitterly opposed. Unfortunately for the liberal party in Germany, Frederick's disease progressed so rapidly that it was in its last stage when he succeeded to the throne on March 9, 1888. He died on June 15, 1888, after a reign of only 91 days. With his death English hopes of friendship ended and Bismarck's policy triumphed, carrying the German people along the road to two world wars.

History might have been different if surgeons had known how to deal with laryngeal cancer then as they do today. The operations of partial and complete extirpation of the larynx have been perfected to the point where the operative mortality in expert hands is less than 10 per cent. Approximately half of those who survive are permanently cured.

Another important advance has been the development of methods of radiation treatment for throat cancer. This is the treatment of choice for cancers of the tonsillar region and the pharynx, for surgery has failed to cure cancer in these regions. The evolution of an effective method of roentgen ray treatment has been to a large extent the work of Henri Coutard, of the Radium Institute of Paris. The method of treatment known by his name involves giving very small doses of the rays daily over a period of months through several different portals of entry. Coutard treated his first case of pharyngeal cancer along these general lines in 1921. In 1932 he was able to report that 212 cases had been treated up to 1926, and that 20 per cent were cured.

We cannot leave the subject of disease of the nose and throat without mentioning bronchoscopy, and the thrilling feats of the bronchoscopists in removing foreign bodies from the bronchi. The laryngeal mirror, that is, *indirect* laryngoscopy, did not permit the laryngologist to do much in the way of instrumentation in the larynx. To overcome this handicap Alfred Kirstein, a young Berlin laryngologist, in 1895 invented a speculum which he called the "autoscope." With this simple device he could get a direct view of the larynx. The instrument was not much more than a specially shaped tongue depressor, over which a source of light was directed, but it sufficed for direct inspection of the larynx. It was from this method of *direct* laryngoscopy that bronchoscopy evolved. Gustav Killian, the distinguished director of the nose and throat clinic at the University of Freiburg, was largely responsible. He modified Kirstein's laryngoscope to make a split tube which gave him a good exposure of the larynx. With the larynx thus exposed, he found that he could pass a long metal tube (he used an esophagoscope at first) far down the trachea into the main bronchi, and see the lumens of the branches of the bronchi to the lobes of the lungs. It was in March, 1897, that he was able to see, by this means, a small piece of bone lodged in the bronchus of a man aged 63, and to remove it successfully by grasping it with a forceps inserted through the tube. This was the first instance of removal of a foreign body from the bronchi, a procedure which has since saved the lives of countless small children. They love to suck buttons, coins, safety pins, etc., and every once in a while swallow one of them. If these objects stick in the throat they are sometimes aspirated through the larynx, lodging in the bronchi. Unless they are removed they usually lead to death, as a result of pulmonary obstruction and infection. An American, Chevalier Jackson, has perhaps done more than anyone else to perfect the technique of bronchoscopy and the removal of these foreign bodies, having extracted some 3,500 of them. The ingenuity required to close and remove a safety pin lodged point upwards far down in the bronchial tree of an infant can be imagined. Today bronchoscopy is so safe that it is used as a matter of routine in the diagnosis of lesions in the bronchi and lungs, permitting the removal of tissue for microscopical examination.

RADIUM

R ADIUM HAS not only had a revolutionary effect on the basic science of physics, but it has also been found to be a useful tool in the surgical attack on cancer. In order to understand its surgical application we need to know something of the story of how radium came to be discovered.

The discovery of radium was an indirect result of the discovery of roentgen rays. In the early roentgen ray tubes the impact of the cathode rays on the glass wall of the tube produced a green fluorescence. This phenomenon suggested that there might be some relationship between visible fluorescence and invisible roentgen radiation. Jules Henri Poincaré, a physicist at the University of Paris, was the first to suggest the desirability of testing ordinary fluorescent or phosphorescent substances to see if they emitted invisible rays similar to roentgen rays. His colleague, Henri Becquerel, undertook a systematic investigation of these substances. They were placed on a photographic plate, which was wrapped in black paper and put aside for some hours. His results were all negative until he tested several uranium salts in this manner. With all of them a distinct photographic effect was obtained. On February 24, 1896, Becquerel reported his discovery at the Academy of Sciences.

At once other physicists began the study of this new phenomenon of radioactivity. Among them were Pierre and Marie Curie, who eventually discovered radium. The story of their discovery is one of the most romantic in modern science. At the time Becquerel made his report, Pierre Curie was teaching physics in the School of Physics and Chemistry of the City of Paris in the rue Lhomond. He was only 35 years old, and had already won an international reputation by his researches in crystalline physics and magnetism, but he was tied down to the job of teaching in his relatively unimportant school. His wife, Marie Slodowska, was a remarkable woman, who became the most distinguished scientist of her sex in the modern world. After six years spent as a governess in provincial families in Poland, she had come to Paris in 1891, determined to devote herself to science. She entered the Sorbonne and passed the examinations for the licentiate in physics three years later. The following year, while she was preparing for the examinations in mathematics, she met Pierre Curie. They were married in 1895, and she began to help her husband at his school in his research with crystals.

The attention of both the Curies was caught by Becquerel's discovery of radioactivity, and Madame Curie undertook to measure the new form of radiation by means of an electrometer designed by her husband. An unheated glassed-in room on the ground floor of the school, which had been used as a storeroom and a machine shop, was fitted up for the work. She at once found that the intensity of the radiation emitted was proportional to the amount of uranium contained in the compound being tested. She searched for such radiation from other elements, and found that thorium was the only other element possessing it. Madame Curie examined a great many compounds in the course of this research, and she found that the radioactivity of a sample of pitchblende from an Austrian mine was particularly marked. This was known to contain uranium and thorium, but Madame Curie's calculations revealed that its radioactivity was much higher than could be accounted for by the content of uranium and thorium alone. Since she knew that no other known chemical elements possessed radioactivity she reasoned that the pitchblende must contain some new unknown chemical element of high radioactivity.

The mystery now became so fascinating that her husband

joined her in the work. Together they carefully separated, by ordinary means of chemical analysis, the different components of pitchblende, and measured the radioactivity of each one. Thus they tracked down, and isolated, a strongly radioactive substance contained in the barium extract from the pitchblende ore. They called the new element *polonium,* in honor of Madame Curie's country. In the barium extract of the ore they soon found another new element, which they called *radium.* They announced the discovery of polonium in July, 1898, and of radium in December of the same year.

The Curies now set out to isolate radium in its pure form. For this purpose they were presented with several tons of pitchblende by the Austrian government. But their facilities for the laborious work of extraction were very crude, and it required over two years of exhausting effort before they obtained a small amount of pure radium chloride.

They found that this new stuff possessed truly remarkable properties. It gave off light, heat, and electricity continuously without suffering any apparent change. Furthermore, it emitted highly penetrating rays even more powerful than x-rays. We know now that the element is spontaneously turning part of its own substance into energy and is, in fact, slowly losing weight. A definite small fraction of all the atoms of radium undergoes disintegration in a given interval of time. Since less than one two-thousandth part of the atoms are changed in one year it will be clear why the loss of weight is not very obvious. Indeed it would take more than a thousand years for a mass of radium to lose one half of its weight. No known chemical or physical process has been found to influence the rate of radiation and disintegration, which proceeds continuously and inevitably.

From the unlucky circumstance of receiving a burn from radium, Becquerel was able to draw attention to the strange physiological properties of radium. In April, 1901, he happened to be using a tube of pure radium and put it in his waistcoat pocket. A fortnight later severe inflammation of the skin beneath developed.

Pierre Curie confirmed this observation by producing on himself in a few hours a burn which took months to heal.

The Curies won the Nobel prize, and a special professorial chair was created for Pierre to continue his important work; but in 1906 the scientific world was shocked to learn that he had been crushed to death under the wheel of a two-horse dray in the streets of Paris. Curie was dead, but his wife lived for many years more to carry on scientific investigations in radium. She died in 1934 from anemia, which was almost certainly due to the destruction of her blood-forming bone-marrow by the constant and relentless action of the rays with which she worked.

As soon as it had been shown that skin burns could be caused by radium, medical men began to experiment in order to find out if malignant growths of the skin could be destroyed by the same agency. Professor Curie intrusted a specimen of the substance to H.-A. Danlos, a dermatologist at the St. Louis Hospital in Paris. Danlos was the first to use radium to treat various lesions of the skin, including cancer. By 1904 he was able to report that it was of value, and recommended important improvements in the methods of applying it. By this time it had been used for skin cancer also in St. Petersburg, where Goldberg and London reported curing epithelioma of the skin of the face with it, and in New York by Morris Manges, who found that he could not influence a melanoma with it, and by Robert Abbe who claimed success in numerous cases of skin epithelioma with it.

Encouraged by these early reports, an institute for the study of the physical and biological properties of radium was organized in Paris in 1906 by a group of workers who were stimulated by the Curies. It was called the Biological Laboratory for Radium. Its staff included the physicist Jacques Danne, the physiologist Henri Dominici, and the clinicians Louis Wickham and Degrais, both of whom were dermatologists. All of these men made important contributions to the new science of radiotherapy. Perhaps the most fundamental were those made by Dominici. Radium emits three types of rays, all invisible, called alpha, beta and gamma rays, respectively. The first two types do not possess much power of penetration but enter the skin deeply enough to produce a sharp reaction in it. Dominici saw that both the alpha and beta rays could be excluded by interposing a primary heavy filter of lead and a secondary filter of paper, allowing only the ultrapenetrating gamma rays to pass. In 1908 he applied gamma radiation of this type to deeply seated tumors and found that the overlying structures showed little change while the deeply seated tumor tissue regressed. This was the first clinical application of the important physical principle of filtration—a principle which has had a profound influence on radiotherapy. Dominici, like so many other of the early workers with radiation, died in 1919 from the effects of excessive exposure to the new rays.

A variety of methods of applying radium were shortly devised. The bromide salt was put into glass tubes which were sealed and then enclosed in an outer tube of silver or platinum that provided filtration. Such tubes could be inserted into hollow cavities like the uterus or the esophagus. It was put into small platinum needles that were inserted directly into the tissues and sutured in place until the required dosage had been given. Plaques were made up of it to be used on the surface of the body. A great variety of special applicators for use in applying radium salt were brought forward. One of the most useful methods of using radium was devised by Giocchimo Failla, physicist to the Memorial Hospital in New York. As it slowly disintegrates radium gives off a gaseous emanation called radon. This gas possesses all the power of affecting tissues that radium itself exhibits, but it loses its radioactivity with comparative rapidity. Half its activity is gone within less than four days and almost all is gone at the end of a month. The physicists who did the early work with radium devised methods of collecting radon and sealing it in small glass tubes. In 1924 Failla worked out a method of sealing it in small sections of very fine gold tubing. These so-called "gold seeds" could be inserted into the tissues like radium-containing needles, but unlike the needles the seeds could be left permanently in place, for their radioactivity was soon exhausted and gold is not a very irritating foreign body in the tissues.

Although laboratories and special institutes for the study of radiation were established in a number of European and American centers of medical teaching early in the century, progress with radium therapy was slow. Soon after the first flush of enthusiasm for the new treatment it was found that most of the cancers which regressed so miraculously with it recurred after a time. The cancer cells, temporarily suppressed and enclosed in scar tissue produced by the radiation reaction, eventually regained their growth vigor and again formed a tumor. Definitive cure could not be assured until several years, preferably five to seven, had elapsed. Moreover, the new form of treatment often left unfortunate sequelae in the form of painful ulcers and bad scars. A feeling of disappointment and reaction against the use of radium developed among the surgeons during the second decade of the century. They saw much harm done with it.

Radium first proved its worth in the specialty of gynecology. In our discussion of uterine cancer we have told how a number of German gynecologists reported encouraging results in cervix cancer with it in 1914, and how its superiority over surgical removal was proved some years later. In the 1920's dependable data began to appear regarding the superiority of radium over surgery for some other forms of cancer. At the Institute of Radium in Paris it was shown that cancers of the tongue, which surgery rarely cured, were not infrequently cured with radium. Cancer of the lip, and some forms of cancer of the skin, gave good percentages of cure with radium.

The technique of using radium for cancer is still evolving, and its ultimate place in the surgeon's armamentarium is not yet settled. Research regarding its biological effects and its clinical use is being carried on in a number of special institutes and laboratories. In several countries the great cost of radium has led to special funds being raised by popular subscription for the purchase of it for their laboratories and clinics. The monarchs of both

Sweden and Britain turned their Jubilee Birthday offerings over to this purpose. The costliness of radium is due chiefly to the labor of separating it from its natural ore. Up to very recently the main sources of this ore have been in Czechoslovakia and the Belgian Congo. In the past it has required about six tons of the richest ore available to obtain one gram of radium. Fortunately new and much richer radium-containing ores have recently been discovered in the Canadian wilderness, and we can look forward to a great reduction in the cost of this precious substance.

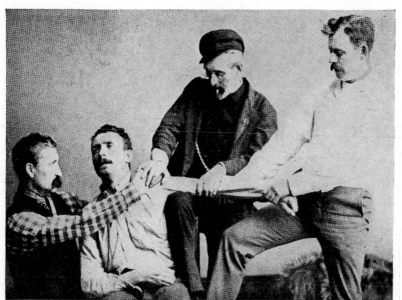

(From Frederick Watson's biography *Hugh Owen Thomas*)

Hugh Owen Thomas Reducing a Dislocated Shoulder, Assisted by Robert Jones

Thomas was a shy and retiring man, and always wore the little peaked cap pulled down over one eye as in this photograph. He smoked cigarettes continuously.

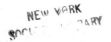

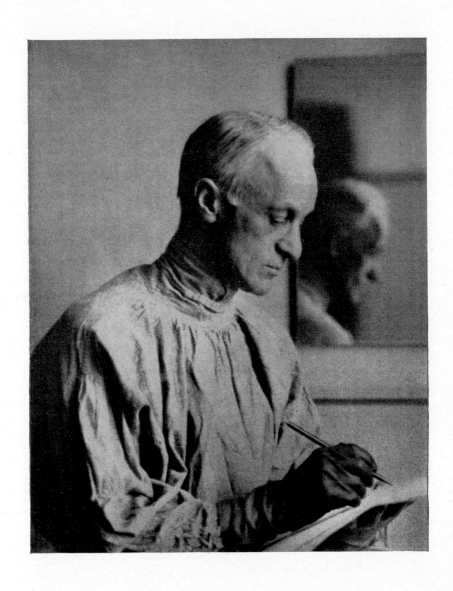

Harvey Cushing Sketching

He spared no effort to make his case records as complete as possible,
and often included impromptu sketches of the operative findings.

TRAINED NURSES

WITH THE enormous growth of medical science which we have been describing, the practical care of the patient has become increasingly complex. The nurses who are responsible for this care must be trained. Florence Nightingale was the first to realize this, and with a kind of religious zeal she devoted her life to reforming hospitals and establishing nursing as a profession.

The hospitals of her day were decidedly not an attractive place for an English lady whose youth had been sheltered by a Victorian environment. Yet in 1851, when she was 31 years old, Florence Nightingale gave up the life of leisure and travel in which she had been reared, and decided to become a nurse. Because she could find no place in England to obtain training, she went for three months to Kaiserswerth in Germany to the Institution for Deaconesses, where there was a school for infants and where some sort of training in nursing was given. How little this was may be judged from her own words: "The nursing there was *nil*. The hygiene horrible. . . . I took all the training there was to be had —there was none to be had in England—but Kaiserswerth was far from having trained me."

Shortly after her return home she became superintendent of a small hospital, The Establishment for Gentlewomen during Illness, in Harley Street, London. During the cholera outbreak of 1854 she left this position to help nurse patients at the Middlesex Hospital.

Her great opportunity came with the Crimean War, and it was

her experience at Scutari, and the magnificent results which she obtained, that supplied the guiding principles in hospital reform. The situation in the war area was horrible indeed before Miss Nightingale began her work. The old army pensioners who had been sent out to nurse the sick and wounded proved quite useless, and in fact spent much of their time nursing one another. The shortage of medical supplies was scandalous. The *London Times* reporter wrote from the battlefield:

"Not only are there not sufficient surgeons—that, it might be urged, was unavoidable: not only are there no dressers and nurses—that might be a defect of system for which no one is to blame: but what will be said when it is known that there is not even linen to make bandages for the wounded?"

It was through Sidney Herbert, who was Minister of War, that Miss Nightingale was asked to undertake the formidable task of organizing the nursing at Scutari. Fired by the revelations in the *Times,* she had offered her services to the Minister in a letter which crossed his in the mail. With his approval, she now rapidly collected a group of thirty-eight women who were to be her staff. She had to choose these with care from hundreds of volunteers who applied, for she saw at once that the women she wanted must not only be able-bodied and tender-hearted but must also have as much previous experience and training as possible. Thus the great experiment began.

It should not be assumed that this was the first experiment in utilizing female nurses for sick soldiers. The French had their Sisters of Charity, and the great Russian surgeon Nikolai Ivano-vich Pirogoff had been induced by the Grand Duchess Helena Pavlovna to use female nurses to care for the wounded in the Crimea in the same campaign.

The state of affairs at Scutari could hardly have been worse when Florence Nightingale arrived there. There were more than seventeen hundred patients in the military hospital, and cholera, dysentery, erysipelas, and gangrene raged among them. Amputations were carried out in the open wards, so that the grisly sight was visible to all. There was a complete breakdown of all medical organization. The food was inedible. There was dirt, confusion, and neglect. The floors of the hospital were rotten and the walls encrusted with filth. There were not enough beds. Vermin and lack of ventilation helped to make the place a stinking inferno. There were not only no medical supplies, but basins, soap, towels, mops, knives, forks, and plates all were wanting. There was no laundry and often not even enough fuel.

Miss Nightingale worked tirelessly to clean the hospital up, to supply the missing necessities, and to organize a rudimentary nursing service. She had to fight against the fierce opposition not only of the military authorities but of some of the medical men themselves. Her success is best shown by the mortality figures. During the first seven months of the war the mortality among the troops *from disease alone* was 60 per cent per annum—a mortality rate exceeding that of the great plague in London. After she had been at Scutari for six months she was able to report that of the 1,100 patients left in the Barrack Hospital only 100 were in bed, and the death rate had fallen from 42 per cent to 2.2 per cent.

This remarkable result was accomplished by foresight, and by methodical and unremitting hard work. Miss Nightingale had armed herself with medical and household supplies in huge amounts before going to Scutari, in spite of the assurance she had received from the head of the Army Medical Department that nothing was wanting there. Furthermore she had money, both her own fund and that collected by the *Times*. She had also the loyal support not only of the Government through the influence of Sidney Herbert but also of public opinion at home.

Besides her battle with officialdom and etiquette she had to fight mainly against dirt and chaos. She provided a new laundry, and reorganized the kitchen and the cooking. She procured socks, boots, shirts, trousers, and dressing-gowns for the patients. She routed out stores that were hidden away under the munitions in the transports and in the labyrinths of the Turkish Customs House. She even engaged workmen to fit out fresh quarters for the reception of new consignments of sick and wounded. In fact, from being simply the matron of a hospital, she became practically "mistress of a barrack and indeed assistant purveyor to the British army."

It was while all this organizing was in progress that Miss Nightingale developed her idea of what a nursing service should be. Nurses were not to be an entirely separate service of domestics; much less were they to interfere with the work of the doctors. They were to be a "subordinate branch of the medical service under the doctor's orders as to the matter of treatment while under their own superintendent as to matters of discipline." Miss Nightingale introduced uniforms for her nurses to promote cleanliness and to give them a smart and sober appearance and to "disarm criticism and belie the untoward reputation of nurses."

But the strain was great, and finally she became seriously ill with Crimean fever. When she recovered, she refused to leave her mission until all the soldiers were gone from Scutari. Then she returned home to be greeted as a heroine.

Back in England she at once began a fight for reform in nursing and in hospital organization that was to last the rest of her life. She was determined, first of all, to change the organization of the Army Medical Service. She collected statistics that showed that the state of affairs in the army hospitals at home was deplorable. Even among the Guards, who were men of picked physique, the death rate was nearly double what it was in civil life. Armed with figures of this sort she was able to browbeat the Government into appointing a Royal Commission to study the situation. She then wrote out her own ideas in a monumental work, *Notes on the British Army*, which Sidney Herbert used as a guide in the reforms that he forced through. Under this legislation barracks and hospitals were ventilated and warmed, water supplies improved, drainage reconstructed, kitchens remodelled, and an Army Medical School founded. As a result the death rate in the Army was halved between 1859 and 1861.

In 1859 Miss Nightingale published her classical *Notes on*

Nursing. The book found a large public at the time, and has remained justly popular ever since. A large fund in her honor was raised by public subscription, and she used it to establish at St. Thomas' Hospital in London the first training school for nurses. It was appropriately called The Nightingale School, and the first probationers were accepted for a year's training in June, 1860. The fundamental features of the plan were: (1) classroom teaching, including the basic sciences, as well as technical instruction in practical nursing care; (2) provision for a nurses' home where the students lived; (3) control of the school by a matron or superintendent of nurses.

The Nightingale School was an immediate success. Many of its graduates were women of executive and teaching ability who played an important part in organizing schools of nursing throughout the British Isles. The St. Thomas nurses still wear the blue and white dresses and the lace frilled caps, tied under the chin, which Miss Nightingale designed for them.

During the decade following the establishment of The Nightingale School the nurses' training school idea spread widely through the English speaking countries. Training schools were soon organized in most of the larger cities of England and Scotland, as well as in Sydney and in Melbourne, Australia. In 1865 a training school for nurses was opened at the Woman's Hospital in Philadelphia, the first of its kind in America. In 1873 three other training schools were established in the United States, at Bellevue in New York, at the New Haven Hospital in New Haven, and at the Massachusetts General Hospital in Boston. Schools were opened at the Pennsylvania Hospital in Philadelphia in 1875, and at the New York Hospital, the Hartford Hospital, the Boston City Hospital, and the Buffalo General Hospital in 1877. Trained nurses were soon found to be indispensable to good hospital management, and Miss Nightingale's battle was won. She had created a new profession for her sex.

The growth of the nursing profession during the last fifty years has been phenomenal. In the United States, for instance, there was a total of 22 schools of nursing in 1883. They had graduated a total of 600 nurses. In 1940 there were 1,300 accredited schools in which some 80,000 student nurses were enrolled. A total of 300,000 nurses had been graduated since nursing training had been instituted.

As medical care has increased in complexity trained nurses have been given more and more responsibility for the carrying out of elaborate and sometimes difficult therapeutic procedures. Exact recording of the patient's fluid intake and output, management of the complicated gastro-intestinal drainage tubes, and carrying out of more or less elaborate surgical dressings, are examples of some of the things that a modern trained nurse is expected to do. If she is to do them intelligently she must have certain fundamental training in the basic medical sciences.

PART FOUR

New Social Aspects of Medicine

A CENTURY OF PROGRESS

THE 19TH CENTURY was for medicine truly a century of phenomenal progress. At the beginning of this crucial century medicine was not much more than a practical art in which folklore and the beginnings of organized knowledge of disease were intermingled. At its end it had evolved into a highly complex science capable of attacking and controlling some of the most formidable diseases.

Having told some of the story of how this came about, we must attempt to sum up in a crude way at least the accomplishments of medicine. What has been the repercussion on the life of the average man?

Anyone wandering through old New England churchyards cannot fail to be struck by the numbers of headstones of children and of young wives. It was not an uncommon thing for a man at the beginning of the 19th Century to have a score of children by several successive wives and to lose most of them. Queen Anne lost all of her eighteen or nineteen children. The great historian, Gibbon, was the sole survivor of seven children. Smallpox, diphtheria, pneumonia, typhoid fever, cholera and yellow fever swept away the youth of the land periodically, while tuberculosis took its steady toll.

At the beginning of the 19th Century several European students of infant mortality estimated that about one quarter of all children died before they reached two years of age, while more than one half succumbed before the age of ten. The mortality was even higher of course in the great cities. In London, for instance, during the period 1790–1809, 41.3 per cent of all children died before reaching the age of 5 years. The substitution of hand feeding for breast feeding was one of the most important causes of deaths of infants, as is well illustrated by the terrible record of foundling hospitals during this period. Of 10,272 infants admitted to the Dublin Foundling Hospital during the period 1775–1796, for instance, only 45 survived, a mortality of 99.6 per cent. The industrial revolution drove mothers to factory work and made breast feeding impossible. They had to leave their babies in the care of mercenary and neglectful wet nurses or farm them out to be hand fed with such unsuitable preparations as gruel and water-pap, which is moistened and sweetened bread.

As late as 1870, when proper mortality records first began to be kept in New York City, the infant death rate (number of deaths under 1 year per 1,000 live births) was still 383.3. It was at about this time that infant mortality began a sharp decline that has brought it down today to less than one tenth of this figure. The infant welfare movement, which has been chiefly responsible for this improvement, was largely French in origin. It was in 1884 that Firmin Marbeau, mayor of the first arrondissement of Paris, founded the first *crèche* or day nursery, where working mothers could leave their babies to be properly fed and cared for. The idea spread rapidly in England and the United States. The humanitarian spirit in the novels of writers such as Victor Hugo and Charles Dickens reflected the awakening interest of men of good will in poor and abused children. Laws were shortly passed in several European countries to protect infants and mothers. In England the "Life Protection Act" of 1872 provided for the regulation and inspection of all places where infants were farmed out, and in France in 1874 the *Loi Roussel* had a similar purpose. In 1877 Switzerland enacted a law requiring a rest period for mothers of ten weeks before delivery and six weeks afterward. Other European countries soon followed suit. One of the important factors in reducing infant mortality during the last years of this century was the development—chiefly by American pediatricians—of improved formulas for preparing artificial feedings from properly sterilized cow's milk. During this period there were some striking demonstrations of what common sense and attention to detail could do. For instance, M. Morel de Villiers, a physician, mayor of the village of Villiers-le-Duc in the Côte d'Or in France, brought the infant mortality down to zero in his village during the period between 1893 and 1903 by the strict application of hygienic measures. These measures included municipal assurance of free medical aid for all pregnant mothers who needed it, a grant of a small daily sum for all mothers remaining in bed for six days after delivery, compulsory sterilization of milk, careful regulation of all wet nurses, systematic weighing of newborn infants on a municipal weighing machine, and a bonus for every nursing mother whose child was in good health at one year of age.

In the United States the past generation has seen a remarkable reduction in infant mortality. The development of the visiting nurse service to look after sick babies, the opening of free milk stations for the poor, and the pasteurization and careful inspection of milk, have all played a part. In New York City the infant death rate fell to 203.6 per 1,000 births in 1900. In 1915 it was 98.8. By 1930 it had fallen to 57.8, and in 1940 it came down to 35.0, a figure which pediatricians of a generation ago never dreamed of.

This great saving of youthful life has more than doubled the average duration of life. Although vital statistics were rudimentary a hundred years ago, several European countries, notably Holland and the Scandinavian countries, had made a beginning at collecting them. In Sweden the expectation of life at birth for males (always a little shorter than for females) was 33.2 years in 1776. By 1870 it had risen to 42.8 years, and in 1930 it was 61.19 years. In the United States the first life table was drawn up in 1789 by the Reverend Edward Wigglesworth. He compiled it from bills of mortality from scattered seacoast towns of Massachusetts and New Hampshire. Imperfect as it must have been

Wigglesworth's table gave the expectation of life at birth as 28.15 years, a figure not very different from that derived from contemporary European data. In 1855 a Massachusetts life table based on fairly extensive data gave the expectation of life as 39.8 years. By 1901, when official life tables representing a considerable part of the territory of the United States first became available, the expectation of life at birth had risen to 49 years. Today it is over 60 years.

We must not, however, delude ourselves into thinking that these figures mean that the life span has been lengthened. The study of the records of antiquity, as a matter of fact, do not indi-

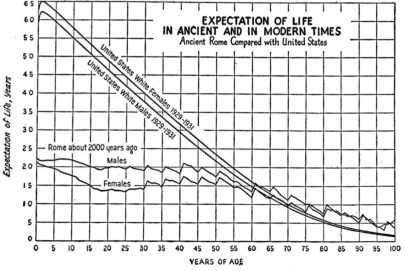

(From *Length of Life* by Dublin and Lotka)

cate that individuals live to be older now than they then did. In ancient Rome it was a common practice to bequeath life annuities, and tables of life expectation were drawn up for making this computation. From these and other data it would appear that a Roman citizen of 2,000 years ago who reached the age of 60 could expect to survive about 15 years more—almost exactly the length of time that a sexagenarian today can hope to survive. The prolongation of life that modern medicine has achieved has all been in the younger age groups.

The net result of the great saving of young lives that we have been describing, plus the effect of a declining birth rate, is that our population in the United States is in the aggregate growing older. This change has been going on for a longer time in European countries, but now the same trend is apparent here. During the last two generations the average age of our population has increased one year each decade. The accompanying chart shows this shift in the age distribution of New York City's population since 1900. It will be seen from it that the proportion of people over 65 years of age has almost doubled since 1900 having increased from 2.8 to 5.5 per cent.

NEW YORK CITY'S AGING POPULATION

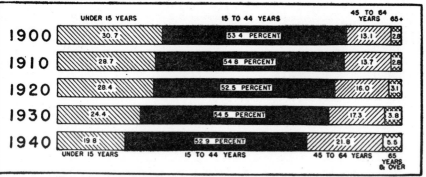

(From *Quarterly Bulletin, Department of Health, City of New York,* 9;55, 1941)

Now this ageing of the population has an important bearing on the relative frequency of different diseases. In 1900 in the United States, pneumonia, tuberculosis, and infantile diarrhea and enteritis—largely diseases of youth—headed the list of the chief causes of death. Today heart disease and cancer—mainly diseases of old age—head the list. The following table made from U.S. Mortality Statistics for 1900 and U.S. Vital Statistics for 1939, shows these changes in a striking manner.

CHANGES IN THE LEADING CAUSES OF DEATH IN THE
UNITED STATES, 1900–1939

*(Figures are for death rates per 100,000 population in the
registration areas of 1900 and 1939)*

	Death Rate per
1900	*100,000 Population*
1. Influenza, pneumonia, bronchitis	252.9
2. Tuberculosis (all forms)	201.9
3. Diarrhea and enteritis	133.2
4. Heart disease	111.2
5. Nephritis	89.0
6. Cerebral hemorrhage	67.5
7. Cancer	63.0
8. Diphtheria	43.3
9. Typhoid fever	35.9

1939	
1. Heart Disease	275.6
2. Cancer	117.8
3. Cerebral hemorrhage	88.0
4. Nephritis	83.0
5. Influenza, pneumonia, bronchitis	82.2
6. Tuberculosis (all forms)	47.2
7. Diabetes	25.6
8. Motor-vehicle accidents	24.8
9. Diarrhea and enteritis	11.5
10. Typhoid fever	1.5
11. Diphtheria	1.5

Thus we see that the actual numbers of cases of heart disease
and cancer are increasing rapidly, not because these diseases are
more frequent but because of the simple fact that they are diseases of older people and there are now more and more older
people to get them. Very careful studies have been made recently
of the incidence of cancer and most authorities agree that only
one form of the disease, namely, cancer of the lung, seems to be
increasing in frequency. The extent to which heart disease and
cancer have a predilection for older people is well shown in the
following chart compiled from 1933 data for the United States:

AGE DISTRIBUTION OF DEATHS
FROM CANCER AND DISEASES OF THE HEART

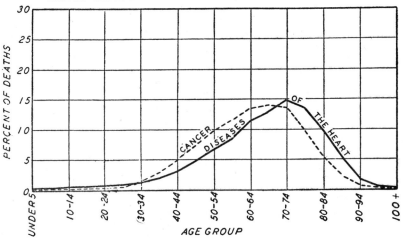

AGE GROUP

(From *U.S. Public Health Reports*, 54:2059, 1939)

Cancer reaches its peak incidence about the age of 65, while heart disease reaches a peak a few years later.

The statistician E. B. Wilson has estimated that the ageing of our population will continue so that by 1950 there will be 40 per cent more persons over the age of 40 years than there were in 1930. Let us see what this means in terms of the frequency of cancer, for instance. Wilson calculates that there actually were in the United States 157,912 deaths from all types of cancer in 1935, and that there will be 212,458 deaths in 1950, and 254,-378 in 1960. Thus the actual number of cases of cancer in 1960 will be almost double what it was in 1935.

A part of the recent increase in the number of cases of cancer reported in vital statistics is no doubt due to the fact that certain types of hidden internal cancer which formerly escaped detection are now diagnosed. With the increasing hospitalization of patients for obscure disease, and particularly the more frequent use of x-ray studies of the gastro-intestinal tract, many unsuspected cancers are brought to light. This is probably the best explanation of why the cancer rate is higher in densely populated, comparatively prosperous areas like the New England states, than in the poor rural areas of the south. In the former the standard of medical practice is high and in the latter medical facilities are poor.

We come to the paradoxical conclusion that although the 19th Century was a century of phenomenal medical progress, the conquests of the diseases of youth that were achieved have left us with more difficult health problems than before—both from the medical and the economic point of view. For the killing diseases of old age—heart disease, cancer, cerebral hemorrhage, and nephritis—are the very ones with which our modern medical science has not made much progress. They are chronic, and in a broad sense usually incurable. Important advances have been made in their palliative treatment. And of course many cases of certain forms of cancer can be permanently cured, although the most frequent type, cancer of the stomach, is still pretty hopeless.

The medical attack on these diseases of old age is more difficult because they fall into what we call, for lack of a better understanding of their causation, the group of *degenerative* diseases. Long standing, profound, and irreversible pathological changes in the tissues are usually present when these degenerative diseases are discovered, and their therapy poses enormously complex problems. No such comparatively simple conquests as the control of certain bacterial diseases with sulfonamide can be hoped for. To get ahead with the control of this group of diseases of old age we shall have to learn a lot more about their fundamental causes, and attempt to prevent their development by detecting and checking the operation of these causes in youth and middle age.

The economic problem presented by these diseases of old age is a staggering one. In Massachusetts the Department of Public Health, under the leadership of the late Dr. George H. Bigelow and Dr. Herbert L. Lombard, carried out an illuminating three-year study of the problem beginning in 1927. A house-to-house canvass of fifty-one cities and towns was made in an effort to determine the actual number of cases of chronic disease and the disability due to it. It was hoped that in this practical way the magnitude of the problem could be assessed.

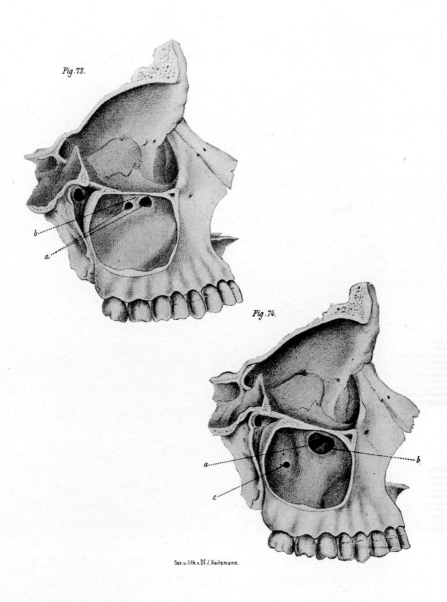

Fig. 73.

Fig. 74.

Ges.u.lith.v.DᵣJ.Heitzmann.

The Maxillary Sinus

Variations in the normal openings of the maxillary sinus as illustrated in two specimens shown in Zuckerkandl's Normale und Pathologische Anatomie der Nasenhöhle, *vol. 1, 1882.*

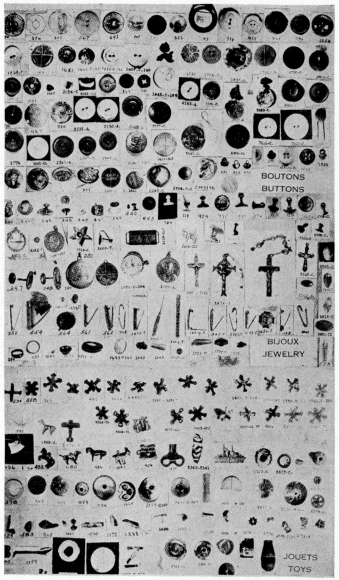

(From Chevalier Jackson's *Autobiography*)

A Collection of Objects Removed by Bronchoscopy

It was found that 29.1 per cent of all persons over 40 years of age were sick with some chronic disease. This means that in the state of Massachusetts alone there are about half a million older people with chronic disease. Of those thus affected, 4.8 per cent were completely disabled and 42.5 per cent partially disabled.

Since the problem of chronic disease in old age concerns not only those diseases that kill, but also those which merely disable, the list of the diseases most frequently encountered includes several that we have not mentioned before. Rheumatism is such a disease. It kills only infrequently yet it is by far the most common of all chronic diseases, affecting about 25 per cent of all those found to be chronically ill in the Massachusetts survey. Heart disease, arteriosclerosis, nephritis, and apoplexy followed in order of frequency in the Massachusetts mortality tables.

These diseases were found to be considerably more frequent in the poor than in the well-to-do. The reasons for this are not fully understood. Be that as it may, the economic burden unfortunately falls where it can least well be borne.

The chronicity of these diseases adds greatly to the economic burden they impose on society. In this Massachusetts survey the median duration of illness in the patients questioned was:

Rheumatism .... 12.0 years
Heart disease .... 7.8 years
Arteriosclerosis .... 5.7 years
Nephritis .... 8.6 years
Apoplexy .... 5.1 years

The average duration of these diseases in patients who died of them, as indicated by Massachusetts mortality data for 1928, is somewhat shorter, but still long as compared with the rapid diseases of youth.

Rheumatism .... 7.0 years
Heart Disease .... 2.9 years
Arteriosclerosis .... 4.2 years
Nephritis .... 3.0 years
Apoplexy .... 0.1 years
Cancer .... 1.7 years

The patient with one of these chronic diseases therefore faces a long and expensive illness. The Massachusetts survey disclosed that only 44.4 per cent of the sick individuals were under the care of a physician, and only 0.8 per cent were receiving care in hospitals. The poorer the patient the less medical care he obtained. These facts make it obvious enough that individuals of limited means cannot afford proper medical care when struck down by one of these chronic diseases. We shall discuss this question in more detail in the following chapter.

Although modern medical science is usually powerless to cure these chronic diseases of old age, it often palliates them and prolongs the patient's life. A study of the duration of chronic illnesses in patients over 50 years of age made in Massachusetts from death certificates indicated that today these patients live 2.6 times as long as they did twenty years ago. Many patients with advanced cancer, for instance, are today given radiotherapy which prolongs life for months and years even when definitive cure is not obtained. Thus it comes about that advances in the medical control of these diseases have increased the economic burden which they impose.

And today, with the population steadily growing older, the proportion of younger wage earners, who bear the social burden, is considerably smaller than it used to be. In 1870, seventy years ago, there were seven persons in the productive ages of twenty to sixty for every one who was over sixty. Today there are only 5.4 persons in this productive age group to share through taxes, philanthropy, and kinship the burden of caring for each aged dependent one.

THE DOCTORS' DILEMMA

THE DOCTORS' dilemma today is how best to utilize our vast modern armamentarium of medical knowledge for the benefit of society. Most doctors realize that the fullest advantage is not being taken of their knowledge, partly because changes in the organization of medical practice have not kept pace with the phenomenal recent growth of medical knowledge, and partly because of the exceedingly complex economic problems which the use of this new knowledge implies. The public has, during the last few years, begun to take an interest in this question. Discussions of various phases of it have appeared in magazines, and several books have been written on the subject.[1] In forming an opinion on this complex question the reader should keep in mind that physicians as a class are as idealistic today as they were in our grandfathers' time, and that there are a great many of them who would welcome any practical plan for improving the organization of medical care. Unfortunately the problem is not an easy one. Let us look at it from the historical point of view.

As recently as fifty years ago the practice of medicine was more of an art than a science. It was largely carried on in the patient's home and in the doctor's office. Only a few simple pieces of equipment were required. A stethoscope, a clinical thermometer (a new gadget in those days), and apparatus for urine analy-

---

[1] The reader who wishes to pursue it in detail will find much that is interesting and provocative in Sir Arthur Newsholme's *Medicine and the State*, Michael Davis' *America Organizes Medicine*, and Hugh Cabot's *The Patient's Dilemma*.

ses were all that were needed. People were born and died in their own homes. Hospitals were places to which the very poor and indigent who had nowhere else to go were carried. Why, after all, should anyone else go there? The only surgical operations that were frequently done were the incision of abscesses and the amputation of diseased or injured limbs, and the average man preferred to have these done in his own home. Even the most serious illnesses required no special medical studies that could not be carried on in the home.

Today adequate medical care is a far more complex and expensive matter. The development of microscopical pathology and bacteriology in the 1860's and 70's transformed our understanding of the fundamental nature of disease. During the next two decades modern surgery was born. Finally, since the turn of the century, a whole series of laboratory methods have been developed for the detection and special study of disease, and these must be available to the competent physician if he is to give his patients the benefit of our modern medical knowledge. They include various methods of x-ray study, chemical analyses of the blood, basal metabolism determination, etc.

Most of these laboratory methods of detecting and studying disease can be carried out only in hospitals. Modern surgery is practised almost exclusively within hospital walls. Thus it has come about that most serious illnesses, and some less important ones, require a period of hospitalization. The modern physician is therefore tied to the hospital: it is his workshop. In former times he was a free and independent agent. Today he is a part of an increasingly complex institutional organization in which laboratory and clinic share in importance.

REFORM IN MEDICAL EDUCATION

There is no better way to follow the course of these great changes than to read of their impact on the lives of the men who lived through this "heroic age" of medicine. We have good biographies of two Americans who played a great part in it, William S. Halsted and William H. Welch.

Welch graduated from the College of Physicians and Surgeons in New York in 1875. His medical course there had consisted of three years' service as assistant to a practicing physician (in Welch's case with his father at Norfolk, Connecticut) and attendance at two yearly courses of lectures, each of five months duration. Except for the usual anatomical dissection his course did not include any laboratory instruction of any sort. The teaching was entirely didactic—lectures, quizzes, and clinics. Welch had, indeed, taken an elective course in pathology under Francis Delafield, the pioneer New York pathologist. In this course Welch did a number of autopsies at Bellevue Hospital and learned something of gross pathology, but his teacher never gave him any instruction in microscopical pathology. Welch had won a microscope as a student prize but he graduated without having learned how to use it!

He went to Germany for post-graduate training in 1875. There he plunged at once into practical laboratory work in histology, pathology, and physiology, for in Germany laboratory methods of teaching had been emphasized for more than a generation. Welch soon became a skilled microscopist. During his second year in Germany, which was spent with the pathologist Julius Cohnheim in Breslau, Welch did a good piece of original research regarding the mechanism of the production of edema of the lungs. All this was a great awakening to an intelligent student like Welch. In his American student background he had known almost nothing of laboratories. Now he found them to be the heart of the new kind of medicine.

German medicine was then leading all the world, and Welch realized from his own experience how this superiority had come about. There were at this period twenty medical schools in Germany, each an integral part of a prominent university. Each medical school had its associated teaching hospital, staffed by the school faculty. Both school and hospital were financed by the state. The staffs of the medical schools held professorial rank and devoted their whole time to teaching and research in the hospital wards as well as in the laboratories. The faculty organization was relatively elastic and provided places for many young assistants who spent years in laboratory and hospital mastering and contributing to the new scientific medicine.

Welch saw that this close association between the laboratories of the medical school and the wards of the hospital was fundamental in the teaching of medicine; that they were inextricably related both in the treatment of disease and in research. He realized the deficiency of American medical education in this respect and the hope was born in him to take a share one day in correcting it.

Full of these new ideas, and thoroughly trained in pathology, Welch returned to New York in 1877 and established a pathological laboratory at Bellevue Hospital. His laboratory was soon recognized as a source of new inspiration for New York medicine and he was offered all sorts of inducements to stay in the city. But when the long hoped for offer to become professor of pathology in the new university medical school being organized at Johns Hopkins came in 1885, Welch accepted. For he saw in it the opportunity to organize medical teaching in the modern way he had observed in Germany. At Hopkins Welch soon became the dominant voice in the group of young men inspired by this common ideal.

One of these young colleagues of his was the great surgeon, William S. Halsted. Halsted's background was similar to Welch's. He had graduated from the College of Physicians and Surgeons in New York in 1877 and after a year's interneship had gone abroad. During the two years that he spent in German surgical clinics he learned Lister's antiseptic methods, which the Germans had been the first to adopt, and he saw these methods transforming surgery. He grasped the importance of attacking surgical problems experimentally in the laboratory, a method which the Germans had used with so much profit. Soon after coming to Hopkins in 1886 Halsted began laboratory experiments regarding thyroid function and intestinal anastomosis which yielded important information.

At the new Johns Hopkins medical school many important contributions were made to medical knowledge during those early years when its faculty included the four truly great physicians painted by Sargent in his famous picture of 1905—Welch, Osler, Halsted, and Kelly. But more important still as regards the development of American medicine was the influence Johns Hopkins had on the teaching in other American medical schools. The German ideal of a university medical school, with high educational requirements for its students, and a faculty devoting their entire time to the care of patients, teaching, and research, in well equipped, university-controlled hospital and laboratories, was fully realized for the first time in America at Johns Hopkins University. University medical schools, as well as other types of university professional schools had not developed in the United States for the simple reason that there were, a century ago, no American universities. The country supported about one hundred and twenty colleges but not a single university. The universities, as they existed in Europe at the time the American educational system was founded under the leadership of Jefferson, were part of a class system of education, and American democracy at first rejected them.

Before the establishment of a university medical school at Johns Hopkins in 1893, important steps had already been taken in this direction at Michigan, Pennsylvania, and Harvard. At Michigan in 1852 President Henry P. Tappan attempted to establish the German university system of higher education, proposing that the college be abandoned and technical and professional schools developed. Although his plan as a whole was not achieved, the medical school, founded as an integral part of the university, was a success from the start. At Harvard, President Eliot, who maintained a deep interest in medical education throughout his whole career, set out to obtain important improvements in the organization of the medical school soon after his inauguration in 1869. In his first annual report he wrote: "The whole system of medical education in this country needs thorough reformation. The course of professional instruction should be a progressive one covering three years; the winter session and summer session should be combined; and the student should give his attendance at lectures and recitations, at hospitals and laboratories during the whole year." This was written at a time when the academic requirements for the M.D. degree consisted merely of attendance at two terms of didactic lectures each lasting five to six months. The candidate for the degree had in addition to prove that he had studied medicine for at least three years as an assistant of some regular practitioner. The medical school at this period was managed almost independently by its faculty, who collected the students' fees and decided questions of policy. Eliot's proposed reforms were bitterly opposed by this old guard, one of whom boldly claimed that "physicians are born not trained." Nevertheless, during the years 1871 and 1872 President Eliot forced his reforms through, and in this process made the medical school a genuine university department. Oliver Wendell Holmes described this change with his usual light touch. He wrote: "Our new President Eliot has turned the whole university over like a flapjack. There never was such a *bouleversement* in the Medical Faculty. The Corporation [of Harvard] has taken the whole management of it out of our hands. We are paid salaries, which I rather like. . . ." President Eliot continued his efforts to improve the training in his medical school, and in 1892 had the satisfaction of seeing the course of study lengthened to four years. He was as successful in obtaining material improvements as he was in raising intellectual standards, for in 1905 he raised a fund of almost five million dollars for the erection of a new school. Pierpont Morgan and John D. Rockefeller each contributed a million dollars. The group of five white marble buildings that rose in Brookline were the finest medical school plant the world had seen.

As time went on the superiority of the university type of medi-

cal school began to prove itself in America by the accomplishments of the graduates from these schools, and a reform in the organization of American medical schools began. This reform movement was given a great impetus by surveys of medical education
in Europe and in the United States and Canada made under the
auspices of the Carnegie Foundation by Abraham Flexner. The
first volume, dealing with medical schools in the United States
and Canada, was published in 1910. In it Flexner pointed out that
among a total of 155 American medical schools—a larger number
than existed in the whole rest of the world—only a small fraction
provided proper medical training. Less than one third were integral parts of universities. Most of the remainder were privately
owned so-called proprietary schools organized chiefly for making
money and staffed by third-rate faculties. They had no proper
hospital or laboratory facilities and accepted students equipped
with only a high school education or less. They were flooding
America with poorly trained so-called physicians.

Flexner's survey laid bare these abuses and specified proper
standards for medical education. Public opinion, and the regula-
tory efforts of the Council on Medical Education of the American
Medical Association and the various state licensing boards, soon
forced many of these proprietary schools out of existence. By 1923
the number of medical schools in the United States had been reduced to 80, just one-half of the number existing before Flexner
made his survey. The beneficent influence of this elimination of
poor schools upon the quality of medical practice in the United
States today can scarcely be over-emphasized.

Another movement of great importance for the improvement
of medical education in the United States during these first decades of the century was the union of medical schools and hospitals.
Medicine is a practical science. If its undergraduate students,
and the hospital internes, fellows, and residents who form its post-
graduate students, are to be properly taught, medical schools
must control the hospitals used for teaching. From the viewpoint
of clinical research this control is even more important. Who are

as well fitted to attack the multitudinous problems of clinical medicine as the medical school faculties who have at their command the laboratories so essential to research? Certainly not the busy private practitioners of medicine who have little time to spare from their arduous task of making a living. American hospitals had developed for the most part as they had in England—as private, voluntarily supported institutions for the care of the sick poor. They were staffed by the private practitioners of the community who gave their services free. Some of these attending physicians, to be sure, held so-called clinical professorships in local medical schools. These were not paid teaching positions, however, and those who held them usually gave but a small part of their time to teaching. Thus at the beginning of the 20th Century medical schools and hospitals in America remained largely independent of each other, and medical training was severely handicapped.

There were a few outstanding exceptions, however. The University of Michigan School of Medicine had had its own hospital since 1869. This teaching hospital, financed by the state, steadily grew in size and distinction, and has now for some years stood as a model of what state medicine can accomplish. In 1874 the University of Pennsylvania Medical School established its University Hospital, and in 1889 the Johns Hopkins Hospital was opened. These hospitals set a new high standard of clinical teaching in the United States and were a strong influence favoring the development of medical-school-controlled teaching hospitals.

It is an interesting fact that the movement received a great impetus from a Baptist clergyman of Montclair, New Jersey, the Rev. Frederick Gates. He was the confidant and financial adviser of John D. Rockefeller. He developed a keen interest in the scientific possibilities of modern medicine from reading Osler's great text book in 1897, and convinced Mr. Rockefeller that there was a great opportunity for him to become a pioneer in endowing medical research. Rockefeller set up a foundation which has given many millions to medical education and research. Under the guidance of an advisory council called the General Education Board, large grants were made to a whole series of American medical schools, enabling them to build or reorganize teaching hospitals and to staff them on a full-time basis. The Washington University School of Medicine in St. Louis with its affiliated Barnes Hospital, and the Yale Medical School with its affiliated New Haven Hospital, received grants in 1914. The Vanderbilt University School of Medicine in Nashville received a large grant in 1919 which made possible the erection of a University Hospital and laboratory building. In 1926 the University of Rochester (New York) Medical School opened its affiliated Strong Memorial Hospital, financed by gifts from the General Education Board, George Eastman, and members of the Strong family.

In the meantime several other American medical schools had acquired their own teaching hospitals as the result of large gifts from other philanthropists. Peter Bent Brigham of Boston left over four and one-half million dollars for a hospital bearing his name which was built in 1913 across the street from the Harvard Medical School and affiliated with it as a teaching hospital, the heads of departments holding professorships in the Medical School. It was the first of a whole group of affiliated teaching hospitals that have since grown up surrounding the Harvard Medical School. In 1917, through the leadership of Dr. Frank Billings, a sum of more than five millions was raised by private contributions to establish a medical school and build a teaching hospital at the University of Chicago. The hospital, appropriately named the Billings Hospital, was opened in 1927. A special hospital for children, the Bobs Roberts Memorial Hospital, was added to the unit in 1930. In 1924 James B. Duke left some four million dollars for the building and equipping of a medical school and hospital at the university bearing his name in Durham, North Carolina. He provided, further, a six million dollar special endowment for the medical school.

In 1921 Columbia University Medical School (The College of Physicians and Surgeons) became affiliated with the Presbyterian

Hospital of New York, and a medical center of a new type was projected. The medical school, the Presbyterian Hospital, and several affiliated hospitals (The Babies Hospital, Sloan Maternity Hospital, Squier Urological Clinic) were to be built as a single unit many stories high. The plan was made possible largely through the generosity of Edward S. Harkness, who gave the site at 168th Street and Broadway and additional gifts totalling many millions. The Medical School contributed an endowment of five and one-half millions left to it by Joseph R. De Lamar. The initial group of buildings cost over three and one half million dollars and were completed in 1928.

A few years later another equally ambitious medical center of the same type was developed in New York as the result of the union of Cornell University Medical School and the New York Hospital. It was made possible by a large legacy from Payne Whitney in 1927, and by gifts from other philanthropists. The main building, 27 stories high, faces 68th Street on the East River and is flanked by three special hospitals, the Lying-in-Hospital, the Children's Clinic, and the Psychiatric Clinic. It was opened in 1932. The striking architectural plan of the main building is reminiscent of the Palace of the Popes in Avignon. It is one of the most beautiful of modern skyscrapers.

Several western state universities had in the meantime acquired teaching hospitals for their medical schools. At the University of Iowa a small general hospital had been maintained since 1898. In 1919 a new unit for pediatrics and orthopaedics was added, and the clinical facilities as a whole considerably enlarged. At the University of Minnesota a general teaching hospital was built in 1911 with a gift from the family of Dr. Adolphus S. Elliott. An eye, ear, nose, and throat hospital (1924), a cancer hospital (1925) and a children's hospital (1929) have since been added to the University of Minnesota Medical Center. At the University of California a new medical school and teaching hospital was built in 1917, placing the clinical work of the school on an academic basis.

In the teaching hospitals that have developed in America during the last generation under the stimulus of the movement to reorganize and improve the teaching of medicine, the staff members holding professorial appointments as heads of departments
in the affiliated medical schools have been for the most part on
full time. By this is meant that they give their entire time to school
and hospital duties and take no private patients at all, or only a
limited number, turning all or a certain part of their earnings from
private patients over to the medical school budget.[1]

Looking back on the great advances in medical education in
the United States achieved during the last generation, the fact
stands out that their cost has largely been borne by private
philanthropy. It is difficult to estimate the total sum which has
been given so generously, but it is certainly many times the
amount that has been spent for medical education in any other
country. Abraham Flexner, who as a member of the General Education Board was concerned with the allocation of the Rockefeller
funds, states in his recent autobiography, "In less than ten years—
between 1919 and 1928—operating with something less than fifty
million dollars, the General Education Board had, directly or indirectly, added half a billion dollars or more to the resources and
endowments of American medical education." Now that the era
of large private fortunes is passing in the United States, it seems
likely that medical education will have to solicit support from the
public purse. With this prospect in view the fact should be emphasized to the public that the leading position in the world
which American medicine holds today is due to a considerable extent to the generous financial support that its medical schools and
teaching hospitals have had. Our hope for progress in medicine
depends upon ample funds for teaching and research.

[1] A warm controversy ensued when the full-time system, long a feature of German and Scandinavian teaching hospitals, was introduced in the United States.
Those interested in reading considered opinions regarding it will find references in
the several writings of Welch on the subject in Chapter XIV of the Flexners' Life
of Welch. An address by Theodore C. Janeway, who resigned in 1917 from the
full-time professorship of medicine at Johns Hopkins, and a letter written by Sir
William Osler, present the other side of this picture.

Following the success of the teaching hospitals organized on the new basis in the United States the idea was adopted to some extent in Canada and in England. In 1924 the Rockefeller Foundation gave half a million dollars to establish a university clinic at the McGill University School of Medicine, the director to be a full-time professor of medicine. In 1919 the University of London began to organize full-time units in medicine, surgery, and obstetrics in its hospital schools: by 1938 a total of ten such units had been established. Lord Nuffield, in 1936, gave two million pounds to Oxford University for the establishment of full-time services in medicine, surgery and gynecology.

Another feature of modern medical education which deserves mention is the follow-up or end result principle. This is simply the principle that the physician's responsibility shall not end when his patient leaves the hospital ward, but that the subsequent course of the patient shall be followed by return visits to the hospital out-patient department, and the ultimate end result of the treatment recorded in the patient's record. In isolated instances physicians have of course kept track of their end results, but the systematic adoption of this follow-up principle as an essential part of the educational contribution of teaching hospitals has been to a large extent an American contribution.

At the beginning of the present century, when surgery was growing so fast in scope and daring, there was little accurate information available as to the permanent value of the new operations that were being devised almost daily. In almost all hospitals the case records describing the events that took place during the patient's stay in the hospital were written out in long hand in consecutive series on the blank pages of bound volumes. Even a final and authoritative diagnosis was often lacking. There was no provision for follow-up. Under these circumstances there was no way of actually proving whether Dr. A's methods were superior to Dr. B's.

The man who was largely responsible for forcing surgeons adopt proper record systems and to institute follow-up clinics was a Boston surgeon named E. A. Codman. A man of truly heroic candor, he sacrificed his own surgical career to put across his conviction of the importance of knowing the end results of surgical treatment. It was in 1910 that he turned the major share of his efforts to this purpose. The climax came in 1914 with his resignation from the staff of the Massachusetts General following a burst of devastating publicity. But his colleagues knew that he was right about his end result idea, and although they excluded him from their circle, they adopted the principle within a short time, and the Massachusetts General became one of the first hospitals to adopt the necessary changes in the case record system, and to institute a systematic follow-up of patients.

Other American hospitals soon followed suit. At the Presbyterian Hospital in New York a plan whereby all surgical patients were brought back for follow-up study was inaugurated in 1916 under the guidance of Dr. James A. Corscaden, who was also a pioneer in emphasizing the necessity of follow-up data.

In these modern case record systems one of the essential features was the introduction of so-called *unit records*. Instead of being written out in bound volumes, the individual records are made on loose-leaf sheets which can ultimately be properly arranged and stitched together to form a unit record that is easily accessible for study. Each case record is given a serial number under which it is filed. The follow-up notes and data regarding subsequent admissions of the patient to the hospital are added to this unit record as the occasion arises.

The ultimate gain of medical education from complete case records of this kind cannot be exaggerated. For these case records form the living text-books of disease which contain far more information than any dusty tome of the past could ever hope to contain. It is upon the basis of the data objectively compiled from them that the decisions of modern physicians are made. They provide the final step in the replacement of the theorist of the past by the realist of today.

SPECIALIZATION

Specialization is another phenomenon of modern medicine. Some degree of specialization has of course existed since the days of the barber surgeons, but during the last fifty years specialists have multiplied at such a rate that the public, and even some members of the medical profession, have begun to talk about the dangers of over-specialization. They overlook the simple fundamental fact that specialization is the direct result of the recent enormous growth of medical knowledge. The available knowledge of disease, and the technical methods of attacking it, are today so complex that it is impossible to cram much more than a small part of what is known into the brain of any one physician.

In the early 19th Century the situation was quite different. Many a man in those days was able to master a number of different aspects of medical knowledge, and make important new contributions in them. Take the case of Sir Jonathan Hutchinson, aptly called the last of the great multi-specialists. He was trained at St. Bartholomew's and became surgeon to the London Hospital in 1859. A skilled surgical pathologist, he interpreted disease wherever he saw it in terms of the gross pathology of his day. In addition he mastered dermatology, ophthalmology, neurology, and general surgery, describing new clinical features of diseases in all of these branches. He was the first to describe, for instance, interstitial keratitis of the eye, notched teeth, and labyrinthine disease (Hutchinson's triad) as signs of congenital syphilis. He identified and made the first adequate descriptions of many of the common diseases of the skin. He made many original observations in surgery, among them the first description of skin cancer caused by the long continued use of arsenic. Today Hutchinson would probably be as nonplussed by the mass of new facts that fill medical text-books as the average medical student. Like our

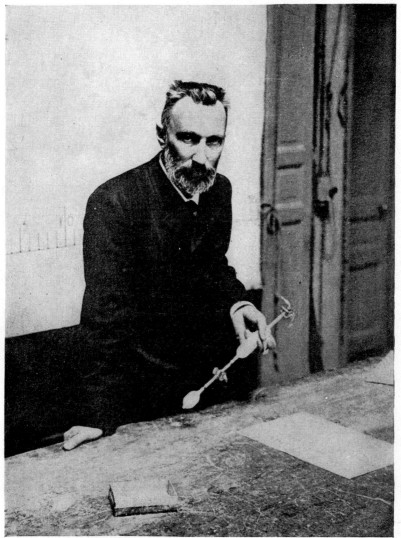

Pierre Curie in His Classroom

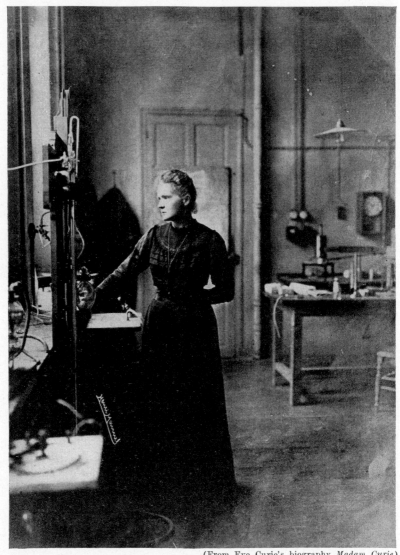

(From Eve Curie's biography *Madam Curie*)

Marie Curie in Her Laboratory

present day students he would no doubt put his teeth into them and try to swallow as many as possible, becoming not a little drugged and confused in the process.

The fact is that it is no longer possible to learn everything in medicine. The specialist has arrived on the stage of modern medicine not because he is fashionable or mercenary—but simply because he is natural and inevitable. Only by concentrating his training and experience in a limited sphere of medicine is it possible for the modern physician to know the myriad facts of chemistry, physiology, and pathology, which must be integrated with the clinical picture of disease if it is to be understood as it can be understood today. As the tree of medical knowledge has grown the specialties have developed like branches from the main trunk. These branches are all nourished by the same basic facts of medicine. But there are as many details of knowledge and experience pertaining to each specialty as there are leaves on a branch. No one branch could bear all the leaves that the tree has developed in its exuberant growth.

No wise physician is ignorant, however, of the truth that the practice of medicine, whether it be in the peasant cottage or in the towering medical center, depends first of all upon the use of sound common sense. A broad general knowledge of the "face of disease" is equally essential. This knowledge, which can come only from actual experience with disease, is just as necessary to the specialist as it is to the general practitioner. And the specialists who have added most to modern medicine have with few exceptions possessed good hospital training in general medicine or surgery before they narrowed their attention to one phase of medicine.

In contrast with Jonathan Hutchinson let us look at the career of a modern specialist—the late Harvey Cushing. When Cushing went to Bern, Switzerland, in 1900 he had already served four years as interne and resident surgeon at Hopkins under Halsted. It was most fortunate that Cushing went to Bern, for the surgical chief there, the great Kocher, believed in specialization. He told

Cushing that "there could be no greater satisfaction for a surgeon than to concentrate on a single problem and study it not only from a strictly operative point of view but from every other possible aspect—physiological, pathological, and chemical." Kocher himself had become the world-wide authority on goiter by attacking the problem in this way.

In this atmosphere Cushing became so absorbed in the experimental pathology of the nervous system that he determined to devote his life to neurological surgery. When the opportunity came to him to do so on his return to Baltimore he mastered *all* phases of the subject, fufilling the ideal that Kocher had dreamed of. He became as expert in the physiology and the pathology of the brain as in the clinical diagnosis of brain lesions and the surgical technique of attacking them. It was precisely because of the breadth of his knowledge of the problem of brain tumors that he made the great advances that he did.

Dr. Cushing's career also illustrates the modern tendency toward realignment of specialties on the basis of special knowledge of disease rather than mere technique of treatment. The old distinction that arose between physicians on the one hand, and surgeons on the other hand, was based largely on the fact that the latter wielded the knife. The *general* surgeon operated on every part of the body. But as time went on and the surgeons attempted ever more serious and drastic procedures, it became apparent to many of them that they must learn all there was to be learned about the particular disease they were attacking—especially the altered physiology and pathology. This knowledge, the intelligent surgeon knows, has saved many more lives than mere facility at cutting and tying. The pursuit of this comprehensive knowledge of a disease has led the surgeon to learn as much about it as his internist colleague. Thus internal medicine and surgery have drawn closer together until today specialists in *diseases* have to a considerable extent replaced specialists in *technique*. The specialist may be an internist or a surgeon depending upon the circumstance of whether or no operative therapy is used for the special disease he works with. Thus thyroid diseases are assigned in larger hospitals to the care of the surgical specialist because surgery is often required, while diseases of the heart go to the medical specialist in cardiac disease because the therapy is medical. This realignment of specialization has already progressed to the point where in some larger teaching hospitals the department of medicine includes specialists in heart disease, tuberculosis, rheumatism, diabetes, allergy, pneumonia, diseases of the blood, and gastro-intestinal disease, while the department of surgery includes specialists in thyroid disease, thoracic surgery, cancer of the stomach and bowel, cancer of the breast, plastic surgery, and fractures. There is as yet a fluidity about these specialty groupings of disease. They are not accepted in some medical circles, for the old traditions die hard. And medicine is growing so rapidly that new specialties are constantly developing. It is new knowledge that makes them—not administrative policy. And since this new knowledge saves lives, specialization is as certain to go forward as truth is to prevail.

We would not give the impression that the importance of the general practitioner of medicine has diminished as a result of the development of specialization. The general practitioner still has to bear the main burden of medical practice everywhere. His is the most difficult task in all medicine—that of knowing the important diagnostic features of all the great diseases, and being able to distinguish them from the trivial ailments that bring most people to a doctor. Having detected serious disease the general practitioner must often treat it as best he can, alone. When complex diagnostic or therapeutic procedures are required he may send his patient to a specialist if one is available, but the skills of the specialists are of no avail unless the general practitioner knows how and when to utilize them. His judgment is therefore the rock upon which the edifice of sound medicine is based.

One of the dangerous tendencies of today is for the layman, when he falls sick, to substitute *his* judgment for that of the general practitioner in this matter of the utilization of specialists. The prominence which specialists so easily acquire as compared with general practitioners often makes them known to laymen who have no general practitioner or family doctor in whom they are accustomed to place their trust. Thus they are tempted and often do go directly to the specialist whose services they think they need. This plan is perhaps without much hazard when the nature of the disease is perfectly obvious, like a fractured leg. But most disease is subtle in its manifestations and difficult of diagnosis, and the layman often gets involved in a money-consuming, time-wasting chain of circumstances if he attempts to diagnose his own illness and select his own specialist. This is the proper function of the general practitioner or internist. In his hands the patient will receive a thorough general examination and a careful consideration of his problem as a whole.

The general practitioner who bears this heavy responsibility has a harder lot than his specialist colleagues. He works longer hours, if indeed it can be said that he is ever off duty, and he is less well paid. But if the general practitioner today is asked as to what he needs most he does not think first of these personal needs. He wants more than anything else better facilities for making modern medical care available to his patients, particularly the help of diagnostic laboratories, the services of expert consultants, and hospital facilities. He cannot provide these things single-handed, and many of his poorer patients cannot afford them unaided by some form of voluntary communal effort or by governmental provision. The knowledge that his patients go without them hangs heavy on his heart.

WHAT PRICE MEDICAL CARE?

This brings us to another feature of the modern medicine that we have been describing, namely, its cost. It is a disturbing but inescapable fact that laboratories and hospitals with their large personnel and expensive equipment, the prolonged training required for adequate preparation for the medical career, the time that physicians today devote to the problems of the individual patient, and finally the research that must go on if progress is to be achieved—all cost money. Medical care which can be classed as adequate in terms of present day standards has become exceedingly expensive. It is in fact so expensive today in the United States that the great bulk of the people *can no longer afford it.*

This question has been carefully studied in America under the auspices of the Committee on the Costs of Medical Care. Roger I. Lee, a distinguished Boston physician, and Lewis W. Jones, estimated the incidence of various types of disease in relation to family groups, and then tabulated the amount and character of medical services which they considered would be required to provide what they regarded as "good medical care." Samuel Bradbury used these tabulations as a basis for estimating the actual cost of this type of medical care, using minimum fees for the various services involved as shown by the fee table of the Chicago Medical Society. Bradbury's "average" family of 4.1 persons would have an average of 4.6 illnesses per year, requiring physicians' services of all types costing $120.96 per year, and other services, including hospital, nursing, and laboratory services, and medicines, amounting to $139.37 per year. Preventive medical services added another $50 per year, bringing the total cost per family to $310 per year. There is every reason to believe that this estimate is fairly accurate for 1933. The cost of adequate medical care of this kind would probably be somewhat lower in rural communities and considerably higher in the largest cities.

It must be kept in mind that this figure of $310 a year is an estimate of what adequate medical care would cost if the American family could buy it—it is not the amount that the American family *actually spends* for medical care. This is a considerably smaller amount. The studies of the Committee on the Costs of Medical Care showed that during the years 1928–1931 it averaged $108.14. The average annual expenditure in families of different income groups was as follows:

Income Group	Average Charge
Under $1,200	$ 49.17
$1,200 to 2,000	66.81
$2,000 to 3,000	94.84
$3,000 to 5,000	137.92
$5,000 to 10,000	249.35
$10,000 and over	503.19
All incomes	$108.14

These two figures—$310 for the estimated cost of adequate medical care, and $108 actually spent for medical care in the average family—leave only one possible inference. It is that the average family does not receive adequate medical care, because it is prohibitively expensive. That this is indeed a fact most of those of us who care for the sick realize full well from practical experience. In the great cities we see the indigent and the poor receiving adequate medical care free or at a limited cost in the wards of the municipal and voluntary charity hospitals. In the private pavilions of these hospitals we see the well-to-do provided with similarly adequate medical care (plus some frills) at a high cost. But we know that the great majority of people with limited and moderate incomes have no way of securing adequate medical care. They usually do not wish to enter as ward patients in the charity hospitals. This privilege is moreover available to them only in a very limited way, for such hospitals exist only in the larger cities and accept ward patients only from lower income groups. And they cannot possibly afford the charges for private care when serious illness strikes them. In the smaller communities the costs of private care are not so high, but they are still far too high for families with lower incomes.

The situation becomes clearer when we consider what the average family income in the United States amounts to. At the time the studies which we have been quoting were made, 48.2 per cent of American families had incomes of $1800 per year or less, while 76.8 per cent had incomes of $3,000 or less. It seems reasonable to say that $310 a year for medical care is too high an expenditure for even this $3,000 a year income group. It is certainly beyond the reach of the $1,800 a year income group. About 70 per cent of the income of this group is spent for items of food, shelter and clothing. An expenditure of more than 15 per cent of income for medical care is out of all reasonable proportion.

This then is the doctor's dilemma in our modern world. He has provided a kind of medical care which costs so much that most of the people cannot buy it. Our modern medical knowledge, which can so often accomplish what in a previous century would be regarded as miraculous, is only partly used. Well trained young physicians sit in their private offices and wait for patients who do not come, and about 30 per cent of the beds in general hospitals are vacant. Meanwhile the average citizen delays going to see his doctor about that sharp twinge he gets over his heart when he climbs stairs, or puts off the necessary gallbladder operation, and almost always neglects to have his teeth attended to, because these things cost too much. It doesn't do much good to tell him that in the long run neglect of these things will cost him dearly, that it is actually cheaper to have the needed operation now if it will add years to his earning capacity. As long as adequate medical service costs as much as it does people will go without it, for it is one of the things that *can* be put off. The penalty for doing so is subtle and remote.

Then the unexpected happens. An acute and serious illness strikes a family of moderate means. The husband develops a coronary thrombosis and requires a month or more of absolute rest in the hospital, followed by a long period of convalescence at home, or the wife's gallbladder that has been grumbling along for several years flares up and an immediate operation is required. Such a calamity may leave a family with a debt amounting to anywhere from a couple of hundred to a thousand dollars. To pay it savings are wiped out, money is borrowed from friends or relatives, and the family budget is put out of balance for years.

A clergyman acquaintance of ours in Richmond, Virginia, who is a keen student of social problems and who works hard to help his parishioners with their difficulties, tells us that of all the trying situations he is called upon to meet, this problem of a large debt contracted for serious illness is one of the most frequent and distressing. His parishioners are largely people of moderate means who lived quiet and useful lives on tree-shaded streets. This clergyman raises the question whether the mental depressions and the maladjustments that often develop when such a debt hangs over a family may not sometimes be as painful as the illness itself that led to it.

The magnitude of the charges for acute diseases requiring hospitalization is suggested by some of the studies reported by the Committee on the Costs of Medical Care. The charges for an operation for appendicitis averaged $167.66, while they averaged $341.51 for the treatment of cancer. In the larger cities they were larger, occasionally reaching the thousand dollar level.

Apropos of expenditure for medical care in larger cities, it must be kept in mind that a good many individuals in such communities get free medical care in the out-patient clinics and wards of municipal and charity hospitals. In Philadelphia a survey showed that 40 per cent of all hospital care was free. The Committee on the Costs of Medical Care studies indicated that at least one fourth of all general hospital care is provided without direct charge to the patient or his family. It is of course chiefly the lowest income groups who make use of this privilege. In families with an annual income of less than $1,200, fifty-two per cent of illnesses requiring hospitalization were cared for free; in the $1,200 to $2,000 income group 22.8 per cent were free; while in the $2,000 to $3,000 group 7.9 per cent were free. There is no doubt a certain amount of abuse of this privilege by the unscrupulous of the higher income groups. The physicians on the hospital staffs give their services gratis for all of this free ward work. The hospital, however, balances its own budget either with subsidies from the state or municipality or by voluntary gifts from the public. In a very real sense therefore the hospital is repaid out of the public purse for its contribution but the physician is not. Of course physicians enjoy giving their services free, but unfortunately they can not live on gratitude. Their custom in the past has been to charge the well-to-do heavily to compensate for their free services to the poor, but this has disadvantages, the chief among which is the fact that the man of moderate means is apt to be squeezed in the process.

MEDICAL INSURANCE SYSTEMS ABROAD

While physicians ponder their modern dilemma a new voice is heard. It is the social consciousness of a new individual right, the right to the adequate medical care that we have been describing. Sir Arthur Newsholme, the distinguished authority on public health, summarized this new voice in the opening paragraphs of his book *Medicine and the State,* as follows: "Civilized communities have arrived at two conclusions from which there will be no retreat, though their full realization in experience has nowhere been completely achieved.

"In the first place, *the health of every individual is a social concern and responsibility;* and secondly, as following from this, *medical care in its widest sense for every individual is an essential condition of maximum efficiency and happiness in a civilized world.*"

And how is adequate medical care for all to be obtained? Certain European governments have been trying to achieve it by various methods for over a century and a half. Careful study of their experiences might make it possible to avoid some of their errors. It was with this aim in mind that the directors of the Milbank Memorial Fund of New York in 1928 commissioned Sir Arthur Newsholme to make a detailed study of medical work as related to public administration in the chief European countries.

The results were embodied in three volumes published in 1931, which should be read by all who are seriously interested in this complex problem.

There are two main aspects to this problem. The first is concerned with the support of hospitals. The second is concerned with sickness insurance. Both are closely related, for a successful insurance plan can contribute a considerable share of the cost of hospitalization.

In the British Isles and in the United States and Canada general hospitals have been largely supported by voluntary gifts. Special hospitals for the tuberculous and the insane, however, have been provided by the state as the need for them has developed. In the United States during recent years many general hospitals for veterans of the First World War, and for members of the armed forces, have been established by the federal government. There were only 71 such federal hospitals in 1909, while in 1941 there were 428. We in the United States are apt to underestimate the extent to which our hospitals are today supported by the government. The fact is that the 1941 hospital census of the American Medical Association showed that some 1,864, or almost one-third of American hospitals, were governmental. In these were 965,511 of the total of 1,324,381 hospital beds. Thus 73 per cent of hospital beds in the United States are today provided for by public funds. It must be pointed out, however, that the remaining 27 per cent of beds include almost all of those in the larger teaching hospitals where the greatest part of research is centered. This group of teaching hospitals, financed in the past largely by generous gifts from private philanthropy, faces a crisis today. The millions that they have been given have come for the most part from very large fortunes, many of them acquired through inheritance. There seems little doubt but that taxation will soon destroy all such large fortunes, and hospitals will no longer be able to depend upon voluntary gifts. The group of teaching hospitals, which have contributed so much to placing American medical science in the position that it holds today, must be subsidized with public funds in some way that will not be deleterious to their independence and efficiency.

In continental Europe governmental support of hospitals began in France at the time of the Revolution. The municipal governments took over all the hospitals, for the people were determined to apply their new humanitarian ideals to medical care. The management of these hospitals is centered in each municipality in a bureau called *L'Assistance Publique*. In general it must be admitted that this administration has been bureaucratic, rigid, and inefficient. The standard of hospital care has been low and the hospitals often overcrowded and inadequate. The attending physicians and surgeons are appointed by competitive examination, on the whole honestly conducted, but theoretical and rigid in nature. Under this system mediocrity prevails. A chief has no voice in the selection of his assistants and internes. Teamwork, the essence of modern medical care, is lacking. The medical and surgical staffs control medical matters but have no authority in other aspects of hospital administration, over which they are continually at odds with the bureaucrats of *L'Assistance Publique*.

Since the Napoleonic era most German hospitals have been supported by public funds. The municipalities and the state have shared in this burden. Many of the best of these tax-supported hospitals have been associated with the university medical schools, and the clinical appointments in them have been controlled by the academic faculties even though salaries came out of public funds. This feature was certainly an important one, and responsible for a large share of the distinction that German medicine achieved during the last century.

In the Scandinavian countries the hospitals have long been supported by the state. The King of Denmark in 1806 ordered the establishment and maintenance at public cost of from one to three hospitals in each of Denmark's seventeen counties. From this beginning Denmark evolved what today is probably the best hospital system in the world. Newsholme wrote regarding Denmark: "Its general hospitals, with special departments, attain a very high standard, and are probably more readily available and more completely utilized by the population than are their hospitals by any other people outside Scandinavia." In 1931 Denmark had 10.3 hospital beds for 1,000 inhabitants. Even the most remote communities are served by modern hospitals. All of these, with the exception of the Rigshospital or University Hospital in Copenhagen, which is a state institution, have been erected and are supported by the local communities which they serve. Sickness insurance payments meet about one-tenth of the cost of maintenance, payments from private patients provide a small proportion, and the local government contributes the rest. The hospital physicians are state officers, on whole time or part-time, living within the hospital grounds and devoting most of their time to hospital patients. The management of the hospitals is in the hands of local Hospital Boards, which include the senior attending surgeons and physicians, public health officers, and municipal officers. The medical profession in Denmark, including private practitioners as well as those engaged on salary, appear satisfied with these hospital arrangements and achieve a high degree of cooperation.

In Norway and Sweden the hospital systems have a general resemblance to that of Denmark. Practically all the hospitals are supported by municipality, county, or state. There, as in Denmark, a high standard of hospital care has been achieved, and political interference in medical matters kept at a minimum.

In Russia, of course, all medical care has been a function of the state since the 1917 Revolution. All hospitals are state institutions and all doctors are state officials paid by the state. In Czarist times there were relatively few hospitals, and these were chiefly for the well-to-do. The U.S.S.R. has made a special effort to guard the health of its workers, and has provided large numbers of dispensaries and hospitals throughout the country. In 1913 there were but 127,000 beds in Russian hospitals, while in 1932 there were 350,000 hospital beds. This is of course still a comparatively limited number of beds in terms of western standards. Newsholme and Kingsbury, who have written what is probably the best study of medical care in modern Russia, state that the standard of hospital treatment in these institutions appeared to be good. As might be expected, the Russian system has led to a concentration of medical practice in dispensaries and hospitals. Home visits are made when required, but illness of any consequence brings the patient at once into the hospital. The proportion of obstetrical cases, for instance, cared for in hospitals is higher in Russian villages than it is in London, according to Newsholme and Kingsbury.

The second aspect of the problem of providing adequate medical care that demands our attention is sickness insurance. The insurance principle is beyond doubt the best way of meeting the cost of medical care, because it makes saving money for this purpose compulsory, and because it distributes among the many who are insured the excessive and fortuitous burden of large medical expense that falls upon the few. The studies of the Committee on the Costs of Medical Care showed that in families with incomes between $1,200 and $2,000 about one half had to meet an average charge of only $60 per year. Yet 1.5 per cent of these families faced charges of between $400 and $700 for the year, and four in a thousand families had medical bills from $700 to more than $1,000 per year. Such a hit and miss distribution of charges is obviously best met by insurance.

Sickness insurance may be either voluntary or compulsory, but the latter form has now been generally adopted in Europe. Sickness insurance was first instituted on a wide scale in Germany by private industrial concerns, among others at the Krupp works. Bismarck became convinced of its advantages and in 1883 forced the adoption of compulsory sickness insurance throughout Germany. In subsequent years the number of classes insured and the benefits were enlarged, and in 1911 the various acts covering sickness, invalidity, and accident insurance were incorporated into a single Federal Insurance Code. The insurance was entrusted to autonomous, legally authorized sickness funds or societies, supervised by the state. At the beginning only about 10 per cent of the population was included, but by 1928 the proportion of the total population insured had been increased to 33 per cent. The insurance not only provides for all costs of illness, but it provides in most instances monetary benefits to family dependents during illness, and disability benefits.

When the first sickness insurance law was drawn up in Germany the medical profession was not consulted. This was the beginning of a controversy between the insurance societies and the physicians which has continued ever since. The societies contract with physicians to provide home and office care for the insured at so much a head per year. In 1928 the sum was 14 marks (about $3.40) in Berlin. The cost of diagnostic laboratory procedures, the services of specialists, and hospital treatment when required are also paid for by the insurance societies. Dental care is included, being provided by dentists employed by the insurance societies. Although there is general agreement that in Germany sickness insurance has greatly benefited the insured, and has made modern medical knowledge more generally available to the people, some serious disadvantages of the German system of providing it are apparent. The inadequate remuneration of the doctor compels him to resort to hurried and inadequate methods: as many as 50 patients may be seen in a day's consulting hours. A second disadvantage of the German system has been the excessive cost of its administration. The number of officials employed in the insurance societies has almost equalled the number of physicians engaged in this work. The doctors are snowed under with paper work and red tape. German physicians on the whole are dissatisfied with the workings of sickness insurance; they see private practice dwindling to little or nothing while they are held in bondage by the insurance societies.

The Scandinavian countries, particularly Denmark, provide a cheering contrast. There sickness insurance has been a success

from the point of view of both the people and the medical profession. In Denmark participation was for a long time voluntary
—an expression of the spirit of thrift and mutual helpfulness
which has made all sorts of cooperatives thrive in the Scandinavian countries. Beginning in a small way in the 1880's the sickness
insurance clubs in Denmark rapidly grew to include 65 per cent
of the whole population in 1928. The movement was, to be sure,
aided by certain indirect penalties laid by the state upon all who
did not join the sickness insurance clubs. A citizen without such
insurance who had to accept medical aid from public institutions
lost his right to vote, he could not marry without the consent of
the public authorities, and he forfeited his claim to old age pension. The insurance clubs are local cooperative organizations,
carefully regulated by state supervision. The insurance provides
complete medical care, including hospitalization, and also pays
family benefits during illness. The premiums paid by the members
meet only a part of the total cost of the insurance, the remainder
being met by subsidies from the national government, and by
smaller contributions from the local government. In 1933 sickness
insurance was made compulsory in Denmark.

Danish physicians seem to be satisfied with their business arrangements with the insurance clubs, for which they serve under
contract to provide home and office care at so much per member
per year. In a representative community this sum was 7.20 Kroner
($1.95) in 1928. The cooperation between health officers, hospital physicians, insurance doctors, and private physicians in achieving a good standard of medical care for the people as a whole is of
a high order. It must be admitted that the number of physicians in
Denmark is relatively small, there being only one for each 1,400
inhabitants, and that their training is uniform and of a high
standard. Quackery has been almost completely abolished, and
sickness insurance has been an important influence in its suppression.

In Sweden and Norway sickness insurance was also generally
adopted, and on the whole functions successfully. In Sweden it is

on a voluntary basis. The insurance societies are cooperatives organized by the people themselves, and subsidized by the state to the extent of about one-half of the cost of the medical care which they provide. In Norway sickness insurance has been compulsory since 1911 for those with an income below 5,200 kroner per year (approximately $1,500). The insured person pays six-tenths, the employer one-tenth, the community one-tenth, and the state two-tenths of the cost of the insurance. The insured has a free choice of doctor, who is paid according to the service rendered rather than a fixed yearly sum per patient as in the other insurance systems that we have described. This brings up the question of which system of payment is best for the health of the patient. This, of course, should be the deciding point in this as in all questions regarding the organization of medical care. Norwegian physicians maintain that their system results in a higher standard of medical care, but recognize that it is an expensive system. In England and in Germany, where the capitation system of payment is used, it has been claimed that hurried and imperfect medical work results. The question is far from settled, but it is fair to say that any system that pays physicians so poorly that they have to attempt to care for more patients than they can properly attend to will inevitably result in poor medicine.

In Russia compulsory sickness insurance for all workers was inaugurated in December, 1917. Although its aim is to include all workers it does not yet include the peasants, who form the vast majority of the population. It purposely excludes all those who have been deprived of their civil rights, a not inconsiderable group consisting of former landlords, merchants, kulaks, and Czarist officials. The insurance provides not only for all the costs of illness, but for permanent incapacity, maternity care, unemployment, old age, and burial. Full wages are paid during illness. The Russian insurance system differs from those in all other countries in that the workers themselves do not contribute anything to its cost, the whole being borne by the factory or institution employing them. In each such organization there is a Social In-

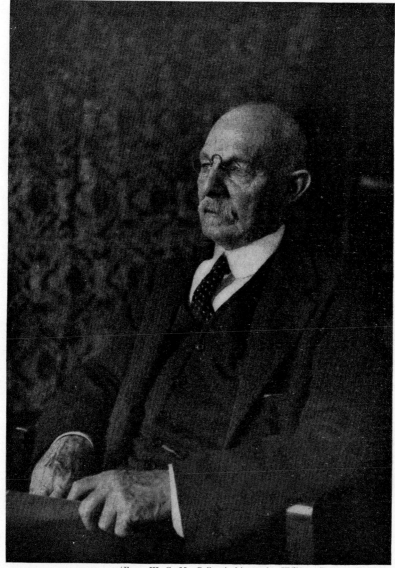

William Stewart Halsted

The extraordinary attention to detail which characterized Halsted's surgery was reflected also in his personal life. For years he had his shirts sent to Paris to be laundered because he could not get it done to his satisfaction in Baltimore. He was a perfectionist in everything.

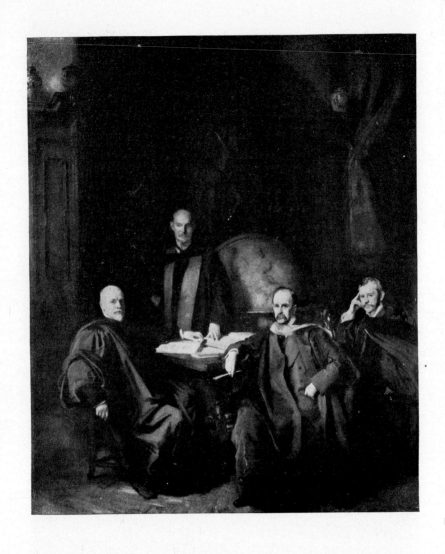

Sargent's Portrait "The Four Doctors" Welch, Halsted, Osler, and Kelly

surance Bank in which contributions from the employer are deposited. The bank is controlled by a committee of workers. The extensive benefits of this system require vast funds. The total contributions of industry vary according to the wages paid, but represent an average tax of 18 per cent of the total wages. Newsholme and Kingsbury found many features in the Russian organization of medical care that they admired. They concluded that the U.S.S.R. "with lightning speed has instituted in its best organized cities provisions for medical care . . . which are more complete and freer from inhibitions to readily accessible help than hold good in any country known to us."

The English system of sickness insurance deserves careful study because the English medical traditions and her hospital system are closer to the American than any other. Voluntary sickness insurance gained a firm hold among English working men in the last decade of the 19th Century. The so-called "friendly societies" organized for this purpose had 5,700,000 members by 1904. These societies contracted with local physicians to provide ordinary home medical care for their members at the rate of somewhat less than a dollar a year per member. The medical work under these conditions was underpaid and usually poorly done.

In 1911 the Liberal Government, with Lloyd George as Chancellor of the Exchequer, passed the National Health Insurance Act which made sickness insurance compulsory for all employed persons, men and women, over the age of 16, whose salary was not over £250 (about $1,250) a year. In 1931 this included some 15 million persons. According to the terms of this act, the employer and the employee each contribute equal amounts weekly (about 18 cents). The state is also a partner, paying one-seventh of the total cost of the benefits and the cost of the central administration. The act also provided for widows and orphans, and for old age pensions, maternity benefits, disability benefits, and sickness allowances.

Unfortunately, in England, as in most other countries where

sickness insurance has been enacted, the medical profession was not taken into partnership in planning it. The result was that serious mistakes were made. In the first place, the medical fee was set at too low a level, namely six shillings ($1.50) per head per year. The British Medical Association, which could justly claim to represent the view of the general practitioner, maintained that the payment should be larger. The Government increased its offer to nine shillings ($2.25), but the doctors thought that this also was too small, and more than 27,000 of them signed an agreement to support the British Medical Association in its determination to fight the government by withholding their services. Prolonged negotiations failed to provide a compromise, and Lloyd George finally broke the doctors' strike in 1913 when the British Medical Association was compelled, by large-scale secessions from its ranks, to release the members from their promises. The doctors, however, had protested to some purpose, for some of their more reasonable demands, such as the free choice of doctor and increase in the capitation fee, had been granted.

Today more than 15,000 general practitioners are working under the sickness insurance scheme, better known as the "panel" system. They serve about one-third of the population. Any physician can become a panel doctor, and the Minister of Health alone can remove him from the panel, and only for some very good reason. The patient has complete freedom of choice of doctor, being limited only by geographical distances, but no one physician may take more than 2,500 panel patients.

Much criticism has been levelled at this system. Yet the preponderant view of English physicians, as represented by a resolution passed at the 1922 annual meeting of the British Medical Association, is that the medical service provided by the panel system, although incomplete, is so satisfactory that it should be continued. The official evidence of the British Medical Association before the Royal Commission on National Health Insurance in 1926 states: "The evidence as to the incidence of sickness benefit

does point to the fact that the scheme has almost certainly reduced national sickness . . ."

The chief indictment of the system has been that some doctors—especially those with large panels—give inferior service. It
has been charged that their offices are crowded during limited
hours, and that a perfunctory interview and a prescription for a
bottle of medicine are all that the patient receives. In answer it
can only be said that such an authority as Newsholme has written
that "the majority of panel doctors give honest and competent
service within the prescribed limits."

The most important defect of the English plan is no doubt the
fact that the medical service that it provides is very incomplete.
There is no provision for hospital care, for the fees of surgeons or
other specialists, or for the cost of special laboratory procedures
such as x-ray examination, so important in modern medicine.
Moreover, the insurance does not cover illness of other dependent
members of the employee's family. Thus the occurrence of serious
illness requiring hospital care in his family leaves the employee
still dependent upon the charity of his local voluntary hospital,
and of the physicians who staff its ward services. Dependence
upon charity for so vital a need is certainly not in keeping with
our democratic ideal of equality of opportunity.

In Britain the organization of medical care has recently been
studied by a Medical Planning Commission representing the British Medical Association and the various Royal Colleges. This
Commission has drafted an Interim Report, which was published
in the June 20th, 1942, number of the *British Medical Journal*. It
is a document that should be read by all who are interested in the
problem.

The report acknowledges the main defects of the present
health insurance system, particularly its failure to include dependents of wage earners, and the inadequate character of the medical care which the general practitioner is able to provide single-
handed. It states: "The days when a doctor armed only with his

stethoscope and his drugs could offer a fairly complete medical service are gone. He cannot now be all-sufficient. For efficient work he must have at his disposal modern facilities for diagnosis and treatment, and often these cannot be provided by a private individual . . . He must also have easy and convenient access to consultant and specialist opinion, whether at hospital or elsewhere, and he must have opportunities for real collaboration with consultants."

The report recommends a comprehensive national health policy embracing the establishment of a responsible ministerial department, headed by a physician, in the national government, and the further development of the National Health Insurance system to provide complete medical care for all persons with incomes within the limits of the present insurance system and for their dependents, in effect for about 90 per cent of the population.

Two fundamental changes in the character of the medical care provided by the health insurance system are suggested. The first of these is the development of *group practice* to end the general practitioner's isolation from consultant and specialist help and from hospital services. This is borrowing an American principle of which we shall write more later on. The group of co-operating health insurance physicians would carry on their work in a communal *health center* where x-ray and certain other laboratory facilities would be available. The patient would still retain the privilege of selecting his doctor from among the 6 to 12 physicians in the group.

The second suggestion is for a unified national hospital system, organized on a regional basis in such a way that all parts of the country would be provided with adequate hospital facilities. The existing voluntary hospitals would be incorporated into this new plan along with the so-called council hospitals already maintained by the local county councils and district councils at public expense. The consultants and specialists of various kinds staffing these regional hospitals would be employed on a whole time or a part-time basis. Their services would be available to all persons in the region coming under the National Health Insurance plan, as part of the complete medical service provided for them. These regional hospitals would be administered by a Regional Council including representatives of the central governmental authority and the local medical profession. Under this plan the differences between voluntary and public hospitals which now exist would be done away with.

It is significant that in Britain, where social security has long been more highly developed than in any other country except the Scandinavian ones, democratic forces have been so stimulated by the war effort that a plan for providing complete medical care for 90 per cent of the population has been put forward by the physicians themselves. Their plan is not a radical departure but a soundly conceived extension of the health insurance system under which British physicians have worked for three decades.

We have written at some length of the history of hospital economy and of sickness insurance in European countries in the hope that careful study of the experience abroad will help us in the United States to avoid defects in the plans for a better distribution of medical care which must soon develop here. We in America will certainly feel the stimulus, before the war is won, of the same democratic forces which are now stirring Britain. Freedom from lack of adequate medical care will be, it is hoped, one of the fundamental freedoms of our future democracy.

NEW DIRECTIONS IN AMERICA

In any plan that is presented for improvement of the distribution of medical care in the United States two innovations in the organization of medical care which are indigenous to this country should be included. Both of these innovations give immediate promise of improving the quality of medical care and of reducing its cost for the hard pressed American family of limited means. These are: (1) the Baker Memorial Hospital plan for patients of moderate means, and (2) group practice of medicine.

The trustees of the Massachusetts General Hospital and its director, Frederic A. Washburn, were the first to do something about the high cost of private hospital care. In 1924 friends of the hospital gave about two million dollars for the construction of a special hospital building for patients of moderate means. It was named the Baker Memorial and was opened in March, 1930. The Baker Memorial, being an integral unit of the Massachusetts General Hospital, served by the same staff and sharing the scientific facilities of the mother hospital, provides medical care of a very high standard. By avoiding the luxuries of private hospital service it has been possible to keep the cost down. The rates vary from $4.50 to $6.50 per day, depending upon the size of the room and the degree of privacy. About half of the rooms are single, while the others contain two or four beds. These rates include nursing care, which is provided by graduate nurses assigned to each floor. Special nurses are allowed only when attending physicians think them really necessary. The charges for laboratory and other special services are kept low. A maximum limit of $150 is set for the total fee of the attending physician, this to include all consultant's fees. This medical fee is collected by the hospital along with its own charges.

Dr. Haven Emerson has recently analyzed the experience of the first ten years of operation of the Baker Memorial. The experiment has been a striking success both from the viewpoint of the patients it has served and the medical profession of Boston. The average individual income of the patients it has served has been slightly over $2,000. The average patient paid a total of $100.19 for all hospital services, and $66.06 for medical fees. Any patient who has had to pay for private care in a typical American hospital will at once realize that these charges are remarkably low. Eighty-four per cent of the hospital's 242 beds have been occupied, and since 1937 the hospital has operated without a deficit.

Another way of lowering the cost of medical care, as well as of improving the quality, is for physicians to form groups. In such a group each member can devote himself to the special aspect of medicine for which he is best trained, and the combined abilities of all offer the patient the advantages of modern medical knowledge in a more readily available and therefore a more economical form than the individual private practitioner can provide. Duplication of laboratory equipment is avoided. Consultants are immediately at hand. Such groups, if they are to function adequately, must be organized in close association with, if not actually within the walls of, a good hospital, for we have seen that the hospital is the workshop of the modern physician. The members of such a group usually pool their earnings, and function as a corporate unit that pays salaries.

The Mayo Clinic at Rochester, Minnesota, was the prototype of this kind of medical organization. Today several hundred similar medical groups exist in the United States. This kind of organization offers the adequately trained young hospital graduate his best opportunity to put his training to immediate use. If he attempts to enter a special field of practice as an individual, he usually faces a long period of sterile inactivity.

The success of group medical practice has led to several interesting experiments in which group clinics have offered the public, or a limited section of the public, complete medical care on the pre-payment or insurance basis. For instance, the Ross-Loss Clinic in Los Angeles has provided complete medical care to employed persons at $24 per year. A slightly different arrangement is exemplified by that which has developed at Baton Rouge, Louisiana, where the employees of the Stanocola Corporation have formed a cooperative consumers medical and hospital association, and organized a group clinic to provide complete medical care at the cost of $36 per year to individual members. Schemes of this sort can provide relatively complete medical care of good quality at about $70 per year per family, it would seem. This sort of insurance plan has one very important advantage over the panel system of compulsory sickness insurance as it has been developed abroad, namely, that the quality of the medical care rendered by a competent group clinic is apt to be better than that which the individual practitioner under the panel system can provide. And when the $70 per year cost is compared with the estimated cost of $310 per family per year for adequate medical care under our present system of individualistic private practice, it would seem that there is also a great economic advantage.

Various objections have been raised to the principle of group practice of medicine. A section of opinion within the American Medical Association has vigorously opposed it. Much of this opposition comes from staunch individualists whose concept of medical practice dates from a past generation. Of the arguments against group practice which need seriously concern us there are two that deserve mention. The first is that physicians are too individualistic to form group clinics on a sufficiently large scale to supply less expensive private medical care to the great section of the public that needs it. That this is not a fact is proven by the history of voluntary charity hospitals in the English speaking countries. In these hospitals, during past centuries, as today, physicians have practiced group medicine in the best sense of our definition of it, providing it free to the sick poor. Having achieved this kind of cooperation for the poor, physicians should find it less effort to achieve it for private patients of limited means.

Another objection to group practice is that it destroys the confidential patient-physician relationship that has been a cherished part of the tradition of medicine. This objection is again best refuted by the experience of those who have served on the staffs of voluntary hospitals. They will recall countless patients whom they have cared for in the wards with whom trust has been as well reciprocated as with any private patient. For the spirit of medicine goes beyond these shallow economic distinctions. It is the stuff of life itself that physicians deal with—and this is too precious a material to be given or taken away on a monetary basis. It is because most people know this that there is hope that they will one day succeed in making adequate medical care available to everyone.

BIBLIOGRAPHY

CHAPTER 1

GARRISON, F. H., *Introduction to the History of Medicine*, 4th edition, Philadelphia, 1929.

NEUBURGER, M., *History of Medicine*. Translated by E. Playfair. Vol. I, 1910. Vol. II, Part 1, 1925. London (Oxford Medical Publications).

OSLER, SIR WM., *The Evolution of Modern Medicine* . . . , New Haven, 1922.

WHIPPLE, A. O., "Role of the Nestorians . . ." *Ann. M. Hist.*, 8:313–323, 1936 (also *Bull. New York Acad. Med.*, 12:446–462, 1936).

CHAPTER 2

BAAS, J. H., *Outlines of the History of Medicine and the Medical Profession*. Translated by H. E. Handerson, New York, 1889.

HAEHL, R., *Samuel Hahnemann, His Life and Work*. Translated by M. L. Wheeler and W. H. R. Grundy, London, 1923.

CHAPTER 3

BARON, J., *The Life of Edward Jenner, M.D.*, 2 vols., London, 1827–38.

BURTON, W., *An Account of the Life and Writings of Herman Boerhaave*, London, 1743.

MEAD, R., *A Short Discourse Concerning Pestilential Contagion and the Methods to Be Used to Prevent It*, 2nd edition, London, 1720.

PAGET, S., *John Hunter, Man of Science and Surgeon (1728–1793)*, London, 1898 (Masters of Medicine).

CHAPTER 4

TILANUS, C. B., *Surgery a Hundred Years Ago* . . . ', edited by H. T. Deelman, London, 1925.

POOL, E. H., AND McGOWAN, F. J., *Surgery at the New York Hospital One Hundred Years Ago*, New York, 1930.

CHAPTER 5

ABRAHAM, J. J., *Lettsom: His Life, Times, Friends and Descendants*, London, 1933.

BRIDGES, R., "An Account of the Casualty Department," *Saint Bartholomew's Hospital Reports*, 14:167–182, 1878.

CLAY, R. M., *The Mediæval Hospitals of England*, London, 1909.

COOK, E. T., *A Short Life of Florence Nightingale*, abridged by R. Nash, New York, 1925.

ERICHSEN, SIR J. E., *On Hospitalism and the Causes of Death After Operation*, London, 1874.

HOWARD, J., *The State of Prisons in England and Wales . . .* , Warrington, 1777.

———, *An Account of the Principal Lazarettos in Europe . . .* , Warrington, 1789.

SIMPSON, SIR J. Y., *Anaesthesia, Hospitalism, etc.*, Edinburgh, 1871 (*Works of Sir James Y. Simpson*, Vol. II)

TENON, M., *Mémoires sur les Hôpitaux de Paris*, Paris, 1788.

CHAPTER 6

CHADWICK, SIR E., *The Health of Nations. A Review of the Works of Edwin Chadwick with a Biographical Dissertation*, by B. W. Richardson, 2 vols., London, 1887.

Citizens' Association of New York, Council of Hygiene and Public Health, *Report on the Sanitary Condition of the City*, New York, 1865.

DICKENS, CHARLES, *American Notes*, London, 1842.

Great Britain, Parliament, Commissioners for Inquiring into the State of Large Towns and Populous Districts, *Report*, London, 1844. *Second Report*, London, 1845.

Great Britain, Poor Law Commissioners, *Sanitary Condition of the Labouring Population of Great Britain*, London, 1842.

GRISCOM, J. H., *The Sanitary Condition of the Laboring Population of New York*, New York, 1845.

HAMMOND, J. L. LE B., AND B., *The Age of the Chartists, 1832–1854 . . .* , London, 1930.

WINSLOW, C. E. A., *The Evolution and Significance of the Modern Public Health Campaign*, New Haven, 1923.

CHAPTER 7

BATEMAN, T., *Reports on the Diseases of London . . .* , London, 1819.

BUER, M. C., *Health, Wealth and Population in the Early Days of the Industrial Revolution*, London, 1926.

FARR, W., Vital Statistics . . . (In J. R. McCullough's *A Statistical Account of the British Empire*, London, 1837. Vol. 2, Chap. IV, pages 567–601).

KOREN, J., *The History of Statistics . . .* , New York, 1918.

PEARL, R., *Introduction to Medical Biometry and Statistics*, Philadelphia, 1923.

CHAPTER 8

CREIGHTON, C., *A History of Epidemics in Britain*, Vol. I, *From A.D. 664 to the Extinction of the Plague*, Cambridge, 1891.

———, *A History of the Epidemics in Britain*, Vol. II, *From the Extinction of the Plague to the Present Time*, Cambridge, 1894.

GREENWOOD, M., *Epidemics and Crowd Diseases . . .* , London, 1935.

HIRSCH, A., *Handbook of Geographical and Historical Pathology*, translated by Charles Creighton, 3 vols., London, 1883.

PACKARD, F. R., *History of Medicine in the United States*, 2 vols., New York, 1931.

RIESMAN, D., "American Contributions to Nosography," (Shattuck Lecture), *New England J. Med.*, 219:591–611, 1938.

SMITH, G., *Plague on Us*, New York, 1941.

WEBSTER, N., *A Brief History of Epidemic and Pestilential Diseases, etc.*, 2 vols., Hartford, Conn., 1799.

CHAPTER 9

BALL, J. M., *The Sack-'em-up Men . . .* , Edinburgh, 1928.

COOPER, B. B., *The Life of Sir Astley Cooper, Bart . . .* , 2 vols., London, 1843.

CHAPTER 10

HABERLING, W., *Johannes Müller, das Leben des rheinischen Naturforschers*, Leipzig, 1924.

LONG, E. R., *A History of Pathology*, Baltimore, 1928.

———, *Selected Readings in Pathology, from Hippocrates to Virchow*, Springfield, Ill., 1929.

NORDENSKIÖLD, E., *The History of Biology, a Survey*, translated by L. B. Eyre, New York, 1928.

POSNER, C., *Rudolf Virchow*, Vienna, 1921.

CHAPTER 11

BROWN, P., *American Martyrs to Science through the Roentgen Rays*, Springfield, Ill., 1936.

CANNON, W. B., "Early Use of the Roentgen Ray in the Study of the Alimentary Canal," *J. A. M. A.*, 62:1–3, 1914.

CHRISTIAN, H. A., "Tribute to Professor Folin," *Science*, 81:37–38, 1935.

GLASSER, O., *Wilhelm Conrad Röntgen and the Early History of Roentgen Rays*, Springfield, Ill., 1934.

GRAHAM, E. A., COLE, W. H., COPHER, G. H., AND MOORE, S., *Diseases of the Gall Bladder and Bile Ducts* . . . , Philadelphia, 1928.

SCHAEFFER, P. A., Obituary of Otto Folin, *Science*, 81:35–37, 1935.

TILDEN, SIR W. A., *Famous Chemists, the Men and their Work,* London, 1921.

WUNDERLICH, C. A., *On the Temperature in Diseases* . . . , translated by W. B. Woodman, London, 1871.

CHAPTER 12

BULLOCH, W., *The History of Bacteriology,* London, 1938.

BURTON, E. F., AND KOHL, W. H., *The Electron Microscope,* New York, 1942.

VALLERY-RADOT, R., *The Life of Pasteur,* translated by Mrs. R. L. Devonshire, 2 vols., London, 1902.

CHAPTER 13

DE KRUIF, P., *Microbe Hunters,* New York, 1926.

———, *Men Against Death,* New York, 1932.

GORGAS, M. C. D., AND HENDRICK, B. J., *William Crawford Gorgas, His Life and Work,* Garden City, N. Y., 1924.

HOWARD, S. in collaboration with DE KRUIF, P., *Yellow Jack,* New York, 1934.

KELLY, H. A., *Walter Reed and Yellow Fever,* New York, 1906.

MANSON-BAHR, P. H., AND ALCOCK, A., *The Life and Work of Sir Patrick Manson,* London, 1927.

MEGROZ, R. L., *Ronald Ross, Discoverer and Creator,* London, 1931.

SNOW, J., *On the Mode of Communication of Cholera,* 2nd edition, London, 1855.

SOPER, G. A., "The Curious Career of Typhoid Mary," *Bull. New York Acad. Med.*, 15:698–712, 1939.

ZINSSER, H., *Rats, Lice and History* . . . , Boston, 1935.

CHAPTER 14

TOPLEY, W. W. C., AND WILSON, G. S., *The Principles of Bacteriology and Immunity,* 2nd edition, Baltimore, 1936.

ZINSSER, H., AND BAYNE-JONES, S., *A Textbook of Bacteriology* . . . , New York, 1939.

CHAPTER 15

JACOBS, M. S., "Paul Ehrlich and his Relation to Modern Chemotherapy," *Bull. Hist. Med.*, 8:956–964, 1940.

LAZARUS, A., *Paul Ehrlich,* Vienna, 1922.

LONG, P. H., AND BLISS, E. A., *The Clinical and Experimental Use of Sulfanilamide, Sulfapyridine and Allied Compounds,* New York, 1939.

CHAPTER 16

BOWDITCH, H. I., *The Young Stethoscopist, or the Student's Aid to Auscultation,* New York, 1846.

BROWN, L., *The Story of Clinical Pulmonary Tuberculosis,* Baltimore, 1941.

JACKSON, J., *A Memoir of James Jackson, Jr., M.D. . . . ,* Boston, 1835.

LONG, E. R., "The Decline of Tuberculosis, with Special Reference to its Generalized Form," (William Snow Miller lecture), *Bull. Hist. Med.,* 8:819–843, 1940.

TRUDEAU, E. L., *An Autobiography,* New York, 1916.

CHAPTER 17

NOTE: There is no comprehensive recent review of the vitamins to which we can refer the reader. The studies referred to here are so many in number that we can not include references to them all. We shall therefore limit ourselves to listing a few of the older reviews and some individual papers of special historical interest.

American Medical Association Council on Food, *The Vitamins—A Symposium,* Chicago, 1939.

BOWLES, G. T., *New Types of Old Americans at Harvard and at Eastern Women's Colleges,* Cambridge, Mass., 1932.

DE KRUIF, P., *Hunger Fighters,* New York, 1928.

FUNK, C., *The Vitamines,* Baltimore, 1922.

HESS, A. F., *Scurvy, Past and Present,* Philadelphia, 1920.

JOLLIFFE, N., McLESTER, J. S., AND SHERMAN, H. C., "The Prevalence of Malnutrition," *J. A. M. A.,* 118:944–950, 1942.

MOZOLOWSKI, W., "Jedrzej Sniadecki (1768–1838) on the Cure of Rickets," *Nature,* 143:121, 1939.

PALM, T. A., "The Geographical Distribution and Aetiology of Rickets," *Practitioner,* 40:270–321, 1890.

VOGEL, K., "Scurvy—The Plague of the Sea and the Spoyle of Mariners," *Bull. New York Acad. Med.,* 9:459–483, 1933.

CHAPTER 18

MINOT, G. R., AND MURPHY, W. P., "Treatment of Pernicious Anemia by a Special Diet," *J. A. M. A.,* 87:470–476, 1926.

MINOT, G. R., "The Development of Liver Therapy in Pernicious Anemia," (Nobel Lecture), *Lancet,* 1:361–364, 1935.

CHAPTER 19

BANTING, F. G., "The History of Insulin," *Edinburgh M. J.*, 36:1–18, 1929.

BARON, M., "The Relation of the Islets of Langerhans to Diabetes with Special Reference to Cases of Pancreatic Lithiasis," *Surg., Gynec., & Obst.*, 31:437, 1920.

BEST, C. H., Obituary of F. G. Banting, *Canad. M. A. J.*, 44:327–328, 1941.

CHAPTER 20

ALLBUTT, T. C., *Diseases of the Arteries Including Angina Pectoris*, 2 vols., London, 1915.

BOUILLAUD, J. B., *Traité Clinique des Maladies du Coeur . . .* , 2 vols., Paris, 1835.

CHEADLE, W. B., *The Various Manifestations of the Rheumatic State*, London, 1889.

Obituary, *Lancet*, 1:962–965, 1910.

DRUMMOND, J. C., AND WILBRAHAM, A., *The Englishman's Food*, London, 1940.

GOLDBLATT, H., LYNCH, J., HANZAL, R. F., AND SUMMERVILLE, W. W., "Studies on Experimental Hypertension, I—The Production of Persistent Elevation of Systolic Blood Pressure by Means of Renal Ischemia," *J. Exper. Med.*, 59:347–379, 1934.

HERRICK, J. B., *A Short History of Cardiology*, Springfield, Ill., 1942.

ROGER, H., "Du rhumatisme articulaire et viscéral chez les enfants et spécialement de leurs rapports avec la chorée," *Arch. gén. de méd.*, 2:641–665, 1866.

TROUSSEAU, A., *Clinique médicale de l'Hôtel Dieu de Paris*, 2 vols., Paris, 1861–1862.

WATERSTON, D., ORR, J., AND CAPPELL, D. F., "Sir James Mackenzie's Heart," *Brit. Heart J.*, 1:237–248, 1939.

WHITE, P. D., *Heart Disease*, New York, 1937.

WILLIAMS, F. H., *The Roentgen Rays in Medicine and Surgery*, New York, 1901.

WILLIUS, F. A., AND KEYS, T. E., *Cardiac Classics*, St. Louis, 1941.

WILSON, R. M., *The Beloved Physician, Sir James Mackenzie*, London, 1926.

CHAPTER 21

BOWMAN, W., "On the Structure and Use of the Malpighian Bodies of the Kidney," *Royal Society of London Philosophical Trans.*, pages 57–80, 1842.

BRIGHT, R., *Original Papers of Richard Bright on Renal Disease*, edited by A. A. Osman, London, 1937.

CHRISTISON, R., *On Granular Degeneration of the Kidneys . . . ,* Philadelphia, 1839.

FISHBERG, A. M., *Hypertension and Nephritis*, 4th edition, Philadelphia, 1939.

HENLE, J., *Zur Anatomie der Niere*, Göttingen, 1862.

JOHNSON, SIR G., *On Diseases of the Kidney*, London, 1852.

MAJOR, R. H., *Classic Descriptions of Disease*, 2nd edition, Springfield, Ill., 1939.

PETERS, J. P., AND VAN SLYKE, D. D., *Quantitative Clinical Chemistry*, Vol. 1, *Interpretation*, Baltimore, 1931.

RICHARDS, A. N., "Physiology of the Kidney," *Bull. New York Acad. Med.*, 14:5, 1938.

STRAUSS, H., *Die chronischen Nierenentzündungen in ihren Wirkungen auf die Blutflüssigkeit . . . ,* Berlin, 1902.

THAYER, W. S., "Richard Bright: The Man and the Physician," *Brit. M. J.*, 2:87–93, 1927.

VOLHARD, F., AND FAHR, T., *Die Brightsche Nierenkrankheit*, Berlin, 1914.

WIDAL, F., AND JAVAL, A., "La chlorurémie et la cure de déchloruration dans les mal de Bright," *J. de physiol. et de path. gén.*, 5:1107–1123, 1903.

CHAPTER 22

FLEXNER, J. T., *Doctors on Horseback*, New York, 1937.

SCHACHNER, A., *Ephraim McDowell, "Father of Ovariotomy" and Founder of Abdominal Surgery*, Philadelphia, 1921.

CHAPTER 23

BIER, A., "Bemerkungen zur Cocainisierung des Rückenmarks," *München. med. Wochenschrift*, 47:1226, 1900.

BIGELOW, H. J., "A History of the Discovery of Modern Anaesthesia," In: *A Century of American Medicine, 1776–1876*, Philadelphia, 1876.

CORNING, J. L., "On the Prolongation of the Anaesthetic Effects of the Hydrochloride of Cocaine when Subcutaneously Injected," *New York Med. J.*, 42:317–319, 1885.

FLEXNER, J. T., *Doctors on Horseback*, New York, 1937.

GRIFFITH, H., "John Snow, Pioneer Specialist in Anesthesia," *Current Res. in Anes. and Anal.*, 13:45–51, 1937.

KEYS, T. E., "The Development of Anesthesia," *Anesthesiology*, 2:552–574, 1941, 3:11, 282, and 650, 1942.

KNAPP, H., *Cocaine and its Use in Ophthalmic and General Surgery*, New York, 1885 (Reprinted from *Arch. of Ophth.*, 13:402–448, 1884).

420   BIBLIOGRAPHY

LUNDY, J. S., "Intravenous Anaesthesia," *Am. J. Surg.*, 34:559–570, 1936.
MacCALLUM, W. G., *William Stewart Halsted, Surgeon*, Baltimore, 1930.
ORÉ, L. L. G., "Nouvelle note sur les injections intra-veineuses de chloral," *Bull. Soc. de Chir. de Paris*, 3rd series, 1:350 and 400, 1872 and 1873.
TAYLOR, F. L., *Crawford W. Long and the Discovery of Ether Anesthesia*, New York, 1928.
WATERS, R. M., "Carbon Dioxide Absorption from Anaesthetic Atmospheres," *Proc. Roy. Soc. Med.*, 30:11–22, 1936.

CHAPTER 24

FINNEY, J. M. T., *A Surgeon's Life*, New York, 1940.
———, "Changing Conditions in Surgery Since the Time of Henry Jacob Bigelow," *New England J. Med.*, 206:263–276, 1932.
GODLEE, SIR R. J., *Lord Lister*, London, 1917.
KEEN, W. W., "Before and after Lister," *Science*, 41:845, 1915.
KOCH, R., *Untersuchungen über die Aetiologie der Wundinfectionskrankheiten*, Leipzig, 1878.
MALLOCH, A., "Biographical Sketch and Memorabilia of Lister," *Bull. New York Acad. Med.*, 4:133–147, 1928.
MARCY, H. O., "The Semi-Centennial of the Introduction of Antiseptic Surgery in America," *Tr. South. Surg. Assoc.*, 33:1 and 25, 1921.
MIKULICZ, J., "Das Operieren in sterilisierten Zwirnhandschuhen und mit Mundbinde . . . ," *Zentralblatt f. Chir.*, 24:713–717, 1897.
VON NUSSBAUM, J. N., *Leitfaden zur antiseptischen Wundbehandlung* . . . , Stuttgart, 1879.
ROBB, H., *Aseptic Surgical Technique*, Philadelphia, 1894.

CHAPTER 25

HALSTED, W. S., "The Operative Story of Goitre," *Johns Hopkins Hosp. Rep.*, 19:71–257, 1920.
———, "Ligature and Suture Material: the Employment of Fine Silk in Preference to Catgut and the Advantages of Transfixing of Tissues and Vessels in Control of Hemorrhage," *J. A. M. A.*, 60:1119–1126, 1913.
POWER, D'ARCY, "Eponyms—Spencer Wells' Forceps," *British J. Surg.* 14:385–387, 1927.

CHAPTER 26

New York (City), Presbyterian Hospital, Surgical Service, *Wound Healing Report*, 1939 (mimeographed).
New York (City), Presbyterian Hospital, *Annual Report, 21st*, 1889.

Appendicitis

COPE, Z., *Pioneers in Acute Abdominal Surgery,* London, 1939.

FITZ, R. H., "Perforating Inflammation of the Vermiform Appendix, with Special Reference to its Early Diagnosis and Treatment," *Am. J. M. Sc.,* new series, 92:321–346, 1886.

KELLY, H. A., *Appendicitis and other Diseases of the Vermiform Appendix,* Philadelphia, 1909.

McBURNEY, C., "Experience with Early Operative Interference in Cases of Disease of the Vermiform Appendix," *New York M. J.,* 50:676–684, 1889.

PARKER, W., "An Operation for Abscess in the Appendix Vermiformis Caeci," *Med. Rec. (New York),* 2:25–27, 1867.

PARKINSON, J., "Case of Diseased Appendix Vermiformis," *Med. Chir. Tr.,* London, 3:57, 1812.

Gallbladder Disease

BOBBS, J. S., "Case of Lithotomy of the Gallbladder," *Tr. Indiana State Med. Soc.,* 1868, page 68.

COURVOISIER, L. G., *Casuistisch-statistische Beiträge zur Pathologie und Chirurgie der Gallenwege,* Leipzig, 1890.

HALSTED, W. S., "Contributions to the Surgery of the Bile Passages, Especially of the Common Bile-Duct," *Boston Med. & Surg. J.,* 141:645–654, 1899.

LANGENBUCH, C., "Ein Fall von Exstirpation der Gallenblase wegen chronischer Cholelithiasis. Heilung," *Berlin. klin. Wochenschrift,* 19:725–727, 1882.

MacCALLUM, W. G., *William Stewart Halsted, Surgeon,* Baltimore, 1930.

McBURNEY, C., "Removal of Biliary Calculi from the Common Duct by the Duodenal Route," *Ann. Surg.,* 28:481–487, and 517–525, 1898.

SIMS, J. M., "Cholecystotomy in Dropsy of the Gallbladder," *Brit. M. J.,* 1:811–815, 1878.

THUDICHUM, J. L. W., *A Treatise on Gallstones,* London, 1863.

Hernia

BASSINI, E., *Nuovo metodo operativo per la cura dell'ernia inguinale,* Padova, 1889.

BULL, W. T., "On the Radical Cure of Hernia with Results of 134 Operations," *Medical News,* 57:5–13, 1890 (also *Tr. Am. Surg. Asso.,* 8:99–117, 1890).

——, "Notes on Cases of Hernia which have Relapsed after Various Operations for Radical Cure," *New York M. J.*, 53:615–617, 1891.

COOPER, SIR A. P., *Observations on Inguinal and Congenital Hernia*, London, 1803.

——, *On Hernia, Part 1. The Anatomy and Surgical Treatment of Inguinal and Congenital Hernia*, London, 1804.

——, *On Hernia, Part 2. The Anatomy and Surgical Treatment of Crural and Umbilical Hernia*, London, 1807.

HALSTED, W. S., "The Radical Cure of Inguinal Hernia in the Male," *Bull. Johns Hopkins Hosp.*, 4:17–26, 1893 (also *Ann. Surg.*, 17:542–556, 1893).

SOCIN, A., "De la valeur de la cure radicale des hernies au point de vue de la guérison définitive," *Rev. de Chir.*, 8:264–274, 1888.

Goiter

GULL, SIR W. W., "On a Cretinoid State Supervening in Adult Life in Women," *Tr. Clinical Soc. London*, 7:180–185, 1874.

HALSTED, W. S., "The Operative Story of Goitre," *Johns Hopkins Hosp. Rep.*, 19:71–257, 1920.

KENDALL, E. C., "The Isolation in Crystalline Form of the Compound Containing Iodin which occurs in the Thyroid; its Chemical Nature and Physiological Activity," *J. A. M. A.*, 64:2042, 1915.

KOCHER, T., "Ueber Kropfexstirpation und ihre Folgen, "*Arch. f. klin. Chir.*, 29:254–337, 1883.

MAGNUS-LEVY, A., "Ueber den respiratorischen Gaswechsel unter dem Einfluss der Thyreoidea sowie unter verschiedenen pathologischen Zuständen," *Berlin. klin. Wochenschrift*, 32:650–652, 1895.

MARINE, D., AND KIMBALL, O. P., "Prevention of Simple Goitre in Man," *Arch. Int. Med.*, 25:661–672, 1920.

MAYO, C. H., "Goiter, with a preliminary report of 300 operations on the thyroid," *J. A. M. A.*, 48:273–277, 1906.

MEANS, J. H., *The Thyroid and Its Diseases*, Philadelphia, 1937.

MÜLLER, F., "Beiträge zur Kenntnis der Basedow'schen Krankheit," *Deutsches Arch. f. klin. Med.*, 51:335–412, 1892 and 1893.

MURRAY, G. R., "The Life-history of the First Case of Myxoedema Treated by Thyroid Extract," *Brit. M. J.*, 1:359, 1920.

PARRY, C. H., *Collections from the Unpublished Medical Writings . . . ,* London, 1825, Vol. 1, page 478.

PLUMMER, H. S., "Results of Administering Iodine to Patients Having Exophthalmic Goiter," *J. A. M. A.*, 80:1955, 1923.

TROUSSEAU, A., *Lectures on Clinical Medicine . . . ,* Lecture XIX, Exophthalmic Goiter or Grave's Disease, London, 1868, Vol. 1, page 587.

Cancer of the Breast

BARDELEBEN, A., *Lehrbuch der Chirurgie und Operationslehre*, 4th edition, 1866, vol. 3, page 598.

COOPER, W. A., "The History of Radical Mastectomy," *Ann. M. Hist.*, 3:36–54, 1941.

GROSS, S. W., *A Practical Treatise on Tumors of the Mammary Gland*, New York, 1880.

HALSTED, W. S., "The Results of Operations for the Cure of Cancer of the Breast Performed at the Johns Hopkins Hospital from June, 1889, to January, 1894," *Ann. Surg.*, 20:497–555, 1894.

MOORE, C. H., "On the Influence of Inadequate Operations on the Theory of Cancer," *Medico-Chirurgical Tr.*, 50:245–280, 1867.

PAGET, SIR J., *Lectures on Surgical Pathology . . .* , London, 1870, page 651.

THIERSCH, C., *Der Epithelialkrebs namentlich der Haut*, Leipzig, 1865.

VOLKMANN, R., *Beiträge zur Chirurgie*, Leipzig, 1875.

WALDEYER, W., "Die Entwicklung der Carcinome," *Virchows Arch. f. path. Anat.*, 55:67–159, 1872.

WILSON, L. B., "Method for Rapid Preparation of Fresh Tissues for Microscope," *J. A. M. A.*, 45:1737, 1905.

Cancer of the Stomach and Bowel

ABBOTT, W. O., "Indications for Use of the Miller-Abbott Tube," *New England J. Med.*, 225:641–646, 1941.

BILLROTH, T., "Offenes Schreiben an Herrn L. Wittelshöfer," *Wien. med. Wochenschrift*, 31:161–165, 1881.

———, *Billroth und Brahms im Briefwechsel* (edited by O. Gottlieb-Billroth), Berlin, 1935.

CZERNY, V., "Zur Darmresection," *Berlin. klin. Wochenschrift*, 17:637 and 683, 1880.

HALSTED, W. S., "Circular Suture of the Intestine," *Am. J. M. Sc.*, new series, 94:436–461, 1887.

JONES, D. F., "A Two-Stage Combined Abdominal-sacral Operation for Carcinoma of the Rectum," *J. A. M. A.*, 65:757–764, 1915.

KRASKE, P. K., "Zur Exstirpation hochsitzender Mastdarmkrebse," *Arch. f. klin. Chir.*, 32:563–573, 1886.

LEMBERT, A., "Mémoire sur l'entéroraphie," *Répert. gén. d'anat. et de physiol.*, 2:100–107, 1826.

LISFRANC, J. L., "Mémoire sur l'excision de la partie inférieure du rectum devenue carcinomateuse," *Mém. de l'acad. de méd.*, 3:291–302, 1833.

MILES, W. E., *Cancer of the Rectum*, London, 1926.

RANKIN, F. W., AND GRAHAM, A. S., *Cancer of the Colon and Rectum,* Springfield, Ill., 1939.

REYBARD, J. F., "Mémoire sur une tumeur cancéreuse affectant l'S iliaque du colon; ablation de la tumeur et de l'intestin; réunion directe et immédiate des deux bouts de cet organe, guérison," *Bull. de l'acad. de méd.* 9:1031–1043, 1844.

SCHINDLER, R., *Gastroscopy,* Chicago, 1937.

CHAPTER 27

ANNAN, G. L., "An Exhibition of Books on the Growth of our Knowledge of Blood Transfusion," *Bull. New York Acad. Med.,* 15:622–632, 1939.

CANTANI, A., *La Cura del Cholera mediante l'ipodermoclisi e l'enteroclisi,* Naples, 1884.

CRILE, G. W., *An Experimental Research into Surgical Shock,* Philadelphia, 1899 (Cartwright Prize Essay for 1897).

———, *Hemorrhage and Transfusion,* New York, 1909.

GLADSTONE, E., "Johann Sigismund Elscholtz (1623–1688)," *California & West. Med.,* 38:432, and 39:45, 119, and 190, 1933.

GUTHRIE, G. J., *Commentaries on the Surgery of the War in Portugal, Spain, France and the Netherlands, from the Battle of Roliça in 1808, to that of Waterloo in 1815; with additions relating to those in the Crimea in 1854–1855,* Philadelphia, 1862.

HUSTIN, A., "Principe d'une nouvelle méthode de transfusion muqueuse," *J. méd. de Brux.,* 19:436–439, 1914.

KEYNES, G., *Blood Transfusion,* London, 1922.

KIMPTON, A. R., AND BROWN, J. H., "A New and Simple Method of Transfusion," *J. A. M. A.,* 61:117, 1913.

LANDOIS, L., *Die Transfusion des Blutes,* Leipzig, 1875.

LANDSTEINER, K., "Ueber Agglutinations-Erscheinungen normalen menschlichen Blutes," *Wien. klin. Wochenschrift,* 14:1132–1134, 1901.

LATTA, T., "Malignant Cholera . . . ," *Lancet,* 2:274–277, 1832.

LE DRAN, H. F., *A Treatise, or Reflections Drawn from Practice on Gunshot Wounds,* Translated from the French original, London, 1743.

LEWISOHN, R., "A New and Greatly Simplified Method of Blood Transfusion," *Med. Rec.,* 87:141–142, 1915.

LINDEMAN, E., "Simple Syringe Transfusion with Special Cannulas," *Amer. J. Dis. Child.,* 6:28–32, 1913.

MATAS, R., "A Clinical Report on Intravenous Saline Infusion," *New Orleans M. & S. J.,* new series, 14:1 and 81, 1891 and 1892.

———, "The Continued Intravenous 'Drip,' " *Ann. Surg.,* 79:643–661, 1924.

Scudder, J., *Shock*, Philadelphia, 1940.

Zimmerman, L. M., and Howell, K. M., "History of Blood Transfusion," *Ann. M. Hist.*, 4:415, 1932.

CHAPTER 28

Deutsche Gesellschaft für Gynäkologie. 15. Versammlung. Sitzungsberichte. 16 Mai, 1913. Vorträge über Strahlentherapie, *Verhand. d. deutsch. Gesellsch. f. Gynäk.*, 15:384–454, 1914.

Fraenkel, L., "Die Function des Corpus luteum," *Arch. f. Gynäk.*, 68:438–545, 1903.

Freund, W. A., "Eine neue Methode der Exstirpation des ganzen Uterus," *Samml. klin. Vortr.* No. 133. Gynäk., 41:911–924, 1878.

Gordon, A., *A Treatise on the Epidemic Puerperal Fever of Aberdeen*, London, 1795.

Gordon, H. L., *Sir James Young Simpson and Chloroform*, New York, 1898.

Irving, F. C., *Safe Deliverance*, Boston, 1942.

Kelly, H. A., "History of American Gynecology: A Brief Outline," (In Curtis, A. H., editor, *Obstetrics and Gynecology*, Philadelphia, 1933, Vol. 2, page 473).

Kerr, J. M. M., *Maternal Mortality and Morbidity*, Edinburgh, 1933.

Lynch, F. W., "Radical Obstetrics and National Maternal Mortality," *Surg., Gynec. & Obst.*, 66:423–426, 1938.

Osler, Sir W., "Oliver Wendell Holmes," *Bull. Johns Hopkins Hosp.*, 5:85–88, 1894.

Spencer, H. R., *The History of British Midwifery*, London, 1927.

Stadfeldt, A. S., "Ueber prophylaktische Uterusausspülung mit Karbolwasser post partum," *Centralblatt f. Gynäk.*, 4:145–147, 1880.

Thoms, H., *Classical Contributions to Obstetrics and Gynecology*, Springfield, Ill., 1935.

Wertheim, E., *Die erweiterte abdominale Operation bei Carcinoma Colli Uteri . . .* , Berlin, 1911.

CHAPTER 29

Albarran, J., *Les Tumeurs de la Vessie*, Paris, 1891

Beer, E., "Removal of Neoplasms of the Urinary Bladder," *J. A. M. A.*, 54:1768, 1910.

Brown, J., "Catheterization of the Male Ureters," *Bull. Johns Hopkins Hosp.*, 4:73, 1893.

Desnos, E., "Histoire de l'urologie," Paris, 1914 (*Encyclopédie française d'urologie*, Vol. 1).

Kelly, H. A., and Burnam, C. F., *Diseases of the Kidneys, Ureters and Bladder*, 2 vols., New York, 1914.

McGill, A. F., "Hypertrophy of the Prostate and its Relief by Operation," *Lancet*, 1:215–217, 1888.

Nitze, M., *Lehrbuch der Kystoskopie. Ihre Technik und klinische Bedeutung*, Wiesbaden, 1889.

Simon, G., *Chirurgie der Nieren*, Stuttgart, Part 1, 1871; Part 2, 1876.

Socin, A., and Burckhardt, E., *Die Verletzungen und Krankheiten der Prostata*, Stuttgart, 1902 (Deutsche Chirurgie, Vol. 53).

Stevens, A. R., "Cystoscopy and Uretheroscopy," (*Nelson New Loose-leaf Surgery*, Vol. 6, pages 773–804, 1927).

Voelcker, F., and Lichtenberg, A., "Pyelographie (Röntgenographie des Nierenbeckens nach Kollargolfüllung)," *München. med. Wochenschrift*, 53:105–107, 1906.

Young, H., *Hugh Young, A Surgeon's Autobiography*, New York, 1940.

CHAPTER 30

Aitkin, D. M., *Hugh Owen Thomas—His Principles and Practice*, London, 1935.

Bérenger-Féraud, L. J. B., *Traité de l'immobilisation directe des fragments osseux dans les fractures*, Paris, 1870.

Bick, E. M., *Source Book of Orthopaedics*, Baltimore, 1937.

Keith, Sir A., *Menders of the Maimed*, London, 1919.

Osgood, R. B., *The Evolution of Orthopaedic Surgery*, St. Louis, 1925.

Valentin, B., *Orthopädie vor 100 Jahren . . .* , Stuttgart, 1935.

Watson, F., *Hugh Owen Thomas—A Personal Study*, London, 1934.

———, *The Life of Sir Robert Jones*, Baltimore, 1934.

CHAPTER 31

Bailey, P., and Cushing, H., *A Classification of the Tumors of the Glioma Group upon a Histogenetic Basis*, Philadelphia, 1926.

Bennett, A. H., "A Case of Cerebral Tumour. The Surgical Treatment by R. Godlee," *Med. Chir. Tr.*, 68:243–275, 1885 (also *Brit. M. J.*, 1:988, 1885).

Bramwell, Sir B., *Intracranial Tumours*, Edinburgh, 1888.

Bramwell, E., "Alexander Hughes Bennett and the First Recorded Case in which an Intracranial Tumour was Removed by Operation," *Edinburgh M. J.*, 42:312–315, 1935.

Cushing, H., "Surgery of the Head," (in *Keen's System of Surgery*, Philadelphia, 1908, Vol. 3, pages 17–276).

———, *Tumors of the Nervus Acusticus*, Philadelphia, 1917.

———, *Intracranial Tumours*, Springfield, Ill., 1932.

Cushing, H., and Bailey, P., *Tumors Arising from the Blood-vessels of the Brain*, Springfield, Ill., 1928.

CUSHING, H., AND EISENHARDT, L., *Meningiomas,* Springfield, Ill., 1938.

FERRIER, SIR D., *Functions of the Brain,* London, 1876.

GIGLI, L., "Zur Technik der temporären Schädelresektion mit meiner Drahtsäge," *Centralblatt f. Chirurgie,* 25:425, 1898.

HORRAX, G., "Harvey Cushing, 1869–1939," *Surg., Gynec., & Obst.,* 69:828–834, 1939.

PAGET, S., *Sir Victor Horsley,* London, 1919.

CHAPTER 32

BRUNN, H., "The Technique of Lobectomy in One Stage," *Surg., Gynec., & Obst.,* 55:616–626, 1932.

FLICK, J. B., "The Evolution of Thoracic Surgery," *Tr. & Stud. Coll. Physicians, Philadelphia,* 2:113–138, 1934.

FRIEDRICH, P. L., "The Operative Treatment of Unilateral Lung Tuberculosis by Total Mobilization of the Chest Wall by Means of Thoracoplastic Pleuro-Pneumolysis," *Surg., Gynec., & Obst.,* 7:632–638, 1908.

GRAHAM, E. A., "Pneumonectomy with Cautery," *J. A. M. A.,* 81:1010–1012, 1923.

——, *Some Fundamental Considerations in the Treatment of Empyema Thoracis,* St. Louis, 1925 (Samuel D. Gross prize essay, 1920).

——, "Some Accomplishments of Thoracic Surgery and its Present Problems," *Surgery,* 3:485–505, 1938.

GRAHAM, E. A., AND SINGER, J. J., "Successful Removal of an Entire Lung for Carcinoma of the Bronchus," *J. A. M. A.,* 101:1371–1374, 1933.

GROSS, R. E., AND HUBBARD, J. P., "Surgical Ligation of a Patent Ductus Arteriosus," *J. A. M. A.,* 112:729–731, 1939.

HEIDENHAIN, L., "Ausgedehnte Lungenresection wegen zahlreicher eiternder Bronchiectasieen in einem Unterlappen," *Arch. f. klin. Chir.,* 64:891–898, 1901.

HEUER, G. J., "The Development of Lobectomy and Pneumonectomy in Man," *J. Thoracic Surg.,* 3:560–572, 1934.

NISSEN, R., "Exstirpation eines ganzen Lungenflügels," *Zentralblatt f. Chir.,* 58:3003–3006, 1931.

PAGET, S., *The Surgery of the Chest,* London, 1896.

SHENSTONE, N. S., AND JANES, R. M., "Experiences in Pulmonary Lobectomy," *Canad. M. A. J.,* 27:138–145, 1932.

WANGENSTEEN, O. H., "Observations on the Treatment of Empyema with Special Reference to Drainage and Expansion of the Lung" *J. Thoracic Surg.,* 4:399–413, 1935.

CHAPTER 33

Ophthalmology

HIRSCHBERG, J., "Geschichte der Augenheilkunde," (Graeffe-Saemisch, *Handbuch der gesamten Augenheilkunde*, Berlin, 1911–1918 Vols., 13 to 15).

SORSBY, A., *A Short History of Ophthalmology*, London, 1933.

Otology

POLITZER, A., *Geschichte der Ohrenheilkunde*, 2 Vols., Stuttgart, 1907–1913.

———, *The Membrana Tympani in Health and Disease*, Translated by A. Mathewson and H. S. Newton, New York, 1869.

SCHWARTZE, H., "Studien und Beobachtungen über die künstliche Perforation des Trommelfells," *Arch. f. Ohrenheilkunde*, 2:24–35 and 239–267, 3:281–298, 1867.

SCHWARTZE, H., AND EYSELL, "Ueber die künstliche Eröffnung des Warzenfortsatzes," *Arch. f. Ohrenheilkunde*, n. f. 1:157–187, 1873.

TOYNBEE, J., *The Diseases of the Ear*, Philadelphia, 1860.

WILDE, SIR W. R. W., *Practical Observations on Aural Surgery, and the Nature and Treatment of Diseases of the Ear*, Philadelphia, 1853.

"Zur Erinnerung an Friedrich Hofmann," *Zeitschrift f. Laryngol.*, 4:237–242, 1911.

Rhinology and Laryngology

CALDWELL, G. W., "Diseases of the Accessory Sinuses of the Nose, and an Improved Method of Treatment for Suppuration of the Maxillary Antrum," *New York M. J.*, 58:526–528, 1893.

COUTARD, H., "Un cas d'épithélioma spino-cellulaire de la région latérale du pharynx, avec adénopathie angulo-maxillaire, guéri depuis six mois par la röntgenthérapie," *Bull. Assoc. franc. p. l'étude du cancer*, 10:160–168, 1921.

CZERMAK, J. N., *Der Kehlkopfspiegel und seine Verwertung für Physiologie und Medizin*, Leipzig, 1860.

DESCHAMPS, J. L., *Dissertation sur les maladies des fosses nazales et leurs sinus*, Paris, 1804 (Thesis, Univ. of Paris).

FRAENKEL, E., "Beiträge zur Pathologie und Aetiologie der Nasennebenhöhlen Erkrankungen," *Virchows Arch. f. path. Anat.*, 143: 42–98, 1896.

HAJEK, M., *Pathologie und Therapie der entzündlichen Erkrankungen der Nebenhöhlen der Nase*, Leipzig, 1899.

HARTMANN, A., "Supraorbitalneuralgie, hervorgerufen durch Empyem der Nebenhöhlen der Nase," *Berlin. klin. Wochenschrift,* 19:732–734, 1882.

———, "Abscessbildung in der Orbita nach acutem Schnupfen," *Berlin. klin. Wochenschrift,* 21:325–327, 1884.

———, "Ueber Empyem der Oberkieferhöhle," *Deutsche med. Wochenschrift,* 15:190, 1889.

JACKSON, C., *Tracheo-Bronchoscopy, Esophagoscopy, and Gastroscopy,* St. Louis, 1907.

———, *Life of Chevalier Jackson, An Autobiography,* New York, 1938.

KIRSTEIN, A., *Die Autoscopie des Kehlkopfs und Luftrohrs,* Berlin, 1896.

KOLLOFRATH, O., "Entfernung eines Knochenstückes aus dem rechten Bronchus auf natürlichem Wege und unter Anwendung der directen Laryngoskopie," *München. med. Wochenschrift,* 44:1038, 1897.

MACKENZIE, M., *The Use of the Laryngoscope in Diseases of the Throat,* Philadelphia, 1865.

MIKULICZ, J., "Zur Operativen Behandlung des Empyems der Highmorshöhle," *Arch. f. klin. Chir.,* 34:626–634, 1886.

TÜRCK, L., *Klinik der Krankheiten des Kehlkopfes,* Vienna, 1866.

WRIGHT, J., *The Nose and Throat in Medical History,* St. Louis, 1898.

ZUCKERKANDL, E., *Normale und pathologische Anatomie der Nasenhöhle,* Vienna, Vol. 1, 1882, Vol. 2, 1892.

CHAPTER 34

CURIE, E., *Madame Curie,* a Biography, New York, 1938.

CURIE, M., *Pierre Curie,* New York 1923.

CHAPTER 35

COOK, E. T., *A Short Life of Florence Nightingale,* abridged by R. Nash, New York, 1925.

LEE, E., *History of the School of Nursing of the Presbyterian Hospital, New York, 1892–1942,* New York, 1942.

GOODNOW, M., *Nursing History,* 7th edition, Philadelphia, 1942.

CHAPTER 36

BIGELOW, G. H., AND LOMBARD, H. L., *Cancer and Other Chronic Diseases in Massachusetts,* Boston, 1933.

DUBLIN, L. I., AND LOTKA, A. J., *Length of Life,* New York, 1936.

GARRISON, F. H., "History of Pediatrics," (*Abt's Pediatrics,* Philadelphia, 1923, Vol. 1, pages 1–170).

VAN INGEN, P., "The History of Child Welfare Work in the United States," (Ravenel, M. P., Editor, *A Half Century of Public Health,* New York, 1921, pages 290–322).

WILSON, E. B., AND BURKE, M., "The Statistical Situation in Cancer," *Bull. Am. Soc. Control Cancer,* 23:4–6, 1941.

CHAPTER 37

CABOT, H., *The Doctor's Bill*, New York, 1935.

——, *The Patient's Dilemma*, New York, 1940.

CODMAN, E. A., *The Shoulder* . . . , Boston, 1934.

Committee on the Costs of Medical Care, Publications.

    FALK, I. S., KLEM, M. C., AND SINAI, N., *The Incidence of Illness and the Receipt and Costs of Medical Care Among Representative Families,* Chicago, 1933 (No. 26).

    FALK, I. S., ROREM, C. R., AND RING., M.D., *The Costs of Medical Care,* Chicago, 1933 (No. 27).

    LEE, R. I., AND JONES, L. W., *The Fundamentals of Good Medical Care,* Chicago, 1933 (No. 22).

    REED, L., *The Ability to Pay for Medical Care,* Chicago, 1933 (No. 25).

CORSCADEN, J. H., "Follow-up System," (Rockefeller Foundation, Division of Medical Education, *Methods and Problems of Medical Education,* 4th series, New York, 1926, pages 27–32).

COWLEY, W. H., "The War on the College," *The Atlantic Monthly,* 169:719–726, (June), 1942.

DAVIS, M. M., *America Organizes Medicine*, New York, 1941.

EMERSON, H., *The Baker Memorial*, New York, 1941.

FLEXNER, A., *Medical Education*, New York, 1925.

——, *Medical Education in Europe*, New York, 1912 (Carnegie Foundation for the Advancement of Teaching, Bulletin No. 6).

——, *Medical Education in the United States and Canada*, New York, 1910 (Carnegie Foundation for the Advancement of Teaching, Bulletin No. 4).

——, *I Remember*, New York, 1940.

FLEXNER, S., AND FLEXNER, J. T., *William Henry Welch and the Heroic Age of American Medicine*, New York, 1941.

HARRINGTON, T. F., *The Harvard Medical School*, 3 vols., New York, 1905.

JANEWAY, T. C., "Outside Professional Engagements by Members of Professional Faculties," *Assoc. Amer. Univ. Annual Conference, 19th, 1917. Proceedings,* pages 72–80.

NEWSHOLME, SIR A., *Medicine and the State*, London, 1932.

——, *International Studies on the Relation between the Private and Official Practice of Medicine*, 3 vols., London, 1931.

NEWSHOLME, SIR A., AND KINGSBURY, J. A., *Red Medicine*, New York, 1933.

OSLER, SIR W., *Whole-Time Clinical Professors, A Letter to President Remsen, Johns Hopkins University*. Privately Printed, 1911.

RORTY, J., *American Medicine Mobilizes*, New York, 1939.

INDEX

ACKNOWLEDGMENTS

The Publishers wish to thank the following publishers and authors for their kind permission to reprint the illustrations listed below for which they hold copyright:

THE SCIENCE PRESS for portrait of Gerhard Domagk which appeared in January 1940 issue of Scientific Monthly published by American Association for the Advancement of Science.

LEA & FEBIGER for picture of "The Little Red" and portrait of Edward Livingston Trudeau from *"An Autobiography"* by Edward Livingston Trudeau, M.D. Copyright 1915 by Lea & Febiger.

J. B. LIPPINCOTT COMPANY and MRS. AUGUST SCHACHNER for picture of the house where McDowell performed the first ovariotomy from *"Ephraim McDowell, Father of Ovariotomy and Founder of Abdominal Surgery"* by August Schachner, M.D. Copyright 1921 by J. B. Lippincott Company.

DOUBLEDAY, DORAN COMPANY, INC. for photographs of Pierre Curie and Marie Cure from *"Madame Curie: A Biography"* by Eve Curie, copyright 1937 by Doubleday, Doran Company, Inc.

THE MACMILLAN COMPANY for photograph of a collection of objects removed by bronchoscopy from *"The Life of Chevalier Jackson,"* Copyright 1938 by the Macmillan Company.

The RONALD PRESS COMPANY, LOUIS I. DUBLIN, and ALFRED J. LOTKA for Table from *"Length of Life,"* Copyright 1936 by The Ronald Press.

The WILLIAMS & WILKINS COMPANY for photograph of Anthrax Bacilli from *"A History of Pathology"* by Esmond P. Long, PH.D., M.D., Copyright 1928 by the Williams & Wilkins Company.

The JOHNS HOPKINS PRESS and W. G. MACCALLUM, M.D. for portrait of William Stewart Halsted from *"William Stewart Halsted, Surgeon"* by W. G. MacCallum, M.D., Copyright 1930 by The Johns Hopkins Press.

HARCOURT, BRACE & COMPANY, INC. for photograph of "Dog 33" from *"Men Against Death"* by Paul de Kruif, Copyright 1932 by Harcourt, Brace & Company, Inc.

JOHN WYETH & BROTHER, INC. for permission to reproduce painting "The Conquerors of Yellow Fever" by Dean Cornwell.

444